# Translational Pain Research, Volume 2: Comparing Preclinical Studies and Clinical Pain Management. Lost in Translation?

# Translational Pain Research, Volume 2: Comparing Preclinical Studies and Clinical Pain Management. Lost in Translation?

Jianren Mao
Editor

Nova Biomedical Books
New York

Copyright © 2006 by Nova Science Publishers, Inc.

**All rights reserved.** No part of this book may be reproduced, stored in a retrieval system or transmitted in any form or by any means: electronic, electrostatic, magnetic, tape, mechanical photocopying, recording or otherwise without the written permission of the Publisher.

For permission to use material from this book please contact us:
Telephone 631-231-7269; Fax 631-231-8175
Web Site: http://www.novapublishers.com

**NOTICE TO THE READER**

The Publisher has taken reasonable care in the preparation of this book, but makes no expressed or implied warranty of any kind and assumes no responsibility for any errors or omissions. No liability is assumed for incidental or consequential damages in connection with or arising out of information contained in this book. The Publisher shall not be liable for any special, consequential, or exemplary damages resulting, in whole or in part, from the readers' use of, or reliance upon, this material.

Independent verification should be sought for any data, advice or recommendations contained in this book. In addition, no responsibility is assumed by the publisher for any injury and/or damage to persons or property arising from any methods, products, instructions, ideas or otherwise contained in this publication.

This publication is designed to provide accurate and authoritative information with regard to the subject matter cover herein. It is sold with the clear understanding that the Publisher is not engaged in rendering legal or any other professional services. If legal, medical or any other expert assistance is required, the services of a competent person should be sought. FROM A DECLARATION OF PARTICIPANTS JOINTLY ADOPTED BY A COMMITTEE OF THE AMERICAN BAR ASSOCIATION AND A COMMITTEE OF PUBLISHERS.

**Library of Congress Cataloging-in-Publication Data**
Translational pain research / Jianren Mao (editor).
    p. ; cm.
Includes bibliographical references and index.
ISBN 1-60021-206-9 (v. 1) -- ISBN 1-60021-205-0 (v. 2)
1. Pain. 2. Pain--Pathophysiology. 3. Pain--Treatment. I. Mao, Jianren.
[DNLM: 1. Pain--physiopathology. 2. Pain--therapy. WL 704 T772 2006]
RB127.T73                                                                                                   2006
616'.0472--dc22
                                                                                                              2006014114

*Published by Nova Science Publishers, Inc.* ✣*New York*

# Contents

| | | |
|---|---|---|
| **Preface** | | vii |
| **Chapter I** | Understanding Central Mechanisms of Pain and Pain Modulation<br>*Anthony Dickenson, Tansy Donovan-Rodriguez and Elizabeth Matthews* | 1 |
| **Chapter II** | Ion Channel Blockers in Clinical Pain Management<br>*Lucy Chen* | 25 |
| **Chapter III** | Spinal N-Methyl-D-Aspartate Receptor Mechanisms of Central Sensitization and Persistent Pain Following Tissue Injury<br>*Wei Guo, Ronald Dubner and Ke Ren* | 45 |
| **Chapter IV** | NMDA Receptor Antagonists and Clinical Pain Management<br>*Jianren Mao* | 79 |
| **Chapter V** | Plasticity of Signaling Molecules and Their Associations after Chronic Morphine: Altered but Not Lost Opioid Receptor-Coupled Functionality<br>*Alan R. Gintzler and Sumita Chakrabarti* | 87 |
| **Chapter VI** | Opioids for Pain Management<br>*Howard S. Smith and Gary McCleane* | 109 |
| **Chapter VII** | Inflammatory Mediators in the Mechanisms of Nociception - Preclinical Studies<br>*Tarek A. Samad* | 147 |
| **Chapter VIII** | Antiinflammatory Medications in Pain Management<br>*Ezekiel Fink and Gary J. Brenner* | 155 |
| **Chapter IX** | Chronic Pain and the Sympathetic Nervous System: Mechanisms and Potential Implications for Pain Therapies<br>*Amit Sharma and Srinivasa N. Raja* | 169 |

| | | |
|---|---|---|
| **Chapter X** | Mechanisms of Tricyclic Antidepressants in Pain Modulation<br>*Peter Gerner and Ging Kuo Wang* | 189 |
| **Chapter XI** | Antidepressant Medication in Clinical Pain Management<br>*Donna Greenberg* | 207 |
| **Chapter XII** | Developing Pain Pathways and Analgesic Mechanisms – Towards Translational Studies<br>*Maria Fitzgerald* | 221 |
| **Chapter XIII** | Pediatric Pain Management: In Translation<br>*Allyssa LeBel* | 239 |
| **Chapter XIV** | Selective Serotonin Agonists for the Acute Management of Migraine<br>*David M. Biondi* | 253 |
| **Chapter XV** | Gender Differences in Clinical Pain Management<br>*Anita Holdcroft* | 277 |
| **Chapter XVI** | Clinical Management of Cancer Pain<br>*Anca Popescu and E. Daniela Hord* | 295 |
| **Chapter XVII** | Complementary and Alternative Medicine in Pain Management<br>*Lucy Chen* | 317 |
| **Index** | | 331 |

# Preface

Translational pain research is an evolving field that helps bridge the gap between basic science pain research and clinical pain management. Translational pain research has multiple objectives: 1) analyzing similarities and differences between animal "pain" models and clinical pain conditions; 2) examining limitations of preclinical research tools and pharmacological interventions; 3) evaluating the relevance of basic science research to clinical pain management; and 4) guiding clinical use of bench information and providing feedback information to preclinical studies.

Despite significant progresses in basic science pain research, clinical pain management remains a daily challenge. A major deficiency of current pain research is the lack of effective communications between basic scientists and pain clinicians. It would be helpful to discuss preclinical information and its application in clinical pain management from the perspectives of both basic scientists and clinicians. For example, the discussion by basic scientists on the function of major ion channels and its relation to the mechanisms of nociception would help clinicians to understand why and how the clinically available ion channel blockers might work or not work for various pain conditions. On the other hand, the discussion by pain clinicians on how the clinically available ion channel blockers are being used for pain management (e.g., indications, side effects) would help basic scientists to understand how bench information is being applied properly or improperly in clinical pain management.

Chapters in this volume are organized in such a way that pairs of chapters (whenever applicable) written by basic scientists and pain clinicians will provide both preclinical and clinical information, respectively, on those topics highly relevant to daily clinical pain management. These chapters provide critical reviews on preclinical and clinical data and offer constructive views on the relevance and deficiency of current pain research and pain management. The readers, including basic scientists, clinicians, psychologists, pharmacologists, graduate students, clinical residents and fellows, and other healthcare professionals, will find exceptionally refreshing information from these chapters and have a unique opportunity to compare and contrast the similarities and differences in the scope of bench information, the intended clinical use, and actual application of such information in clinical pain management.

The topics covered in this volume are carefully selected and directly related to the daily practice of pain medicine. These topics include 1) central mechanisms of pain and pain modulation (Dickenson, Donovan-Rodriguez, Mattews) and clinical use of ion channel blockers (Chen); 2) spinal glutamatergic mechanisms (Guo, Dubner, Ren) and issues related to glutamate receptor antagonists in pain management (Mao); 3) basic science of opioid analgesics (Gintzler, Chakrabarti) and clinical opioid use (Smith, McCleane); 4) inflammatory cytokines (Samad) and clinical use of anti-inflammatory drugs (Fink, Brenner); 5) role of the sympathetic nervous system in pain mechanisms and its relation to clinical pain management (Sharma, Raja); 6) preclinical studies on tricyclic antidepressants (Gerner, Wang) and clinical use of antidepressants in pain management (Greenberg); 7) developing pain pathways and analgesic mechanisms during the developmental stage (Fitzgerald) and challenges of pediatric pain management (Lebel); 8) basic science mechanisms of serotonin agonists and their use in the clinical management of migraine headache (Biondi); 9) clinical research on gender differences in clinical pain and their implications for clinical pain management (Holdcroft); 10) current modalities of clinical cancer pain management (Popescu, Hord); and 11) preclinical and clinical information on alternative medicine (Chen).

I am extremely grateful to the authors for their commitment and contribution to this refreshing volume on the issue of translational pain research. I am also thankful to Nova Science Publishers, Inc for their support and timely publication. I hope this volume will provide our readers with comprehensive and analytic views on many issues directly related to current pain research and clinical pain management and promote translational pain research through understanding the existing gaps between pain research and clinical pain management.

Jianren Mao
March 26, 2006

*Chapter I*

# Understanding Central Mechanisms of Pain and Pain Modulation

*Anthony Dickenson[1], Tansy Donovan-Rodriguez[2] and Elizabeth Matthews[1]*

[1]Dept Pharmacology, University College London, Gower St., London UK
[2]Instituto de Neurociencias, Universidad Miguel Hernández,
San Juan de Alicante, Spain

## Abstract

The pharmacology of pain and analgesia exhibits plasticity in different pain states in that the signalling mechanisms change following physiopathological events. Understanding this plasticity may lead to improved therapies for the two broad major types of pain, neuropathic and inflammatory pain. Cancer pain can be one or the other or a combination. The peripheral mechanisms of these types of pain are very different yet within the central nervous system the signalling systems appear to be more common. This chapter examines how approaches based on ion channel function in peripheral nerves can use central spinal neuronal activity as a marker of the roles of these channels in transmission from the periphery to spinal circuits. The second half of the chapter looks at a model of cancer-induced bone pain. Here, we discuss how peripheral pathophysiology changes the coding properties of spinal neurons and engages descending controls to further modulate the ascending messages to the brain. Studies such as these in integrated systems can shed light on the mechanisms of pain and allow the roles of certain pain targets to be better understood.

## Introduction

The translation of work using animal models of any human disease, disorder or pathological process are critical for understanding both the mechanisms behind the process as well as being essential for the discovery of new therapeutic targets. In terms of pain research, the use of animal models allows a whole raft of approaches to be used to understand how the peripheral and central nervous systems transduce, transmit and modulate these incoming sensory messages. Thus comparisons can be made between pain transmission under normal circumstances and events that occur after pathological damage so guiding us towards understanding those systems that alter in models of human pain states. This may allow targets to be defined that play a unique or enhanced role in the abnormal pain condition so that therapy may allow this to be damped down whilst sparing normal function. A major step forward in translating from animals to patients is the development of imaging techniques such as fMRI since both activity and drug effects can be observed in normal humans and circuits active in the human central nervous system defined.

In the case of pain, the ability to apply a defined stimulus where the consequences for human perception is known (e.g. brush, prod, thermal or chemical stimulation etc) is a major advantage in translating from animals to patients compared to other animal models of higher functions or disorders where links are more tenuous. But this also leads to one of the major problems with pain translation. Although humans are similar in many genetic, molecular and neuronal pathways to other mammals, and species differences can be clearly defined, the human pain experience is exactly that. Animals cannot inform us of the affective (emotional) aspects of pain such as anxiety and depression, nor the role of memory, the implications of the pain for social function and how coping strategies are brought into play. These are not easily amenable to study although attempts are being made to better understand these aspects of supraspinal processing and again, the imaging studies in humans can guide the basic science to the neural systems involved.

Another issue is the duration of the pain state, which due to the control of animal experimentation quite rightly, is invariably much shorter than the human chronic pain state. Finally, when considering therapy for pain, the effects of many drugs and other manipulations in basic science can really only inform on efficacy and marked side effects. Subtle effects of drugs on cognitive processing and arousal in humans will be very hard to gauge in animals.

The point about efficacy also needs to be tempered by what is being measured in animals. Behavioural studies study the response to a stimulus that is defined by the withdrawal of the animal at a certain intensity of the stimulus. This will be close to the threshold for "pain" and so will be far from the severe pains, often rated as 6-7 on a visual analogue scale that patients have. Thus a drug may have reasonable efficacy against a pain of 1-2 on this scale but lose effectiveness at higher pain levels. One way around this problem would be to use neuronal recordings in vivo (although potentially complicated by general anaesthesia) where responses of defined sensory neurones, for example in spinal cord or thalamus or other areas with somatosensory inputs, can be quantified using stimuli that would be above the threshold. Effects on threshold and suprathreshold responses can therefore be revealed. In a similar way, immunohistochemcial approaches such as c-fos labeling can also be used (but at a defined time point only) to study responses to suprathreshold stimuli.

What follows is an account of two very different approaches to translation from animals to patients, namely genetic studies and then an overview of the recently developed models of cancer induced bone pain (CIBP), a major clinical pain state.

## Ion Channels in Pain

Primary afferent neurones transmit sensory information from the periphery to the spinal cord from where modulation occurs before transmission to the higher centres of the brain and the final perception is established. The peripheral terminals of sensory neurones permit the discrimination of various modalities such as mechanical, thermal and chemical stimuli via a number of different ion channels that convert modality into electrical impulses. Critical to this are voltage-gated sodium channels (VGSCs) as they initiate and propagate action potentials that travel the length of the axons and thus control neuronal excitability. These mechanisms are fundamental to normal sensation whether it is signaling everyday tactile or thermal innocuous stimuli, and also acute painful stimuli, in which case it serves as a warning to protect. However in pathological pain states, for example resulting from peripheral or central nerve damage due to disease or trauma, these same mechanisms malfunction such the system becomes hyperexcitable and sensory transmission persists, generally not reflective of the evoking stimulus, and often spontaneous in nature.

Preclinical experimental studies have been, and continue to be, invaluable in uncovering both physiological and pathophysiological mechanisms responsible for sensory signaling and chronic pain conditions, respectively. However it still remains a challenge to translate such findings to clinically observed symptoms and possible therapeutic strategies [1]. Blockade of VGSCs are a major target in current clinical practice in several therapeutic areas including epilepsy, arrhythmias and pain, and a number of studies have highlighted sodium channels as important mediators in neuropathic pain see [2]. Widely used local anaesthetics, such as lidocaine, act as sodium channel blockers, and this is a good reflection on the potential for specifically targeting these channels as analgesics. In neuropathic pain patients, microneurographic recordings also demonstrate aberrant electrical activity in peripheral nerves, which interestingly can be reduced in parallel with a reduction in symptoms after local anaesthetic nerve block [3, 4]. Within the nervous system, at least nine subtypes, defined by their pore-forming a-subunit, each with individual functional and expression characteristics, are expressed [5] with most DRG neurones expressing most types [6]. Therefore without specificity of action or use-dependency, block of sodium channels per se runs the risk of complete sensory anaesthesia and intolerable side effects due to potential ubiquitous block of cardiac and brain electrical activity. Indeed, sodium channel blocking drugs (local anaesthetics, anticonvulsants, antiarrhythmics) used clinically for pain indications, show some degree of use-dependency in that normal low frequency neuronal firing is not affected whereas pathological high frequency patterns of activity are reduced [7, 8].

Despite ongoing attempts to identify VGSC subtype-specific ligands, currently no such agents exist. This means that differential physiological roles of individual sodium channel subtypes cannot be studied in vivo by pharmacological means. Fortunately, in animals other methodological approaches can be employed such as genetic modifications to knockout specific sodium channel subtypes and oligodinucleotide (ODN) antisense knockdown protocols. Although non-specific sodium channel blockers can be examined clinically, more specific investigations cannot be conducted at this level and thus progress in this therapeutic area is dependent on translation of findings from animal studies. In order for this to be of any

## Voltage-Gated Sodium Channels and Pain

Based on knowledge acquired so far with regard to the role of VGSCs in pain transmission, the analgesic efficacy of broad-spectrum sodium channel blockers, translates well from what is observed in animal studies into what is observed clinically, and vice versa. The nature of the majority of this data is behavioural animal testing in models of neuropathic pain or inflammation where assessment of pain like behaviours can be related to clinically observed symptoms characteristic of chronic pain states.

Damage to peripheral nerves, whether a result of trauma, disease or tissue inflammation is associated neuronal membrane hyperexcitability often characterised by spontaneous and/or evoked neuronal impulses [9]. Abnormal peripheral nerve activity, such as that mediated by injury-induced changes in sodium channels, can generate an ongoing barrage of input into the spinal cord that has been shown to lead to central sensitisation [10]. Central sensitisation is manifest as hyperexcitability of dorsal horn neurones, expanded peripheral receptive fields and altered stimulus-response relationships and results in hyperalgesia and allodynia [11, 12]. Therefore alterations to peripheral sodium channel expression and function are likely to impact upon dorsal horn neuronal activity.

$Na_v$ 1.8

Experimentally it has been demonstrated that after nerve injury that there is decrease in Nav 1.8 protein, particularly in small diameter DRG cell bodies alongside elevation of Nav 1.8 immunoreactivity at distal axons and nerve terminals, reflective of a redistribution of Nav 1.8 to the site of damage creating a localised area of hyperexcitability [13]. Similarly, such injury-evoked alterations to Nav 1.8 expression is also observed in tissue samples taken from patients with various chronic pains [14-16]. Further, what makes this sodium channel subtype of interest from a therapeutic angle is that unlike the other sodium channels it is only expressed in sensory ganglia of predominantly small diameter, a pattern demonstrated in both rodents and human [15, 17]. Such a restricted expression pattern indicates that were a drug specific for Nav 1.8 available then the side-effect profile would likely be minimal, as CNS-related problems associated with other sodium channel blockers would be avoided. Since such pharmacological agents are not available, in vivo physiological investigations into the role of Nav 1.8 in sensory signaling have been furthered by the generation of a Nav 1.8 knockout mouse [18] and knockdown of Nav 1.8 using antisense ODNs [19, 20]. Initial reports demonstrated that Nav 1.8 KO mice show a lack of spontaneous activity in saphenous nerve fibres after experimental neuroma [21], and antisense Nav 1.8 ODNs diminish experimental inflammation-induced hyperalgesia in a manner reversed on termination of antisense administration [19]. Similarly knockdown of Nav 1.8 at the time of spinal nerve ligation prevents the development of mechanical allodynia and thermal hyperalgesia, which can subsequently develop then diminish on termination and restoration of antisense application, respectively [20]. Further, in experimental models of visceral pain, Nav 1.8 knockout animals show reduced pain behaviours [22]. These studies indicate that accumulation of Nav 1.8 is likely involved in generation of aberrant firing, spontaneous or evoked, that results in persistent pain behaviours and symptoms.

## Behavioural and In Vivo Electrophysiological Investigative Approaches

So it appears from these behavioural studies that there is a very real role for Nav 1.8 in pathological sensory transmission. But what is its importance in normal physiology? Behavioural assessment of the Nav 1.8 KO mouse shows that these animals appear similar to littermate controls in terms of thresholds to non-noxious mechanical and noxious thermal stimulation, yet display deficits in responses to noxious mechanical pressure [18, 23]. However, although behavioural assessment of the physiological function of channels or proteins implicated in pain pathways is extremely useful, it does possess limitations. Given that the endpoint for von Frey testing is a withdrawal threshold, intensities above this cannot be tested, such that only sub-threshold punctate mechanical intensities can be assessed. In the case of thermal stimulation latency to withdrawal to some degree permits testing of suprathreshold stimuli. Therefore in the absence of a chronic pain state where allodynia and hyperalgesia are not evident such that mechanical and thermal thresholds are not altered, it may be difficult to comprehensively assess the complete physiological function of a channel. Additionally, assessments of supra-threshold stimulus intensities are important since they represent the intensities of pain that are encountered in the clinic. It must also be taken into consideration that the nociceptive withdrawal response is not solely under the control of the sensory system. It is also dependent on the motor system and affected by motivation and sedation that may be altered in transgenic mice where the target gene is not exclusive to sensory pathways. Further, it has also been demonstrated that animal behavioural responses are influenced by many environmental factors [24, 25].

Some of these limitations can be addressed using an in vivo electrophysiological approach. In intact anaesthetised mice the evoked activity of single dorsal horn neurones to a wide range of electrical and natural stimuli can be recorded such that neuronal responses to a full range of modalities and intensities, including suprathreshold stimuli can be characterised. This extends information that can be attained from transgenic studies beyond the scope of the behavioural phenotype. In this setting the effect of deletion of a channel on neuronal responses can be studied in a manner that focuses predominantly on the sensory pathways, relatively independent of influencing environmental factors.

Nav 1.8 knockout mice show marked deficits in the evoked activity of spinal dorsal horn neurones in response to mechanical stimuli, whether it be brush, von Frey or pinch [26]. Further, the more noxious the stimulus is, the greater the deficit. Given the reported distribution of Nav 1.8 channels predominantly in small diameter nociceptive fibres over non-noxious stimuli-sensing large diameter fibres, the comparative reductions fit well with the location of the channel on mainly noxious small-diameter afferents. However, no such reductions in neuronal activity were observed to thermal stimuli over the warm and noxious heat range. Thus deletion of Nav 1.8 reveals a stimulus-defined role for this VGSC in the transmission of sensory stimuli from the periphery to the spinal cord via predominantly nociceptive primary afferents as its distribution dictates. It may be that $Na_v$ 1.8 VGSCs are localised to a population of mechanosensitive fibres, or possibly associated with another transducer responsible for mechanosensation. (Figure 1).

Interestingly, this modality specificity in the physiological role of sodium channels is also observed clinically where the use of sodium channel blockers to manage chronic pain, appears only to be effective on mechanically-evoked pains, such as dynamic and punctate mechanical allodynia, yet not on thermally-evoked symptoms see [27]. As mentioned earlier, clinically used sodium channel blockers are not subtype selective and many have additional modes of action, therefore from clinical pharmacological studies it cannot be determined if a particular sodium channel subtype is associated with a particular symptom, however from preclinical and clinical data it seems to concur that sodium channels are certainly important in mechanosensation. It is interesting to note that pains, dysesthesia and paraesthesias that are under the umbrella of 'mechanically-evoked symptoms', show differential susceptibilities to the various sodium channel-blocking drugs clinically.

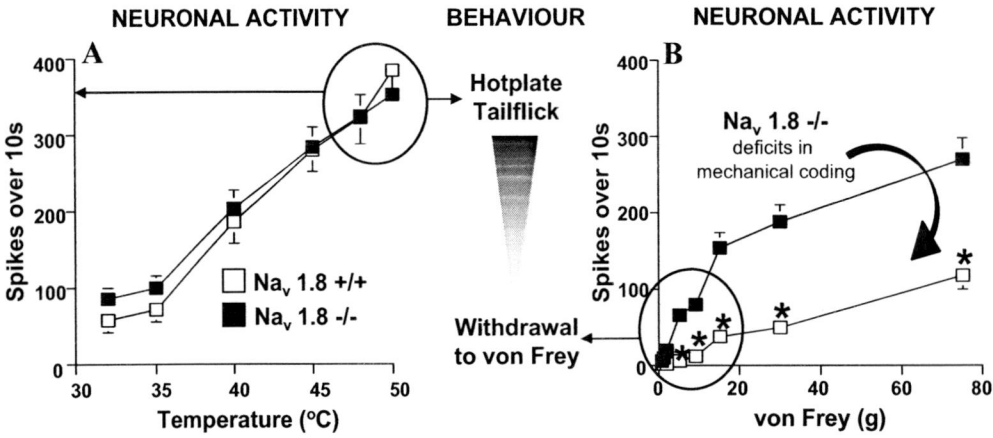

Figure 1. $Na_v$ 1.8-null mice display marked deficits in mechanically-evoked dorsal horn neuronal activity. Wide dynamic range neurones recorded from $Na_v$ 1.8 -/- (n = 30) show similar activity to thermal stimuli compared to littermate control $Na_v$ 1.8 +/+ (n = 45) mice (A) yet significantly reduced activity to punctate mechanical von Frey stimuli (B). This graph further highlights that the levels of neuronal activity evoked to thermal stimuli of intensities that cause the behavioural withdrawal reflex (circled) are much greater than that to mechanical stimuli (circled)

For example lidocaine, mexilitine and phenytoin alleviate punctate and dynamic mechanical allodynia arising from various aetiologies [28-30], whereas lamotrigine has little effect [31, 32]. Carbamazepine has shown useful against evoked paroxysms and spontaneous pain in trigeminal neuralgia [33]. With regards to thermal-evoked symptoms only a handful of studies exist exploring the effects of sodium channels on thermal allodynia or hyperalgesia. In such cases lidocaine was shown to be without effect [34, 35] and this included cold-allodynia that is certainly an important clinical need. The converse is the case for lamotrigine, however, which has been demonstrated to be useful against cold allodynia [31, 32].

## Na$_v$ 1.7

Nav 1.7 is another VGSC that has been of interest in terms of sensory transmission. This subtype of sodium channel is expressed in sympathetic and sensory ganglia, and localised to nerve terminals of sensory neurones in any cell type [6, 36] with week expression in the CNS [37, 38]. A pathophysiological role for Nav 1.7 is observed in inflammation. Global deletion of the Na$_v$ 1.7 gene leads to death shortly after birth. However a nociceptor-specific knockout of the Nav 1.7 gene has been generated and this results in a behavioural phenotype exhibiting dramatic deficits in inflammatory pain models [23]. Recently, a human heritable pain condition, primary erythermalgia, has been shown to map to Nav1.7 where burning pain is experience in response to warm stimuli or moderate exercise [39]. In contrast to the deficits seen in the nociceptor-specific Nav 1.7 knockout, this is a gain of function mutation presented clinically as chronic inflammation and associated pain.

Acutely this Nav 1.7 deletion, similar to Nav 1.8, show deficits in mechanosensation, but not thermal, though only in the noxious range observed behaviourally to noxious pressure, and to noxious von Frey stimulation as assessed from electrophysiological study of dorsal horn neuronal activity [23]. In the acute situation, this further promotes a link between sensory sodium channels and mechanosensation.

An interesting observation from the use of in vivo dorsal horn neuronal recordings in knockout mice is the differing levels of spinal cord activity necessary to drive the behavioural withdrawal response to mechanical and thermal stimuli. In the range of von Frey intensities that evoke a nociceptive withdrawal response in mice, the corresponding evoked neuronal responses are at around 4-fold less than the activity corresponding to the temperature range required to elicit a withdrawal. Variation in modality-specific responsiveness of spinal neurones to peripheral stimuli may reflect differential control of the primary afferent central terminals. It also poses the question as to what drives the withdrawal response and how this may vary between evoking modality.

## Na$_v$ 1.9

The expression pattern of Nav 1.9 highlights this channel as one for consideration in the pain research field as a potential therapeutic target since it is expressed within the DRG and trigeminal ganglia and predominantly in nociceptors of several classes [40]. However few studies exist investigating its role in pain pathology and these have not been particularly promising since, for example, neuropathic pain behaviours induced by nerve injury remained unaltered after Nav 1.9 knockdown with antisense ODN infusion [20]. The kinetic properties of the channel are the likely reason behind this disappointment since this channel may modulate the response of nociceptors to subthreshold stimuli since it is active at resting membrane potentials [41].

$Na_v$ 1.3

Nav 1.3 is also interesting from a pain perspective, as it is not expressed in the adult human peripheral nervous system yet widely expressed in the CNS. In the rat there is a developmental decline of Nav 1.3 such that by adulthood its expression in low in both peripheral and central nervous systems [36]. Experimentally, Nav 1.3 exhibits a striking re-emergence in sensory neurones after peripheral nerve damage [42-44], in a manner reversed by exogenous GDNF application, simultaneous with reduction in ectopic activity and neuropathic pain behaviours [45]. Further ODN knockout down of upregulated Nav 1.3 in dorsal horn neurones in a model of spinal cord injury, reverses associated pain behaviours [43] and more recently in the ventroposterior lateral nucleus of the thalamus [46]. Such pathological alterations in Nav 1.3 expression have yet to be demonstrated in humans and if so its therapeutic potential may be hindered by side effects given its known distribution in the adult human brain.

Many of the drugs that possess sodium channel blocking ability also show other modes of action, for example lamotrigine is thought to modulate calcium and potassium currents [47], and tricyclic antidepressants, which are first and foremost monoamine uptake inhibitors, are commonly employed in pain clinics where their analgesic effects may be via sodium channels [48, 49]. Multiple modes of action for drugs is often associated with poor side-effect profiles, and thus often reports of lack of effect of sodium channel blockers in patients may actually reflect lack of toleration to side-effects such that sufficient analgesic dose cannot be achieved. Although animal studies are useful in identifying causal mechanisms and ion channels or proteins of importance and pharmacological alterations to pain behaviours can be monitored, they are not so useful in predicting unwanted side effects.

## Mechanisms of Cancer-Induced Bone Pain

Translating information from laboratory experiments into useful clinical therapies is a key process in the identification, or improvement, of treatments for chronic pain. Translational research is equally important in the other direction; clinical observations should be used to create or refine specific research goals for basic scientists. In other words, it is essential to translate information from the laboratory to the clinic, and back again. These types of investigations can lead to a better understanding of pain processing. For example, genetic studies in mice have identified factors contributing to gender differences in analgesic mechanisms in humans [50] and as discussed above, genetic manipulation of genes can shed light on roles of their protein products. Research has shown that the melanocortin-1 receptor (Mc1r) gene mediates □-opioid analgesia in female mice. The human MC1R gene is associated with red hair and, in this same study, female redheads with variant MC1R alleles demonstrated higher analgesia with a □-opioid than non-redheads, or males of any hair colour. This study validates the extrapolation of mouse genome data to gene function in humans.

One particular type of translational research that has been important in the area of chronic pain is the use of animal models; we have better knowledge of nociceptive processing at the peripheral, spinal, and higher central level thanks to investigation in animal models of inflammatory and neuropathic pain for example. An area that has received close attention over the past few years is cancer-induced bone pain (CIBP), a class of chronic pain that, in the presence of ongoing illness, is difficult to treat effectively with the drugs currently available. This review focuses on the impact that, in less than a decade, translational research has had on CIBP.

## Cancer-Induced Bone Pain

Here we wish to use the example of a model of an important clinical pain state to tease out the peripheral driving forces behind the pain state and then consider how these peripheral inputs can produce states of central spinal hypersensitivity and how this relates to the abnormal pain behaviours and their modulation.

Improvements in the detection and treatment of cancers have resulted in sufferers surviving longer, but severe pain is often a major contributor to the decreased quality of life endured by many of these patients [51]. Bone metastases are frequently predictive of pain and CIBP is in fact the most common cancer-related pain, with metastatic cancers invading the skeleton in 60-84% of cases [52]. Interestingly, the presence and intensity of CIBP do not correlate with the size or number of active malignancies. Although the majority (up to 80%) of patients with breast cancer have metastatic spread to the bone, about 66% of the metastatic sites are painless but, on the other hand, there may be severe pain reported from a single bone metastasis in the absence of fracture [52]. Patients experience a triad of pain states consisting of background pain, spontaneous pain, and incident pain. The intermittent nature of spontaneous and incident pains makes them hard to treat, and it is very difficult to attain freedom from pain on movement in patients with bone metastases [52].

## Treating Cancer-Induced Bone Pain

Currently, treatment of CIBP involves a number of approaches including radiotherapy, chemotherapy, surgical intervention, and pharmacotherapy. In terms of pharmacotherapy, the main classes of drugs used are bisphosphonates, non-steroidal anti-inflammatory drugs (NSAIDs), and opioids.

Bisphosphonates inhibit osteoclastic bone resorption, these drugs therefore reduce pain in patients by decreasing destruction of the bone [52]. Bisphosphonates have been reported to potentiate the effects of analgesics in treating CIBP, although the effect is modest and does not allow for reduction of the dose of analgesic [52]. Side effects associated with bisphosphonates include gastrointestinal tract toxicity, fever, and electrolyte abnormalities [53].

NSAIDs are the first step on the analgesic ladder for cancer pain relief and even where the severity of pain requires progression to other analgesics, administration of NSAIDs may continue to take advantage of possible additive effects [52]. NSAIDs inhibit the cyclo-oxygenase pathway of arachadonic acid breakdown to reduce the formation of prostaglandins. The rationale for their use in CIBP is based on preventing activation and sensitization of primary afferents by prostaglandins. However, trials of NSAIDs in cancer pain, which include bone metastases, do not specify effects on incident pain and there is a general lack of clinical evidence to support a significant analgesic effect of NSAIDs in CIBP [54]. Side effects associated with NSAIDs include bleeding, gastrointestinal ulceration and renal toxicity [53]. The new class of COX-2 selective antagonists may provide better pharmacological tools for treating CIBP as they have been reported to inhibit cancer cell growth [55].

Opioids remain the mainstay for treatment of severe pain from malignancy in the bone but adverse side effects including constipation, nausea and vomiting, sedation, and respiratory depression are highly problematic at the doses that would be required to combat incident pain.

## Processes Underlying Cancer-Induced Bone Pain

There is a rich supply of sensory nerves to the periosteum, bone marrow, and mineralized bone [56]. Therefore, destruction of bone architecture in regions with sensory innervation will result in direct mechanical damage of these afferent fibres and lead to pain. Furthermore, stretching of the periosteum due to growth of tumour within the bone, or nerve entrapment after pathological fracture or by the invading tumour itself may also result in pain [52].

As well as mechanical damage or distension of primary afferents by tumours invading the bone, pain may arise as a result of stimulation of nociceptors by factors released by tumour cells and the accompanying inflammatory infiltrate. In addition to cancer cells, tumours are made up of a number of cell types including macrophages, neutrophils, and T-cells [53], and release a plethora of growth factors, cytokines, interleukins, chemokines, prostanoids and endothelins [57-59] resulting in activation of primary afferents which express receptors for many of these factors. Furthermore, the local environment of the tumour is made more acidic [60] and this decrease in pH can activate acid sensing ion channels (ASICs) expressed by primary afferents. The vanilloid receptor TRPV1, a cation channel activated by noxious heat and capsaicin and expressed by nociceptors, is also activated by decreases in pH, and protons decrease the temperature threshold for TRPV1 activation [61]. The local acidosis induced by cancers not only causes activation of primary afferents, but in addition facilitates osteoclastic bone destruction; osteoclast formation and activation are reliant on macrophage colony stimulating factor (M-CSF), and the interaction between the receptor activator for nuclear factor κB (RANK - expressed on osteoclast precursors) with the RANK ligand (RANK-L - expressed on various cell types including osteoblasts), in an acidic environment [54]. Osteoblasts secrete a soluble protein called osteoprotegrin (OPG) that acts as a decoy receptor for RANK-L preventing RANK and thus osteoclast activation [62]. It is this interaction between RANK – RANK-L that is disrupted by tumours invading the bone as cancer cells and invading T-cells secrete RANK-L and sequester OPG [54].

## Recent Advances in Animal Models of Cancer-Induced Bone Pain

Previously, systematic investigation of mechanisms underlying CIBP had been hindered as animal models involved systemic injection of carcinoma cells, resulting in unwell animals with multiple randomly sited metastases [63, 64]. Recently however, more suitable models have been developed.

In 1999, a murine model of bone cancer was described that closely resembled the clinical condition but in which the tumour was confined to the femur [65]. The cancer was induced by injecting sarcoma cells (NCTC 2472), which had previously been shown to induce lytic lesions in bone after intramedullary injection [66, 67], into the femur of adult mice. The injection site was then plugged with a bone restorative material confining the tumour to the femur for the duration of the experiment. Over the next 21 days mice showed behavioural signs indicative of pain progressing at the same time as osteoclastic destruction of the bone. In addition, the study showed unique neurochemical and cellular alterations in segments of spinal cord receiving afferent input from the damaged bone: massive astrocyte hypertrophy and elevated expression of dynorphin (pro-hyperalgesic peptide) in the dorsal horn of the spinal cord – changes which were almost exclusive to the side of the spinal cord ipsilateral to the tumour-laden femur. Furthermore, non-noxious palpation of the bone resulted in nocifensive behaviours as well as Substance P (SP) receptor internalisation and increased c-Fos protein expression in lamina I neurones, providing evidence that primary afferent fibres are sensitised after malignant destruction of the bone.

Hypertrophy of astrocytes, increased expression of dynorphin and c-Fos, and internalisation of SP-R have all been reported in models of neuropathic and/or inflammatory pain [68-71]. Conversely, whilst SP levels in primary afferent neurones are elevated in models of inflammation and decreased in models of neuropathy, they are not altered in the murine bone cancer model [65]. Thus, the neurochemical alterations occurring in this model are unique, reflecting a unique pain state but one that shares some features of neuropathy and inflammation. These findings alone starts to give indications as to why current pharmacotherapy is not very effective; although neuropathy and inflammation are clearly contributors to cancer-induced bone pain, the underlying mechanisms show some differences and therefore probably require distinct drug treatments.

The original model has been further developed to involve different bones such as calcaneus [72], humerus [73], and tibia [74], as well as different cell lines – fibrosarcoma [73], melanoma and adenocarcinoma [75]. The latter study showed that the different cell lines caused distinct localisation and extent of bone destruction, type of pain behaviour, and neurochemical reorganisation of the spinal cord demonstrating that multiple mechanisms are involved in generating and maintaining CIBP.

These models were validated further with the description of CIBP in different species, where injection of syngeneic MRMT-1 mammary gland carcinoma cells into the tibia of Sprague-Dawley rats resulted in astrocyte hypertrophy, progressive bone destruction, and pain behaviour thus having parallels to the murine models [76]. The similarities in neurochemical signature and behavioural manifestations of pain in the models indicate that they should be adequate for translational studies. In our laboratory we developed a rat model of CIBP, based closely on the original studies in rat, in order to investigate possible electrophysiological correlates of the pain behaviour. We found a similar development of pain behaviour as described in the previous models and characterization of neurons in the dorsal horn of the spinal cord, an important hub in the network of nociceptive pathways, revealed hyperexcitability [77] in agreement with the idea of an ongoing central sensitization [78]. The dorsal horn neuronal response was not the same as in neuropathy or inflammation, thus in line with the different neurochemical profiles reported between the pain states.

Perhaps the most interesting finding in our investigations was the alteration of the ratio between nociceptive specific (NS) and wide dynamic range (WDR) neurones in the superficial dorsal horn. Compared to sham-operated rats, animals with CIBP had an increased proportion of WDR neurons, which also showed hyperexcitable responses to mechanical, thermal and electrical stimuli. As some of these superficial cells will be NK1-expressing projection neurones this could translate to increased transmission of signals to the brain areas involved in the affective component of pain, as well as access of lower threshold inputs. This does in fact fit with the clinical condition of bone cancer and neuropathy correlating with increased anxiety and depression [52] and the low threshold access may be important in terms of the mechanical allodynia seen behaviourally in the animal models.

This shift in populations was a change that had not been reported previously in any chronic pain model, but the hyperexcitability of WDR neurones we reported has recently been confirmed in a murine model [79] thus demonstrating again the high probability of translational validity of these models. Subsequently, we showed a temporal correlation between the development of pain behaviour and the neuronal alterations in the superficial dorsal horn [80]. Correlates between behavioural and neuronal alterations have not yet been widely studied in chronic pain states, a void that is also present in other areas of neuroscience. Our investigations showing a relationship between behavioural alterations and neuronal responses indicate the latter as the most suitable substrate for pharmacological study, being suprathreshold responses more clinically relevant than the threshold level behavioural responses. Furthermore, the close correlation between the temporal development of pain behaviour and increased dorsal horn excitability suggests that this would be a suitable model in which to study changes in gene expression in hyperalgesia and allodynia. In addition, these investigations contribute to evidence for a major role of superficial dorsal horn neurones in the regulation and behavioural expression of pain sensitivity [81, 82].

Increased excitability may be generated in both spinal and supraspinal pathways. Superficial dorsal horn NK1-expressing neurones have been shown to form the origin of a spino-bulbo-spinal loop which, relaying in the rostroventral medulla (RVM) and having a facilitatory action at spinal 5-HT3 receptors, modulates mechanical and thermal nociceptive transmission and is necessary for full coding of inputs by deep DH neurons [83]. Furthermore, this circuit will receive input from centres such as the parabrachial area and amygdala involved in the affective component of pain (i.e. the fear, anxiety, emotional aspect) to amplify and prolong the sensation to a painful stimulus so that emotional state may alter the perception of pain [84]. In order to assess the role of the descending serotonergic facilitatory pathway in CIBP, we measured the effects of spinally administered ondansetron, a selective 5-HT3 receptor antagonist, on electrical- and natural-evoked DH neuronal responses in MRMT-1-injected and sham-operated rats [85]. We found that ondansetron reduced mechanical- and thermal-evoked dorsal horn neuronal responses in all animals, suggesting that the pathway is normal active, but the effects of ondansetron were significantly greater in animals injected with MRMT-1 (compared to sham-operated rats), suggesting that there is increased activation of this excitatory serotonergic pathway in CIBP. Comparing these results to inflammatory and neuropathic pain models [86, 87] it seems that the effects of ondansetron are only enhanced at longer time points after induction of the model in question when alterations have been reported in dorsal neuronal responses, implying that plasticity in the 5-HT3 descending pathway does not occur immediately after tissue injury and is more likely to be involved in the maintenance rather than the generation of chronic pain.

The translational studies mentioned so far based on behavioural, neurochemical and neuronal characterizations have already shed some light on the mechanisms underlying CIBP, but what have we learned from pharmacological investigations? As mentioned previously, opioids although plagued with severe side effects remain the mainstay for treatment of severe pain from malignancy in the bone and at present represent the most widely studied class of drug in CIBP models [73, 74, 76, 88-94]. The first studies with morphine added to the growing body of evidence suggesting CIBP to be a unique pain state as efficacy of acute systemic administration was far lower than in inflammatory models [73, 90]. These, and subsequent investigations have also shown that with acute opioid administration high doses are necessary to significantly reduce pain behaviour [74, 94]. This is consistent with the clinical problem of high doses of opioids being necessary to combat incident pain as discussed previously, and thus further validation of these as suitable animal models of CIBP closely mimicking the clinical condition.

In our laboratory we used a chronic dosing schedule (bi-daily injection for four days, and a single injection on the morning of the fifth day) in order to monitor the efficacy of morphine over time [93]. We found that from the first dose onwards morphine effectively reduced pain behaviour, but pre- versus post-morphine testing carried out on the final day of morphine treatment showed that there was a significant difference, indicating that the analgesic effects are wearing off between doses. However, it was clear that the analgesic effects did not wear off completely between doses, as pain behaviour in animals with CIBP prior to the final morphine injection was still significantly lower than in cancer animals receiving saline injections. We also found that acute systemic injection of morphine on post-operative day 15 (i.e. equivalent to the last day of treatment in the chronic morphine group) significantly reduced pain behaviour, although not to the same extent as the chronically treated cancer animals at this time point. These data not only support a chronic opioid treatment schedule in CIBP, but may also add to the explanation of why higher doses of systemic morphine were necessary in the other studies to attenuate pain as they were carried out on later post-operative days when the pain has reached a more severe level, and which although was sensitive to acute morphine in this investigation, was less so than with chronic administration.

Electrophysiological characterization in our chronically treated animals revealed that the hyperexcitability of superficial dorsal horn neurones is attenuated although not reversed, and furthermore the abnormally high ratio of wide dynamic range cells remains. This finding, suggesting that even with chronic morphine treatment there is still greater access of low-threshold stimuli to brain regions involved in pain processing, may relate to the problems of controlling incident pain with opioids in the clinic.

Pharmacological studies have also focused on the other two main classes of drug mentioned earlier that are used to combat CIBP - NSAIDs and bisphosphonates. It has been demonstrated in the murine and rat models that chronic bisphosphonate treatment reduces destruction of bone and sensory nerves innervating the bone, as well as movement-evoked bone pain [95, 96]. Selective inhibition of COX-2 (by NS-398) in the murine model has been shown to reduce spontaneous pain, bone destruction, and tumour growth [97] supporting the previously reported evidence for anti-tumorigenic properties of this class of drug [55, 98] and the involvement of prostaglandin sensitisation of primary afferents in this pain state. However, a different study in the murine model [92] showed that whilst non-selective inhibition of COX (with indomethacin) significantly reduced mechanically-evoked pain, inhibition of COX-1 (with SC560) or COX-2 (with celecoxib) was ineffective. The discrepancy between the investigations may be due to differences in effects on spontaneous and evoked pain, or differing selectivity for COX-2. There are similar discrepancies in rat models of CIBP where acute dosing with COX-2 antagonist celebrex has been shown to be ineffective against CIBP [76], whilst another investigation in the same model showed chronic administration of COX-2 antagonists lumiracoxib and valdecoxib to significantly reduce pain behaviour [99]. Here the different findings could be due to acute versus chronic administration regimes or, again, differing selectivity for COX-2. Regardless, it is clear that further investigation is necessary to evaluate the use of this class of drug in CIBP.

Translational studies in rodent models of CIBP have also enabled investigation of potential novel drug treatments. One example is gabapentin, an anticonvulsant with an unknown mechanism of action that is effective against neuropathic and inflammatory pain. Due to its proven effects in these chronic pain conditions and their contribution to CIBP, we decided to test gabapentin in our rat model. We found that chronic (but not acute) treatment with gabapentin significantly reduced pain behaviour and, moreover, normalised the hyperexcitable dorsal horn response and reset the neuronal populations [100]. This contrasts with our findings for morphine where both acute and chronic administration attenuated pain behaviour and to some extent dorsal horn hyperexcitability, but even with chronic administration the abnormally high proportion of wide dynamic range neurones in the superficial dorsal horn remained. Cessation of gabapentin treatment resulted in a return to the uninhibited pain state showing that permanent changes, such as anatomical reorganisation, are unlikely to account for CIBP and that neuronal physiology probably has a more prominent role. The antihyperalgesic effects of gabapentin have also been confirmed in the murine model of CIBP where chronic systemic treatment attenuated ongoing and movement-evoked pains [101]. These finding along with our own imply that for more adequate pain control in CIBP combination therapy of an opioid with gabapentin for example may be useful, particularly if as has been shown to be the case in neuropathic pain there is a synergistic action between morphine and gabapentin [102].

Potential novel targets for attenuating CIBP identified by investigation in these models include the bradykinin B1 receptor[95], TRPV1 receptor[103], and Endothelin receptor[101]. One of the first targets identified in the murine model of CIBP was the RANK ligand (RANK-L). As mentioned previously osteoprotegrin (OPG) acts as a decoy receptor for

RANK-L preventing RANK and thus osteoclast activation [62], and was demonstrated to reduce skeletal destruction, pain and the spinal neurochemical alterations in the model[104]. A human antibody against RANK-L is now undergoing clinical trials [105].

The development of rodent models of CIBP that mimic the clinical condition in terms of disease progression, pain, and also pharmacological response, have added a great deal to our knowledge of mechanisms responsible for generating and maintaining this devastating condition. In doing so they have also highlighted possible new therapies and drug targets for more effective treatment of this type of chronic pain that currently poses a major problem in the clinic. Perhaps the most important pharmacological message from these studies is the need to use combination therapies to target the multiple processes so far identified as contributing to CIBP if we are to treat it effectively: direct destruction of bone by tumour, destruction of bone by factors released by tumour, destruction of sensory fibres innervating bone (neuropathy), inflammation, and central sensitization.

Many of the investigations in the different models come to the same conclusions regarding underlying processes and pharmacological efficacy; this suggests that the results should be successfully extrapolated to humans. Furthermore, where there are contradictory findings in these studies it is always in the presence of differing drug doses, treatment regimes, or types of pain behaviour assessed and methods of doing so. This emphasizes the need to reach a consensus on the most relevant ways of assessing pain behaviour and drug efficacy in these types of studies in order to be able to properly compare and consolidate their findings, and thus identify the most appropriate animal models. There is still much more we need to learn about CIBP, but what all the studies mentioned here show clearly is that translational research a valuable tool in the quest to understand, and thus alleviate, chronic pain.

# References

[1] Jensen, T. S. and Baron, R. (2003). Translation of symptoms and signs into mechanisms in neuropathic pain. *Pain, 102*, 1-8.

[2] Atanassoff, P. G., Hartmannsgruber, M. W., Thrasher, J., Wermeling, D., Longton, W., Gaeta, R., Singh, T., Mayo, M., McGuire, D. and Luther, R. R. (2000). Ziconotide, a new N-type calcium channel blocker, administered intrathecally for acute postoperative pain. *Reg. Anesth. Pain. Med, 25*, 274-278.

[3] Campbell, J. N., Raja, S. N., Meyer, R. A. and Mackinnon, S. E. (1988). Myelinated afferents signal the hyperalgesia associated with nerve injury. *Pain, 32*, 89-94.

[4] Nystrom, B. and Hagbarth, K. E. (1981). Microelectrode recordings from transected nerves in amputees with phantom limb pain. *Neuroscience Letters, 27*, 211-216.

[5] Catterall, W. A. (2000). From ionic currents to molecular mechanisms: the structure and function of voltage-gated sodium channels. *Neuron, 26*, 13-25.

[6] Black, J. A., Dib-Hajj, S., McNabola, K., Jeste, S., Rizzo, M. A., Kocsis, J. D. and Waxman, S. G. (1996). Spinal sensory neurons express multiple sodium channel alpha-subunit mRNAs. *Brain Research Molecular Brain Research, 43*, 117-131.

[7] Balser, J. R., Nuss, H. B., Orias, D. W., Johns, D. C., Marban, E., Tomaselli, G. F. and Lawrence, J. H. (1996). Local anesthetics as effectors of allosteric gating. Lidocaine effects on inactivation-deficient rat skeletal muscle Na channels. *Journal of Clinical Investigation, 98*, 2874-2886.

[8] Willow, M., Gonoi, T. and Catterall, W. A. (1985). Voltage clamp analysis of the inhibitory actions of diphenylhydantoin and carbamazepine on voltage-sensitive sodium channels in neuroblastoma cells. *Molecular Pharmacology, 27*, 549-558.

[9] Devor, M. (2006). Response of nerves to injury in relation to neuropathic pain. In: McMahon, S. B. and Koltzenburg, M., (Eds.), *Wall and Melzack's Textbook of Pain*, (Fifth Edition, pp. 905-928), Elsevier, Churchill Livingstone.

[10] Woolf, C. J. and Mannion, R. J. (1999). Neuropathic pain: aetiology, symptoms, mechanisms, and management. *Lancet, 353*, 1959-1964.

[11] Dickenson, A., Matthews, E. and Suzuki, R. (2002). Neurobiology of neuropathic pain: mode of action of anticonvulsants. *European Journal of Pain, 6*, 51-60.

[12] Suzuki, R., Kontinen, V. K., Matthews, E., Williams, E. and Dickenson, A. H. (2000). Enlargement of the receptive field size to low intensity mechanical stimulation in the rat spinal nerve ligation model of neuropathy. *Experimental Neurology, 163*, 408-413.

[13] Novakovic, S. D., Tzoumaka, E., McGivern, J. G., Haraguchi, M., Sangameswaran, L., Gogas, K. R., Eglen, R. M. and Hunter, J. C. (1998). Distribution of the tetrodotoxin-resistant sodium channel PN3 in rat sensory neurons in normal and neuropathic conditions. *Journal of Neuroscience, 18*, 2174-2187.

[14] Bucknill, A. T., Coward, K., Plumpton, C., Tate, S., Bountra, C., Birch, R., Sandison, A., Hughes, S. P. and Anand, P. (2002). Nerve fibers in lumbar spine structures and injured spinal roots express the sensory neuron-specific sodium channels SNS/PN3 and NaN/SNS2. *Spine, 27*, 135-140.

[15] Coward, K., Plumpton, C., Facer, P., Birch, R., Carlstedt, T., Tate, S., Bountra, C. and Anand, P. (2000). Immunolocalization of SNS/PN3 and NaN/SNS2 sodium channels in human pain states. *Pain, 85*, 41-50.

[16] Shembalkar, P. K., Till, S., Boettger, M. K., Terenghi, G., Tate, S., Bountra, C. and Anand, P. (2001). Increased sodium channel SNS/PN3 immunoreactivity in a causalgic finger. *European Journal of Pain, 5*, 319-323.

[17] Akopian, A. N., Sivilotti, L. and Wood, J. N. (1996). A tetrodotoxin-resistant voltage-gated sodium channel expressed by sensory neurons. *Nature, 379*, 257-262.

[18] Akopian, A. N., Souslova, V., England, S., Okuse, K., Ogata, N., Ure, J., Smith, A., Kerr, B. J., McMahon, S. B., Boyce, S., Hill, R., Stanfa, L. C., Dickenson, A. H. and Wood, J. N. (1999). The tetrodotoxin-resistant sodium channel SNS has a specialized function in pain pathways. *Nature Neuroscience, 2*, 541-548.

[19] Khasar, S. G., Gold, M. S. and Levine, J. D. (1998). A tetrodotoxin-resistant sodium current mediates inflammatory pain in the rat. *Neuroscience Letters, 256*, 17-20.

[20] Porreca, F., Lai, J., Bian, D., Wegert, S., Ossipov, M. H., Eglen, R. M., Kassotakis, L., Novakovic, S., Rabert, D. K., Sangameswaran, L. and Hunter, J. C. (1999). A comparison of the potential role of the tetrodotoxin-insensitive sodium channels, PN3/SNS and NaN/SNS2, in rat models of chronic pain. *Proc. Natl. Acad. Sci. U S A, 96*, 7640-7644.

[21] Roza, C., Laird, J. M., Souslova, V., Wood, J. N. and Cervero, F. (2003). The tetrodotoxin-resistant Na+ channel Nav1.8 is essential for the expression of spontaneous activity in damaged sensory axons of mice. *Journal of Physiology, 550*, 921-926.

[22] Laird, J. M., Souslova, V., Wood, J. N. and Cervero, F. (2002). Deficits in visceral pain and referred hyperalgesia in Nav1.8 (SNS/PN3)-null mice. *Journal of Neuroscience, 22*, 8352-8356.

[23] Nassar, M. A., Levato, A., Stirling, L. C. and Wood, J. N. (2005). Neuropathic pain develops normally in mice lacking both Nav1.7 and Nav1.8. *Mol. Pain, 1*, 24.

[24] Crabbe, J. C., Wahlsten, D. and Dudek, B. C. (1999). Genetics of mouse behavior: interactions with laboratory environment. *Science, 284*, 1670-1672.

[25] van der Staay, F. J. and Steckler, T. (2001). Behavioural phenotyping of mouse mutants. *Behavioural Brain Research, 125*, 3-12.

[26] Matthews, E. A., Wood, J. N. and Dickenson, A. H. (2006). Nav 1.8-null mice show stimulus-dependent deficits in spinal neuronal activity. *Molecular Pain, 2*.

[27] Attal, N. and Bouhassira, D. (2006). Translating Basic Research on Sodium Channels in Human Neuropathic Pain. *The Journal of Pain, 7*, S31-S37.

[28] McCleane, G. J. (1999). Intravenous infusion of phenytoin relieves neuropathic pain: a randomized, double-blinded, placebo-controlled, crossover study. *Anesthesia and Analgesia, 89*, 985-988.

[29] Rowbotham, M. C. and Fields, H. L. (1996). The relationship of pain, allodynia and thermal sensation in post-herpetic neuralgia. *Brain, 119 (Pt 2)*, 347-354.

[30] Wallace, M. S., Magnuson, S. and Ridgeway, B. (2000). Efficacy of oral mexiletine for neuropathic pain with allodynia: a double-blind, placebo-controlled, crossover study. *Reg. Anesth. Pain Med, 25*, 459-467.

[31] Eisenberg, E., Alon, N., Ishay, A., Daoud, D. and Yarnitsky, D. (1998) Lamotrigine in the treatment of painful diabetic neuropathy. *Eur. J. Neurol, 5*, 167-173.

[32] Finnerup, N. B., Sindrup, S. H., Bach, F. W., Johannesen, I. L. and Jensen, T. S. (2002). Lamotrigine in spinal cord injury pain: a randomized controlled trial. *Pain, 96*, 375-383.

[33] Sindrup, S. H. and Jensen, T. S. (2002). Pharmacotherapy of trigeminal neuralgia. *Clinical Journal of Pain, 18*, 22-27.

[34] Attal, N., Gaude, V., Brasseur, L., Dupuy, M., Guirimand, F., Parker, F. and Bouhassira, D. (2000). Intravenous lidocaine in central pain: a double-blind, placebo-controlled, psychophysical study. *Neurology, 54*, 564-574.

[35] Attal, N., Rouaud, J., Brasseur, L., Chauvin, M. and Bouhassira, D. (2004). Systemic lidocaine in pain due to peripheral nerve injury and predictors of response. *Neurology, 62*, 218-225.

[36] Felts, P. A., Yokoyama, S., Dib-Hajj, S., Black, J. A. and Waxman, S. G. (1997). Sodium channel alpha-subunit mRNAs I, II, III, NaG, Na6 and hNE (PN1): different expression patterns in developing rat nervous system. *Brain Research Molecular Brain Research, 45*, 71-82.

[37] Sangameswaran, L., Fish, L. M., Koch, B. D., Rabert, D. K., Delgado, S. G., Ilnicka, M., Jakeman, L. B., Novakovic, S., Wong, K., Sze, P., Tzoumaka, E., Stewart, G. R.,

Herman, R. C., Chan, H., Eglen, R. M. and Hunter, J. C. (1997). A novel tetrodotoxin-sensitive, voltage-gated sodium channel expressed in rat and human dorsal root ganglia. *Journal of Biological Chemistry, 272*, 14805-14809.

[38] Toledo-Aral, J. J., Moss, B. L., He, Z. J., Koszowski, A. G., Whisenand, T., Levinson, S. R., Wolf, J. J., Silos-Santiago, I., Halegoua, S. and Mandel, G. (1997). Identification of PN1, a predominant voltage-dependent sodium channel expressed principally in peripheral neurons. *Proc. Natl. Acad. Sci. U S A, 94*, 1527-1532.

[39] Dib-Hajj, S. D., Rush, A. M., Cummins, T. R., Hisama, F. M., Novella, S., Tyrrell, L., Marshall, L. and Waxman, S. G. (2005). Gain-of-function mutation in Nav1.7 in familial erythromelalgia induces bursting of sensory neurons. *Brain, 128*, 1847-1854.

[40] Fang, X., Djouhri, L., Black, J. A., Dib-Hajj, S. D., Waxman, S. G. and Lawson, S. N. (2002). The presence and role of the tetrodotoxin-resistant sodium channel Na(v)1.9 (NaN) in nociceptive primary afferent neurons. *Journal of Neuroscience, 22*, 7425-7433.

[41] Herzog, R. I., Cummins, T. R. and Waxman, S. G. (2001). Persistent TTX-resistant Na+ current affects resting potential and response to depolarization in simulated spinal sensory neurons. *Journal of Neurophysiology, 86*, 1351-1364.

[42] Dib-Hajj, S., Black, J. A., Felts, P. and Waxman, S. G. (1996). Down-regulation of transcripts for Na channel alpha-SNS in spinal sensory neurons following axotomy. *Proc. Natl. Acad. Sci. U S A, 93*, 14950-14954.

[43] Hains, B. C., Klein, J. P., Saab, C. Y., Craner, M. J., Black, J. A. and Waxman, S. G. (2003). Upregulation of sodium channel Nav1.3 and functional involvement in neuronal hyperexcitability associated with central neuropathic pain after spinal cord injury. *Journal of Neuroscience, 23*, 8881-8892.

[44] Waxman, S. G., Kocsis, J. D. and Black, J. A. (1994). Type III sodium channel mRNA is expressed in embryonic but not adult spinal sensory neurons, and is reexpressed following axotomy. *Journal of Neurophysiology, 72*, 466-470.

[45] Boucher, T. J., Okuse, K., Bennett, D. L., Munson, J. B., Wood, J. N. and McMahon, S. B. (2000). Potent analgesic effects of GDNF in neuropathic pain states. *Science, 290*, 124-127.

[46] Hains, B. C., Saab, C. Y. and Waxman, S. G. (2005). Changes in electrophysiological properties and sodium channel Nav1.3 expression in thalamic neurons after spinal cord injury. *Brain, 128*, 2359-2371.

[47] Grunze, H., von Wegerer, J., Greene, R. W. and Walden, J. (1998). Modulation of calcium and potassium currents by lamotrigine. *Neuropsychobiology, 38*, 131-138.

[48] Bielefeldt, K., Ozaki, N., Whiteis, C. and Gebhart, G. F. (2002). Amitriptyline inhibits voltage-sensitive sodium currents in rat gastric sensory neurons. *Digestive Diseases and Sciences, 47*, 959-966.

[49] Gerner, P., Mujtaba, M., Khan, M., Sudoh, Y., Vlassakov, K., Anthony, D. C. and Wang, G. K. (2002). N-phenylethyl amitriptyline in rat sciatic nerve blockade. *Anesthesiology, 96*, 1435-1442.

[50] Mogil, J. S., Wilson, S. G., Chesler, E. J., Rankin, A. L., Nemmani, K. V., Lariviere, W. R., Groce, M. K., Wallace, M. R., Kaplan, L., Staud, R., Ness, T. J., Glover, T. L., Stankova, M., Mayorov, A., Hruby, V. J., Grisel, J. E. and Fillingim, R. B. (2003). The

melanocortin-1 receptor gene mediates female-specific mechanisms of analgesia in mice and humans. *Proc. Natl. Acad. Sci. U S A, 100*, 4867-4872.

[51] Portenoy, R. K., Payne, D. and Jacobsen, P. (1999). Breakthrough pain: characteristics and impact in patients with cancer pain. *Pain, 81*, 129-134.

[52] Mercadante, S. (1997). Malignant bone pain: pathophysiology and treatment. *Pain, 69*, 1-18.

[53] Mantyh, P. W., Clohisy, D. R., Koltzenburg, M. and Hunt, S. P. (2002). Molecular mechanisms of cancer pain. *Nat. Rev. Cancer, 2*, 201-209.

[54] Urch, C. (2004). The pathophysiology of cancer-induced bone pain: current understanding. *Palliative Medicine, 18*, 267-274.

[55] Sheng, H., Shao, J., Kirkland, S. C., Isakson, P., Coffey, R. J., Morrow, J., Beauchamp, R. D. and DuBois, R. N. (1997). Inhibition of human colon cancer cell growth by selective inhibition of cyclooxygenase-2. *Journal of Clinical Investigation, 99*, 2254-2259.

[56] Mach, D. B., Rogers, S. D., Sabino, M. C., Luger, N. M., Schwei, M. J., Pomonis, J. D., Keyser, C. P., Clohisy, D. R., Adams, D. J., O'Leary, P. and Mantyh, P. W. (2002). Origins of skeletal pain: sensory and sympathetic innervation of the mouse femur. *Neuroscience, 113*, 155-166.

[57] Safieh-Garabedian, B., Poole, S., Allchorne, A., Winter, J. and Woolf, C. J. (1995). Contribution of interleukin-1 beta to the inflammation-induced increase in nerve growth factor levels and inflammatory hyperalgesia. *British Journal of Pharmacology, 115*, 1265-1275.

[58] Sorkin, L. S., Xiao, W. H., Wagner, R. and Myers, R. R. (1997). Tumour necrosis factor-alpha induces ectopic activity in nociceptive primary afferent fibres. *Neuroscience, 81*, 255-262.

[59] Suzuki, K. and Yamada, S. (1994). Ascites sarcoma 180, a tumor associated with hypercalcemia, secretes potent bone-resorbing factors including transforming growth factor alpha, interleukin-1 alpha and interleukin-6. *Bone Miner, 27*, 219-233.

[60] Griffiths, J. R. (1991). Are cancer cells acidic? *British Journal of Cancer, 64*, 425-427.

[61] Tominaga, M., Caterina, M. J., Malmberg, A. B., Rosen, T. A., Gilbert, H., Skinner, K., Raumann, B. E., Basbaum, A. I. and Julius, D. (1998). The cloned capsaicin receptor integrates multiple pain-producing stimuli. *Neuron, 21*, 531-543.

[62] Lacey, D. L., Timms, E., Tan, H. L., Kelley, M. J., Dunstan, C. R., Burgess, T., Elliott, R., Colombero, A., Elliott, G., Scully, S., Hsu, H., Sullivan, J., Hawkins, N., Davy, E., Capparelli, C., Eli, A., Qian, Y. X., Kaufman, S., Sarosi, I., Shalhoub, V., Senaldi, G., Guo, J., Delaney, J. and Boyle, W. J. (1998). Osteoprotegerin ligand is a cytokine that regulates osteoclast differentiation and activation. *Cell, 93*, 165-176.

[63] Kostenuik, P. J., Orr, F. W., Suyama, K. and Singh, G. (1993). Increased growth rate and tumor burden of spontaneously metastatic Walker 256 cancer cells in the skeleton of bisphosphonate-treated rats. *Cancer Research, 53*, 5452-5457.

[64] Sasaki, A., Yoneda, T., Terakado, N., Alcalde, R. E., Suzuki, A. and Matsumura, T. (1998). Experimental bone metastasis model of the oral and maxillofacial region. *Anticancer Research, 18*, 1579-1584.

[65] Schwei, M. J., Honore, P., Rogers, S. D., Salak-Johnson, J. L., Finke, M. P., Ramnaraine, M. L., Clohisy, D. R. and Mantyh, P. W. (1999). Neurochemical and cellular reorganization of the spinal cord in a murine model of bone cancer pain. *Journal of Neuroscience, 19*, 10886-10897.

[66] Clohisy, D. R., Ogilvie, C. M., Carpenter, R. J. and Ramnaraine, M. L. (1996). Localized, tumor-associated osteolysis involves the recruitment and activation of osteoclasts. *Journal of Orthopaedic Research, 14*, 2-6.

[67] Clohisy, D. R., Ogilvie, C. M. and Ramnaraine, M. L. (1995). Tumor osteolysis in osteopetrotic mice. *Journal of Orthopaedic Research, 13*, 892-897.

[68] Abbadie, C., Brown, J. L., Mantyh, P. W. and Basbaum, A. I. (1996). Spinal cord substance P receptor immunoreactivity increases in both inflammatory and nerve injury models of persistent pain. *Neuroscience, 70*, 201-209.

[69] Honore, P., Buritova, J. and Besson, J. M. (1995). Carrageenin-evoked c-Fos expression in rat lumbar spinal cord: the effects of indomethacin. *European Journal of Pharmacology, 272*, 249-259.

[70] Nichols, M. L., Lopez, Y., Ossipov, M. H., Bian, D. and Porreca, F. (1997). Enhancement of the antiallodynic and antinociceptive efficacy of spinal morphine by antisera to dynorphin A (1-13) or MK-801 in a nerve-ligation model of peripheral neuropathy. *Pain, 69*, 317-322.

[71] Wagner, R., DeLeo, J. A., Coombs, D. W., Willenbring, S. and Fromm, C. (1993). Spinal dynorphin immunoreactivity increases bilaterally in a neuropathic pain model. *Brain Research, 629*, 323-326.

[72] Wacnik, P. W., Eikmeier, L. J., Ruggles, T. R., Ramnaraine, M. L., Walcheck, B. K., Beitz, A. J. and Wilcox, G. L. (2001). Functional interactions between tumor and peripheral nerve: morphology, algogen identification, and behavioral characterization of a new murine model of cancer pain. *Journal of Neuroscience, 21*, 9355-9366.

[73] Wacnik, P. W., Kehl, L. J., Trempe, T. M., Ramnaraine, M. L., Beitz, A. J. and Wilcox, G. L. (2003). Tumor implantation in mouse humerus evokes movement-related hyperalgesia exceeding that evoked by intramuscular carrageenan. *Pain, 101*, 175-186.

[74] Menendez, L., Lastra, A., Fresno, M. F., Llames, S., Meana, A., Hidalgo, A. and Baamonde, A. (2003). Initial thermal heat hypoalgesia and delayed hyperalgesia in a murine model of bone cancer pain. *Brain Research, 969*, 102-109.

[75] Sabino, M. A., Luger, N. M., Mach, D. B., Rogers, S. D., Schwei, M. J. and Mantyh, P. W. (2003). Different tumors in bone each give rise to a distinct pattern of skeletal destruction, bone cancer-related pain behaviors and neurochemical changes in the central nervous system. *International Journal of Cancer, 104*, 550-558.

[76] Medhurst, S. J., Walker, K., Bowes, M., Kidd, B. L., Glatt, M., Muller, M., Hattenberger, M., Vaxelaire, J., O'Reilly, T., Wotherspoon, G., Winter, J., Green, J. and Urban, L. (2002). A rat model of bone cancer pain. *Pain, 96*, 129-140.

[77] Urch, C. E., Donovan-Rodriguez, T. and Dickenson, A. H. (2003). Alterations in dorsal horn neurones in a rat model of cancer-induced bone pain. *Pain, 106*, 347-356.

[78] Clohisy, D. R. and Mantyh, P. W. (2003). Bone cancer pain. *Cancer, 97*, 866-873.

[79] Khasabov, S. G., Biorn, C. and Simone, D. A. (2004) Sensitization of spinal dorsal horn neurons in a murine model of cancer pain. In: *Society for Neuroscience 34th Annual Meeting.* San Diego, USA.

[80] Donovan-Rodriguez, T., Dickenson, A. H. and Urch, C. E. (2004). Superficial dorsal horn neuronal responses and the emergence of behavioural hyperalgesia in a rat model of cancer-induced bone pain. *Neuroscience Letters, 360,* 29-32.

[81] Mantyh, P. W. and Hunt, S. P. (2004). Setting the tone: superficial dorsal horn projection neurons regulate pain sensitivity. *Trends in Neurosciences, 27,* 582-584.

[82] Yezierski, R. P., Yu, C. G., Mantyh, P. W., Vierck, C. J. and Lappi, D. A. (2004). Spinal neurons involved in the generation of at-level pain following spinal injury in the rat. *Neuroscience Letters, 361,* 232-236.

[83] Suzuki, R., Morcuende, S., Webber, M., Hunt, S. P. and Dickenson, A. H. (2002). Superficial NK1-expressing neurons control spinal excitability through activation of descending pathways. *Nature Neuroscience, 5,* 1319-1326.

[84] Suzuki, R., Rygh, L. J. and Dickenson, A. H. (2004). Bad news from the brain: descending 5-HT pathways that control spinal pain processing. *Trends in Pharmacological Sciences, 25,* 613-617.

[85] Donovan-Rodriguez, T., Urch, C. E. and Dickenson, A. H. (2006). Evidence of a role for descending serotonergic facilitation in a rat model of cancer-induced bone pain. *Neuroscience Letters, 393,* 237-242.

[86] Rahman, W., Suzuki, R., Rygh, L. J. and Dickenson, A. H. (2004). Descending serotonergic facilitation mediated through rat spinal 5HT3 receptors is unaltered following carrageenan inflammation. *Neuroscience Letters, 361,* 229-231.

[87] Suzuki, R., Rahman, W., Hunt, S. P. and Dickenson, A. H. (2004). Descending facilitatory control of mechanically evoked responses is enhanced in deep dorsal horn neurones following peripheral nerve injury. *Brain Research, 1019,* 68-76.

[88] Baamonde, A., Lastra, A., Juarez, L., Garcia, V., Hidalgo, A. and Menendez, L. (2005). Effects of the local administration of selective mu-, delta-and kappa-opioid receptor agonists on osteosarcoma-induced hyperalgesia. *Naunyn-Schmiedebergs Archives of Pharmacology, 372,* 213-219.

[89] El Mouedden, M. and Meert, T. F. (2005). Evaluation of pain-related behavior, bone destruction and effectiveness of fentanyl, sufentanil, and morphine in a murine model of cancer pain. *Pharmacology, Biochemistry and Behavior, 82,* 109-119.

[90] Luger, N. M., Sabino, M. A., Schwei, M. J., Mach, D. B., Pomonis, J. D., Keyser, C. P., Rathbun, M., Clohisy, D. R., Honore, P., Yaksh, T. L. and Mantyh, P. W. (2002). Efficacy of systemic morphine suggests a fundamental difference in the mechanisms that generate bone cancer vs inflammatory pain. *Pain, 99,* 397-406.

[91] Menendez, L., Lastra, A., Meana, A., Hidalgo, A. and Baamonde, A. (2005). Analgesic effects of loperamide in bone cancer pain in mice. *Pharmacology, Biochemistry and Behavior, 81,* 114-121.

[92] Saito, O., Aoe, T. and Yamamoto, T. (2005). Analgesic effects of nonsteroidal antiinflammatory drugs, acetaminophen, and morphine in a mouse model of bone cancer pain. *J. Anesth, 19,* 218-224.

[93] Urch, C. E., Donovan-Rodriguez, T., Gordon-Williams, R., Bee, L. A. and Dickenson, A. H. (2005). Efficacy of chronic morphine in a rat model of cancer-induced bone pain: behavior and in dorsal horn pathophysiology. *The Journal of Pain, 6*, 837-845.

[94] Vermeirsch, H., Nuydens, R. M., Salmon, P. L. and Meert, T. F. (2004). Bone cancer pain model in mice: evaluation of pain behavior, bone destruction and morphine sensitivity. *Pharmacology, Biochemistry and Behavior, 79*, 243-251.

[95] Sevcik, M. A., Luger, N. M., Mach, D. B., Sabino, M. A., Peters, C. M., Ghilardi, J. R., Schwei, M. J., Rohrich, H., De Felipe, C., Kuskowski, M. A. and Mantyh, P. W. (2004). Bone cancer pain: the effects of the bisphosphonate alendronate on pain, skeletal remodeling, tumor growth and tumor necrosis. *Pain, 111*, 169-180.

[96] Walker, K., Medhurst, S. J., Kidd, B. L., Glatt, M., Bowes, M., Patel, S., McNair, K., Kesingland, A., Green, J., Chan, O., Fox, A. J. and Urban, L. A. (2002). Disease modifying and anti-nociceptive effects of the bisphosphonate, zoledronic acid in a model of bone cancer pain. *Pain, 100*, 219-229.

[97] Sabino, M. A., Ghilardi, J. R., Jongen, J. L., Keyser, C. P., Luger, N. M., Mach, D. B., Peters, C. M., Rogers, S. D., Schwei, M. J., de Felipe, C. and Mantyh, P. W. (2002). Simultaneous reduction in cancer pain, bone destruction, and tumor growth by selective inhibition of cyclooxygenase-2. *Cancer Research, 62*, 7343-7349.

[98] Sheng, G. G., Shao, J., Sheng, H., Hooton, E. B., Isakson, P. C., Morrow, J. D., Coffey, R. J., Jr., DuBois, R. N. and Beauchamp, R. D. (1997). A selective cyclooxygenase 2 inhibitor suppresses the growth of H-ras-transformed rat intestinal epithelial cells. *Gastroenterology, 113*, 1883-1891.

[99] Fox, A., Medhurst, S., Courade, J. P., Glatt, M., Dawson, J., Urban, L., Bevan, S. and Gonzalez, I. (2004). Anti-hyperalgesic activity of the cox-2 inhibitor lumiracoxib in a model of bone cancer pain in the rat. *Pain, 107*, 33-40.

[100] Donovan-Rodriguez, T., Dickenson, A. H. and Urch, C. E. (2005). Gabapentin normalizes spinal neuronal responses that correlate with behavior in a rat model of cancer-induced bone pain. *Anesthesiology, 102*, 132-140.

[101] Peters, C. M., Lindsay, T. H., Pomonis, J. D., Luger, N. M., Ghilardi, J. R., Sevcik, M. A. and Mantyh, P. W. (2004). Endothelin and the tumorigenic component of bone cancer pain. *Neuroscience, 126*, 1043-1052.

[102] Matthews, E. A. and Dickenson, A. H. (2002). A combination of gabapentin and morphine mediates enhanced inhibitory effects on dorsal horn neuronal responses in a rat model of neuropathy. *Anesthesiology, 96*, 633-640.

[103] Ghilardi, J. R., Rohrich, H., Lindsay, T. H., Sevcik, M. A., Schwei, M. J., Kubota, K., Halvorson, K. G., Poblete, J., Chaplan, S. R., Dubin, A. E., Carruthers, N. I., Swanson, D., Kuskowski, M., Flores, C. M., Julius, D. and Mantyh, P. W. (2005). Selective blockade of the capsaicin receptor TRPV1 attenuates bone cancer pain. *Journal of Neuroscience, 25*, 3126-3131.

[104] Honore, P., Luger, N. M., Sabino, M. A., Schwei, M. J., Rogers, S. D., Mach, D. B., O'Keefe P, F., Ramnaraine, M. L., Clohisy, D. R. and Mantyh, P. W. (2000). Osteoprotegerin blocks bone cancer-induced skeletal destruction, skeletal pain and pain-related neurochemical reorganization of the spinal cord. *Nature Medicine, 6*, 521-528.

[105] Goblirsch, M. J., Zwolak, P. and Clohisy, D. R. (2005). Advances in understanding bone cancer pain. *Journal of Cellular Biochemistry, 96,* 682-688.

*Chapter II*

# Ion Channel Blockers in Clinical Pain Management

*Lucy Chen*

MGH Pain Center, Massachusetts General Hospital, Harvard Medical School

## Abstract

This chapter will review the current clinical application of several commonly used ion channel blockers in pain management. While it remains difficult to define the exact mechanisms of many ion channel blockers currently used in clinical pain management because of their complex pharmacological actions, the increasing level of understanding on the role of sodium and calcium channels in transduction, transmission, perception, and modulation of nociception may allow us to distinguish each drug's specific mechanism of action and correlate their actions with the intended clinical use for pain management. In this chapter, clinical data are discussed regarding the efficacy, adverse effects and clinical indications of ion channel blockers. Despite the encouraging progress over the last two decades, there are still significant issues that need to be addressed in order to translate basic research knowledge into clinical application for better pain management.

## Introduction

The current knowledge on pathophysiology of norciceptive and neuropathic pain has led to a better understanding of the mechanisms of action of drugs that have been used to treat different pain disorders. It may also shed light on the future of identifying new medications for clinical pain management. Many anticonvulsants and antidepressants may have analgesic and/or antihyperalgesic effects through a number of mechanisms. These agents may block voltage sensitive sodium channels (VSSC) and/or voltage sensitive calcium channels (VSCC), facilitate opening of chloride channels, increase γ-aminobutyric acid (GABA) system, and modulate substance P and N-mehtyl-D-aspartate (NMDA) system as well as multiple neurotransmitters. Nevertheless, these agents may have common effects on transmission, modulation and perception of norciceptive signals through out the central and peripheral nervous system.

This chapter will review current clinical applications of several commonly used ion channel blockers in pain management, which will be categorized on the basis of their putative mechanisms of action on ion channels (Table 1). While it remains difficult to define the exact mechanisms of many ion channel blockers currently used in clinical pain management because of their complex pharmacological effects on multiple sites of actions on ion channels, the increasing level of understanding on the role of sodium and calcium channels in transduction, transmission, perception, and modulation of nociception may allow us to distinguish each drug's specific mechanism of action and correlate their actions with the intended clinical use for pain management.

**Table 1. Ion channel blockers in clinical pain management**

| Sodium channel blockers: | lidocaine, carbamazepine, oxcarbazepine, lamotrigine, sodium valproate, phenitoin, topiramate |
|---|---|
| Calcium channel blockers: | gabapentin, pregablin, zonisamide, ziconotide levetiracetam, topiramate |

## Calcium Channel Blockers

Calcium ion has been recognized to play an important role in nociception and antinociception processes. Transient changes in cellular calcium ion concentration lead to a key step for neurotransmitter release and the modulation of cell membrane excitability. Calcium ions are also involved in the analgesic effects of opioids. The intracellular calcium concentration may be increased by releasing calcium from its bounding state in an intrinsic process and/or opening the membrane calcium channels to allow the influx of calcium from extracellular compartment. Thus, drugs that reduce the influx of calcium ions into neuronal or glial cells may be used as adjuvants or alternatives to opioids for pain control. Drugs that possess calcium channel blockade as their partial mechanism of action and also produce analgesic effects may include gabapentin, oxacarbazepine, zonisamide, ziconotide, topiramate and levetiracetam.

### Gabapentin

Gabapentin is one of the most commonly used drugs to treat different neuropathic pain conditions in current practice. Although the mechanism of action for gabapentin remains unclear, gabapentin may block the voltage activated calcium current by binding to alpha 2-delta subunit of the membrane calcium channel [1]. This effect results in a significant reduction of the calcium influx. Consequently, it could reduce the glutamate release from primary afferent nerve endings and substance P-related activation of AMPA receptors on noradrenergic synapses, leading to the modulation of neuronal activity. With an increasing number of clinical trials and emerging body of evidence supporting its use in treating different neuropathic pain conditions, gabapentin has been used to treat painful diabetic neuropathy, post-herpetic neuralgia, trigeminal neuralgia, complex regional pain syndrome and other peripheral painful neuropathy caused by variety of diseases such as HIV, cancer, multiple sclerosis and spinal cord injury.

## Diabetic Neuropathy

Painful diabetic neuropathy (PDN) is a common and debilitating complication in patients with longstanding diabetes mellitus. It is estimated that up to about 25% of patient with diabetes may suffer from spontaneous pain, allodynia, hyperalgesia, paresthesias and other symptoms [2]. The treatment strategy for diabetic neuropathy is two-fold: one is to control the underlying disease and the other is to aim at symptomatic pain control. Multiple classes of drugs have been used to treat neuropathic pain symptoms in diabetic patients. Tricyclis antidepressants (TCA), such as amitriptyline, nortrityline, imipramine and desipramine have used as a first-line treatment until new antiepileptic drugs such as gabapentin (neurontin) was developed. While the clinical outcome of using gabapentin remains uncertain, gabapentin has been shown to relieve burning and shooting pain, allodynia, and hyperalgesia caused by PDN.

In a multi-center, double blind, placebo control large clinic trial that included 165 patients, gabapentin was used as a monotherapy to treat neuropathic pain associated with diabetes mellitus. In an 8-week trial, patients in the gabapentin group showed a significant reduction of pain as well as improvement of sleep, mood and quality of life [3, 4]. A similar result also has been observed in another randomized placebo controlled study [5]. Comparing with amitriptyline, gabapentin provided moderate pain relief that was not different from amitriptyline in one study or better pain relief and fewer side effects in another study [6, 7]. In a review of clinical trials of treating diabetic neuropathy, the number-needed-to-treat (NNT) to achieve at least 50% pain relief with antidepressants as compared to placebo was 3.4 and anticonvulsants including gabapentin were 2.7 compared to placebo [8]. There was a little difference in the incidence of minor adverse effects with either antidepressants or anticonvulsants. The number-needed-to-harm (NNH) for major adverse effect and drug related study withdraw was significantly higher with antidepressants (17 compared to placebo), whereas there was no difference as compared to placebo for anticonvulsants [8]. These clinical data demonstrated that although both antidepressants and anticonvulsants have similar efficacy in pain relief and minor adverse effects, major adverse effects causing drug-related withdrawal from the clinical trials were much higher in patients treated with antidepressants for their diabetic neuropathy.

The dosage of gabapentin for optimal therapeutic effects is 1800-3600 mg/day based on current available data [9] with a starting dose of 100-300 mg /day and increasing 100-300 mg every 1-3 days depending on the patient's condition. Adverse effects are usually mild to moderate and typically subside within 7-10 days after the treatment is started. In general, a slow titration process could avoid some of the intolerable adverse effects.

Besides being used a monotherapy, gabapentin can also be used with other neuropathic pain medicines to enhance the analgesic effect. It is a common practice (polypharmacy) that gabapentin is used in conjunction with tricyclic antidepressants (TCA) or other anticonvulsants to treat chronic intractable neuropathic pain syndromes. In a recent trial that compared the efficacy of a gabapentin and morphine combination with either gabapentin or morphine alone for the treatment of diabetic neuropathy or postherpetic neuralgia, it was found that the combination therapy with morphine and gabapentin was favored as compared with the single agent therapy [10]. The combination therapy provided better analgesia, although the maximal tolerable dose of morphine and gabapentin was lower as compared with that of each agent alone. However, at the maximal tolerable dose, the morphine-gabapentin combination therapy resulted in a higher incidence of constipation and dry mouth than each single agent alone [10]

*Postherpetic Neuralgia*

Postherpetic neuralgia (PHN) is another common neuropathic pain syndrome in chronic pain patients. PHN usually follows an acute attack of herpes zoster infection (shingles) with persistent aching, burning, itching and intermittent severe lancinating/shooting pain as well as abnormal sensation such as allodynia and hyperalgesia. The incidence of PHN is estimated around 9-34%, which increases significantly with age. Patients at 60 years or older with acute herpes zoster could have up to a 50% incidence of developing PHN.

Although TCA have been shown to be efficacious in treating PHN, the use of TCA may be limited largely because the elderly patients may be more prone to anticholinergic and cardiovascular side effects from TCA. Recent evidence shows that gabapentin appears to be effective in the treatment of PHN [11]. Gabapentin not only reduced pain symptoms and sleep disturbance but also was well tolerated by patients [12]. With regard to the side effects of gabapentin in the treatment of PHN, common transient side effects of dizziness and somnolence did not increase with the dose titration, although the peripheral edema was increased when gabapentin was titrated to greater than 1800 mg/day [13].

*Other Pain Conditions*

In a number of clinic trials or anecdotal case reports, gabapentin has been shown to be effective in treating other neuropathic pain conditions including complex regional pain syndrome, phantom pain, trigeminal neuralgia, cancer related neuropathic pain, multiple sclerosis, spinal cord injury, HIV associated painful sensory neuropathy, glossopharyngeal neuralgia [14-29]. More randomized control trials would be warranted to further investigate the use of gabapentin in these pain conditions.

Gabapentin was initially approved by FDA as an anticonvulsant agent. Its off label use has now certainly exceeded its initial intended use as an antiepileptic agent. Gebapentin is perhaps the most widely used anticonvulsant (off label) based on one epidemiology investigation in patients receiving Medicaid [30]. Physicians not only have used gabapentin to treat neurapathic pain, but also for other medical conditions. Headache, tinnitus, purities, hot flashes, drug detoxication (opioid, benzodiazepines, sedatives and perhaps alcohol) are just some of these examples that have been treated by using gabapentin. Although the mechanism of these specific effects are still not clear, the reduction of neural hypersensitivity and kindling by gabapentin has been suggested to be an unifying mechanism of gabapentin actions for these conditions [31-36].

Recently, gabapentin also has been used in the postoperative period [37-40]. Some studies have shown improved analgesia, reduced opioid consumption, decreased anxiety, and enhanced early functional recovery with gabapentin following orthopedic surgeries such as knee surgery, spinal surgery and lumber diskectomy [37-40], gynecologic surgeries such as vaginal hysterectomy and abdominal hysterectomy [41-43] as well as some ear-nose-throat surgeries [44]. In addition, the combination use of gabapentin with non-steroidal antiinflammatory drugs (NSAIDs) also has been evaluated in the perioperative period [45]. The result suggested that the combination use of these medications is superior to either single agent alone for postoperative pain, which includes opioid sparing, mood and sleep improvement, increase in peak expiratory flow and decrease in movement-related pain [45]. Similar observations also have been reported in healthy volunteers using a cold pressor test or in subjects with experimental inflammatory pain in which gabapentin enhanced the analgesic effect of morphine [46, 47]. Of interest to note is that while previous preclinical and clinical studies have indicated that gabapentin does not change baseline nociceptive threshold and is unlikely to act as an analgesic itself [1], the new information on the role of gabapentin in perioperative pain management after common surgical procedures may prompt basic science and clinical researchers to examine new mechanisms of action of gabapentin.

In summery, gabapentin is probably the most commonly used anticonvulsant in the clinical management of neuropathic pain. Although gabapentin's exact mechanism of action remains unclear, its reported efficacy in some pain conditions, low incidence of serious adverse events, favorable side effect profile, easy monitoring, and fewer drug-drug interactions may have been some of the important reasons why this drug has been used as a first line treatment option for a variety of clinical pain conditions.

## Pregabalin

Pregabalin is a new anticonvulsant that has a high affinity to the alpha2-delta subunit protein of voltage-sensitive calcium channels similar to gabapentin. Pregabalin decreases the calcium influx and reduces the release of excitatory neurotransmitters including glutamate, substance P and calcitonin gene-related peptide. Pregablin has no activity on GABA or benzodiazepine receptors and no significant drug-drug interactions. This drug has been evaluated in large clinical trials for treating PDN, PHN with clinically and statistically significant therapeutic effects [48-50]. Its onset of effects was fast such that a significant pain reduction could appear on the first day of treatment with pregabalin (300 mg/day) and sleep improvement were observed at one week after the treatment and sustained thereafter. Common side effects are dizziness, somnolence and mild to moderate peripheral edema [48-50]. Of note is that pregabalin has been shown to be effective in fibromyalgia patients with diffuse musculoskeletal pain, sleep disturbance and fatigue. At an average dose of 450 mg/day, pregabalin reduced the pain severity and sleep interference and also improved fatigue and global measures of quality of life [51], suggesting another indication of pregabalin for the clinical management of fibromyalgia patients.

## Zonisamide

Zonisamide inhibits voltage-dependent sodium channels and N-type calcium channels. The drug also influences monoamine neurotransmission and exhibits free radical scavenging properties. These possible mechanisms of action of zonisamide suggest that zonisamide might have a therapeutic effect on neuropathic pain symptoms. In a pilot study [52] on the effect of zonisamide on painful diabetic neuropathy (a randomized, double-blind, placebo controlled design), the drug was titrated over a 6-week period with a mean dose at 540 mg/day. More significant reduction of pain score was observed in the zonisamide group than the placebo group, although these differences did not reach a statistical significance. Tolerability of zonisamide was only fair in this study with a high number of dropouts from the zonisamide group [52]. Zonisamide is often used in polytherapy, making it difficult to assess the importance of its interaction with other anticonvulsant drug. Recently experimental and clinical studies have suggested other new indications of zonisamide, such as mania, Parkinson's disease, central post-stroke pain or migraine prophylaxis [53-55]. Although zonisamide has also been used to treat a wide variety of neuropathic pain conditions, the clinical data is very limited for this new drug. More large size, double blind, placebo controlled randomized trials and peer reviewed reports are needed before the effects of zonisamide on different pain conditions could be fully evaluated.

## Ziconotide

Ziconotide is a new drug with the property of a synthetic peptide analog of the omega-conotoxin deprived from the marine snail, Conus magus. Ziconotide can potently and selectively block N-type voltage-sensitive calcium channels. Interference of these channels may inhibit nociceptive transmission from primary afferent nociceptors. Currently, this drug is approved by the United States FDA only for the intrathecal use in patients who have severe pain and are refractory to other treatment options including systemic analgesics, adjunctive therapies and intrathecal morphine. In early clinical trials, there are frequent and severe central nervous system and psychiatric adverse effects associated with a rapid intrathecal infusion rate (0.4 mcg /h) and frequent dosing titration up [56]. Accordingly, patients with severe psychiatric symptoms may not be proper candidates for this drug therapy. For safety, it is recommended that the initial infusion rate start at 0.1 mcg /h, and slowly titrate up at no more than 2-3 times of the initial dose per week. If the patient is responsive to ziconotide, an implanted intrathecal infusion system is required for the long-term drug delivery [56].

In a recent randomized, double blind, placebo controlled trial through multiple medical centers in several countries, the safety and efficacy of ziconotide in treating cancer and AIDS pain patients were assessed. The result was promising with patients in the ziconotide group showing 53.1% reduction in the VAS score versus 18.1% in placebo group [57]. Dose-related analgesia was observed in another trial for chronic non-malignant pain patients [58]. The higher ziconotide concentrations in cerebral spinal fluid were generally associated with analgesia as well as the increased incidence of adverse neurological effects [58]. In addition, ziconotide has been evaluated for the post-operative pain management in patients undergoing total abdominal hysterectomy, total hip replacement and radical prostatectomy [59]. In this study, patients were given continuous local anesthetic intrathecal injection in combination with either placebo or ziconotide continuous infusion at 48-72 hours postoperatively. Patients in the ziconotide group (up to 0.7 mcg /h) had a lower VAS score and morphine PCA consumption with an acceptable side effects profile.

In summary, ziconotide is a new N-type calcium channel blocker with a favorable risk/benefit ratio. It may provide another option for patients with refractory pain not responsive to opioid or non-opioid treatment. Ziconotide administered intrathecally can produce analgesia by blocking neurotransmitter release from primary nociceptive afferents and prevent nociceptive transmission. Ziconotide may be advantageous over intrathecal morphine in that there is no development of tolerance after a prolonged use of ziconotide. On the other hand, the development of neurological adverse effects will require careful patient monitoring, smaller dose increment, and a slow titration process to avoid systemic toxicity.

## Levetiracetam

Levetiracetam is a new anticonvulsant drug that recently received approval from FDA as an adjunctive epilepsy therapy [60]. It may act via an unknown central binding site and has effects on several neurotransmitter systems, including dopaminergic, glutamatergic, and GABAergic pathways. Levetriacetam also selectively inhibits N-type voltage sensitive calcium channels. In a human study, levetiracetam significantly increased pain tolerance score but had no effect on pain summation thresholds [61]. Besides case reports on the treatment of neoplastic plexopathies and painful peripheral neuropathy [62, 63], there is one small clinical trial of levetiracetam in PHN patients refractory to a first line treatment with an encouraging outcome [64]. Moreover, in a retrospective chart review of the use of levetiracetam for migraine headache prophylaxis [65], 11 out of 20 patients (55%) experienced reduction in frequency, severity and duration of their migraine attack with the efficacy score of 2.65. The dose range was at 500-2000 mg/day, which was well tolerated by these patients with only two patient reporting adverse effects with dry eyes and dizziness [65]. It is anticipated that future large scale, double blind, placebo controlled clinical trials may further evaluate the efficacy of this drug in treating neuropathic pain.

In summery, the data from current basic science research have focused on the antihyperalgesic effects resulting from the blockade of N-type voltage sensitive channels. The $\alpha2\beta$ subunits of calcium channels appear to be the site of action for gabapentin. Given that gabapentin itself may not act as an analgesic agent, it would be of interest to examine whether gabapentin will only be effective when there is an up-regulation of the $\alpha2\beta$ subunit after peripheral nerve injury [66]. It is expected that a growing knowledge of calcium channels and their subunits may promote the search for more effective therapeutic agents for clinical management of neuropathic pain conditions.

# Sodium Channel Blockers

Sodium channels are found in all nerve cells and are primarily involved in nerve signal conduction and transmission. More than nine subtypes of sodium channels have been identified and can be divided into tetrodotoxin (TTX) sensitive (TTX-S) or resistant (TTX-R) sodium channels [67]. While TTX-S sodium channels are mostly expressed in large and medium dorsal root ganglion (DRG) neurons, TTX-R sodium channels are largely expressed in small diameter DRG neurons including C-afferent neurons [68]. The expression of both TTX-S and TTX-R sodium channel expressions can be altered after peripheral nerve injury or axotomy. There is an increase in TTX-R and TTX-S sodium channel currents after nerve injury, which results in abnormal high frequency spontaneous ectopic discharges [69]. These findings suggest a link between specific sodium channels and peripheral mechanisms of neuropathic pain and sodium channel blockers may suppress aberrant action potentials (ectopic discharges) without blocking normal nerve conduction. Despite these preclinical findings, the mechanisms of commonly used sodium channel blockers in clinical neuropathic pain management are yet fully understood. Nonetheless, a large number of clinical trials have been conducted to investigate the role of sodium channel blockers in clinical pain management.

## Lidocaine

The clinical use of lidociane as local anesthetic and anti-arrhythmic agent has a long history, and even the systemic use of lidocaine for pain treatment has been more than four decades. Over the last two decades, intravenous administration of lidocaine as a diagnostic and therapeutic tool for intractable neuropahtic pain has gained its popularity [70]. A number of clinical trials have been done to evaluate the efficacy of such treatment in different pain condition. Intravenous administration of lidocaine has showed the benefit in relieving chronic pain caused by different neurological diseases, post-stroke central pain, chronic neurogenic facial pain and myofascial pain [71-76]. The efficacy varies in these trials, although at least in trial the percent of positive responders reached 78% of all patients who received the intravenous (IV) lidocaine treatment [71].

In order to overcome transient pain relief in some pain patients receiving IV lidocaine due to its short half-life, oral mexiletine, which has a similar structure to lidocaine, has been used to maintain the therapeutic effect after patients have demonstrated beneficial responses to IV lidocaine. The pain reduction sustained for a long time if patients continue to take mexiletine. In diabetic neuropathy patients, IV lidocaine infusion seems to be a new alternative treatment although the duration of effects varies from 3 to 21 days [77]. Oral mexilatine after IV lidocaine is also recommended for patients whose diabetic neuropathy is resistant to other conventional therapies [78, 79].

Sodium channel blockers have the antihyperalgesic effect rather than a simple analgesic action and the impact of this effect is not necessarily influenced by the location of tissue injury (central or peripheral) [80]. Mexiletine alone has also been used to treat phantom pain, a central pain phenomenon, with excellent pain relief in about 58% of study patients [81]. If clonidine, an alpha-2 receptor agonist, was combined with mexiletine, the response rate was increased to 95% of patients in this study [81]. Of interest, IV lidocaine infusion also relieved neuropathic pain caused by spinal cord injury such that spontaneous pain at or below the level of spinal cord injury was significantly reduced by lidocaine in all patients with or without evoked pain [82]. However, IV lidocaine did not reduce cold allodynia, pinprick hyperalgesia and pain evoked by repetitive pinpricks in this study [82]. Of interest to note is that in a different clinical study with small patient samples (10 patients), ketamine (an NMDA receptor antagonist) was effective in reducing pain but not IV lidocaine [83].

Fibromyalgia and myofascial pain are other entities in which lidocaine treatment may have favorable outcomes by either trigger point injection or IV infusion. This treatment has become rather common in current pain management practice. In comparisons between lidocaine injection and Botulinum toxin type A (BTA) injection or dry needling to trigger points in myofascial pain patients, the pain pressure threshold was significantly higher after the lidocaine treatment and pain score was significantly lower in both lidocaine and BTA groups [76]. When the price of both injections was compared, lidocaine injection was much more cost effective than BTA. In addition, IV lidocaine infusion has been extensively used in patients with chronic diffuse myofascial pain and fibromyalgia with some success.

There are anecdotal reports of using IV lidocaine or oral mexiletine to treat primary erythromelalgia [84], hiccup [85], and metastasis bone pain [86], although clinical experience with such applications remains limited. Another application of lidocaine treatment has been in headache treatment. IV lidocaine might be a useful tool in the treatment of chronic daily headaches in patients with a substantial overuse of narcotic analgesic medications. In one study, IV lidocaine infusion (mean 8.7 days) resulted in the discontinuation of the use of other analgesic agents in 97% patients and most patients remained no or improved headache symptoms and free of analgesic agents at the 6 month follow up [87].

## Lidocaine Patch

Topical 5% lidocaine patch is a new agent that provides a local analgesic effect and may reduce allodynia and/or hyperalgesia. Lidocaine patch has been used in patients with neuropathic pain conditions such as diabetic neuropathy, postherpetic neuralgia or other peripheral neuropathy and also in patients with low back pain with some success. In several studies, lidocaine patch effectively reduced the intensity of common pain qualities in patients with moderate to severe chronic pain without reported serious adverse effects [88-92]. Some clinicians have used a combination of topical lidocaine patch with systemic gabapentin to treat chronic pain resulting from diabetic neuropathy, postherpetic neuralgia and low back injury, which allowed them to optimize the therapeutic effect and minimize the adverse effects [93]. Controlled clinical trials are warranted to define the impact of such a combination therapy.

## Carbamazepine and Oxcarbazepine

Carbamazepine's primary mechanism of action on neuropathic pain was thought through the sodium channel blockade, which decreases the spontaneous firing rate of A-delta and C fibers in a hypersensitized state. Carbamazepine is one of the earliest drugs that were approved by FDA to treat trigeminal neuralgia (TN), a neuropathic pain condition with episodic lightning like lancinating, shooting pain. This drug has been used for over four decades. Several randomized, double blind, placebo control, crossover clinical trials have been evaluated the efficacy of this drug. The results have shown that carbamazepine is superior to placebo and up to date remains a treatment of choice for TN with a responsive rate of 89% within 5-14 days after the treatment onset [94-97]. The NNT for carbamazepine to treat TN was 2.6 [98]. It should be noted that the clinical use of carbamazepine was limited by its significant drug-drug interactions, central nervous system side effects, and especially black box warning regarding a low incidence of aplastic anemia and agranulocytosis. Since newer anticonvulsants have become available clinically, neuropathic pain conditions, except for TN, are now treated more often with new anticonvulsants (see above) than carbamazepine.

Oxacarbazepine is an analogue of carbamazepine, which also acts as a sodium channel blocker and stabilizes the hyperexcitable neuronal membrane. Comparing to carbamazepine, oxcarbazepine appears to have fewer drug-drug interactions and side effects. In particular, severe blood dyscrasias have not been reported with this drug. Most common side effects are dizziness, drowsiness, hypotension, nausea, and asymptomatic mild hyponatremia. Similar to carbamazepine, oxcarbazepine has been used to treat TN including intractable TN refractory to other anticonvulsants [99]. With a median dose of 750 mg /day, this new drug has the same efficacy as that of carbamazepine in reducing evoked pain, frequency of attacks and the overall assessment score with much lower incidents of developing side effects in the oxcarbazepine group [100].

Oxacarbazepine as a single agent appears to be an efficacious and safe option for the symptomatic management in painful diabetic neuropathy. Significant improvement in total pain score and pain intensity has been observed with a mean reduction of VAS score of 48.3% [101, 102]. With regard to the treatment of patients with PHN unresponsive to carbamazepine and gabapentin, oxcarbazepine, starting at 150 mg/day and titrating up to a maintenance dose of 900 mg/day, has shown a promising result with a significant reduction in allodynia [103]. Similar results have been observed in patients with complex regional pain syndrome [104]. In addition, oxcarbazepine was well tolerated by these patients and the percentage of responders was closed to 50% [105]. Clinically, this drug may be a therapeutic alternative to other sodium channel blockers for patients with neuropathic pain conditions with a variety of etiologies.

## Lamotrigine

Lamotrigine is another anticonvulsant drug that may have multiple mechanisms of action regarding its therapeutic effect. Lamotrigine blocks voltage-sensitive sodium channels and inhibits the release of excitatory neurotransmitters such as glutamate and aspartate. It may also suppress the calcium influx by blocking calcium channels. Lamotrigine has been shown to be effective in treating TN in patients with multiple sclerosis [106] and in patients who suffered neuralgia after nerve section [107]. With a daily dose of 75-300 mg lamotrigine, the burning and shooting pain intensity was relieved by 33-100% and the frequency of shooting pain attack was reduced by 80-100% [107]. In patients with spinal cord injury, lamotrigine was able to decrease pain below the level of spinal cord injury in patients with incomplete spinal cord injury, but had no significant effect on spontaneous and evoked pain in complete spinal cord injury [108].

Of interest is that some patients with chronic refractory neuropathic pain who developed profound opioid tolerance have shown to regain the opioid analgesic effect after receiving the lamotrigine treatment. The combination therapy of lamotrigine and morphine provided these patients with sustained pain relief for several months [109]. In a recent randomized, double blind clinic trial in HIV patients, lamotrigine has been shown to be efficacious in treating HIV associated neuropathic pain related to neurotoxic antiretroviral therapy and the lamotrigine treatment was well tolerated in this population [110]. Given the fact that most HIV patients receive antiviral medications and a cure for HIV has not been discovered yet, the focus has been placed on improving the quality of life for HIV patients and managing HIV (AIDS)-related symptoms. Thus, lamotrigine may play a significant role in the management of HIV-related neuropathic pain conditions.

The common starting dose for lamotrigine is 25-50 mg/day, increasing slowly in small increments every 14 days to 250-500 mg/day in two divided doses. Due to the slow titration of this drug, with the purpose of minimizing the incidence of rash, the therapeutic effects may not be observed until the range of therapeutic doses has been reached. This may result in a high dropout rate in the treatment course. Poor tolerability at high dose (>300mg) of lamotrigine may be another factor to contribute to high drop out rate in clinic trials [111]. Up to 10% patient may have a rash, which may be an indication of the Stevens - Johnson syndrome with an incidence rate of 3/1000. Other side effects are mild, such as dizziness, somnolence, nausea, and constipation. Most patients can tolerate this medication well with only mild side effects. The current clinical data suggests that lamotrigine may be effective in the clinical management of neuropathic pain, especially for HIV-positive patients.

## Topiramate

Topiramate has multiple mechanism of action, similar to other anticonvulsants. It has been postulated that topiramate may block voltage sensitive sodium channels, potentiate GABA inhibitory action, block voltage sensitive calcium channels, and block subtypes of glutamate receptors. Other than mild side effects similar to other anticonvulsants, topiramate can cause weight loss up to 7% of body weight. In this regard, using topiramate to treat diabetic neuropathy in morbidly obese patients may a preferred choice. In a large multi-center, randomized, double blind clinical trial with 323 patients [112], topiramate was compared with placebo in treating painful diabetic neuropathy. After 12 week treatment with a daily dose equal or more than 400 mg, the topiramate group showed more reduction that the placebo group in VAS scores, the worst pain intensity, and sleep disruption. Topiramate also reduced body weight without disrupting the glycemic control in this same study [113]. However, the open-label extension study (N=205) for a 6 month follow up in these same groups of patients, the VAS score, current pain and sleep disruption scores were not significantly different between the topiramate and placebo groups [113]. Notably, 39.5% patients discontinued from the study mainly due to other side effects [113]. In another large-scale clinical study examining the effect of topiramate on painful diabetic neuropathy with a total of 1259 patients in three study groups, topiramate failed to show a favorable effect as compared with placebo in pain reduction and the authors contributed this failure possibly due to the inadequate study design [114].

In addition to the treatment of neuropathic pain, topiramate has been tried for treating chronic lumber radicular pain in a double blind, randomized, crossover study (N=42). However, the results are not encouraging with little pain reduction, a high dropout rate, and frequent side effects [115]. On the other hand, clinical data have indicated a significant effect of topiramate, superior to placebo, on chronic daily headaches (tension, migraine and cluster) as well as on migraine headache in pediatric and adult patient populations with a success rate up to 87.5% [116-119]. In these studies, topiramate was well tolerated, which significantly decreased the frequency, severity, and duration of the headache attack and improved the global assessment score and disability at a low dose range (30-80 mg/day) [116-119].

## Conclusion

With the improved understanding of pain pathways and pain mechanisms from basic science research, we know clearly now that ion channels play an important role in transduction, transmission, and modulation of the nociceptive input. This opens a new avenue for developing novel therapeutic agents useful for the clinical management of pain in general and neuropathic pain in particular. Despite the encouraging progress, there are significant issues to be addressed when translating basic research knowledge into clinical applications such as 1) different responses to the same agent in human and animal studies, 2) different responses to the same therapeutic agent among patients with a similar pain condition, and 3) the exact mechanism of action of each drug and its therapeutic target at both system and cellular levels.

As discussed in other chapters in this volume, we must consider the fact that pain score is a collective response that reflects not only nociceptive processing and also the perception of the nociceptive input, which can be readily influenced by other conditions (such as mood, affective and cognitive state). While a specific agent may be effective in reducing nociceptive transmission, it does not necessarily alter the pain response that is routinely assessed in the clinical setting using pain scores. Moreover, each patient's social background may also influence a treatment outcome. In this regard, certain therapeutic agents such as sodium or calcium channel blockers discussed in this chapter may only aid the treatment of chronic pain conditions. Nonetheless, it is anticipated that a better understanding of the cellular and molecular mechanisms of ion channel blockers in the field of basic science research is likely to provide new tools in the clinical pain management.

# References

[1] Mao J, Chen L. Gabapentin in pain management. *Anesth. Analg.* 2000; 91: 680-687.

[2] Vinik A. Clinical review: Use of antiepileptic drugs in the treatment of chronic painful diabetic neuropathy. *J. Clin. Endocrinal. Metab.* 2005, Aug; 90 (8):4936-45.

[3] Backonja MM, Beydouon A, Edward KR, et al. Gabapentin for the symptomatic treatment of painful neuropathy in patients with diabetes mellitus; a randomized controlled trial. *JAMA* 1998 Dec 2; 280(21)1831-6.

[4] Backonja MM. Gabapentin monotherapy for the symptomatic treatment of painful neuropathy: a multicenter, double-blind, placebo-controlled trial in patients with diabetes mellitus. *Epilepsia* 1999; 40 Suppl 6:S57-9; discussion S73-4.

[5] Parodowski B, Bilinska M. Gabapentin in the treatment of neuropathic pain in patients with type2 diabetes mellitus. *Pol. Merkuriusz. Lek.* 2003 Jul; 15 (85): 61-4.

[6] Morello CM, Leckband SG, Stoner CP, et al. Randomized double-blind study comparing the efficacy of gabapentin with amitriptyline on diabetic peripheral neuropathy pain. *Arch. Intern. Med.* 1999 Sep13; 159(16):1931-7.

[7] Dallocchio C, Buffa C, Mazzarello P, Chiroli S. Gabapentin V.S Amitriptyline in painful diabetic neurophathy: an open-label pilot study. *J. Pain Symptom Manag.* 2000 Oct; 20 (4): 280-5.

[8] Collins SL, Moore RA, McQuay HJ, Wiffen P. Antidepressants and anticonvulsants for diabetic neuropathy and posherpetic neuralgia: a quantitative systematic review. *J. Pain Symptom Manage.* 2000 Dec; 20(6): 449-58.

[9] Backonja MM, Glanzman RL. Gabapentin dosing for neuropathic pain: evidence from randomized placebo-controlled clinical trials. *Clin. Ther.* 2003 Jan; 25 (1):81-104.

[10] Gilron I, Bailey JM, Tu D, Holden RR, Weaver DF, Houlden RL. Morphine, gabapentin or their combination for neuropathic pain. *N. Eng. J. Med.* 2005 Mar 31; 352(13): 1324-34.

[11] Rowbotham MC, Harden N, Stacey B, et al. Gabapentin for the treatment of postherpetic neuralgia: a randomized control trial. *J. Am. Med. Assoc.* 1998; 280: 1837-1842.

[12] Rice ASC, Mator S. Gabapentin in postherpetic neuralgia: a randomized double blind placebo controlled study. *Pain* 2001; 94: 215-224.

[13] Parson B, Tive L, Huang S. Gabapentin: a pooled analysis of adverse events from three clinical trials in patients with postherpetic neuralgia. *Am. J. Geriatr. Pharmaco. Ther.* 2004 Sep; 2(3): 157-62.

[14] Van de Vusse A, Van den Berg S, Weber A. Randomized controlled trial of gabapentin in Complex Regional Pain Syndrome Type 1. *BMC Neurology* 2004 Sep 29; 4(1):13.

[15] Mellick GA, Mellick LB. Reflex sympathetic dystrophy treated with gabapentin. *Arch. Phys. Med. Rehabil.* 1997 Jan; 78(1):98-105.

[16] Rusy LM, Troshynski TJ, Weisman SJ. Gabapentin in phantom limb pain management in children and young adult: report of seven cases. *J. Pain Symtom. Manage* 2001 Jan; 21(1):78-82.

[17] Cheshire WP Jr. Defining the role for gabapentin in the treatment of trigeminal neuralgia: a retrospective study. *J. Pain* 2002 Apr; 3(2): 137-42.

[18] Solaro C, Messmer M, Uccell A, et al. Low dose gabapentin combined with either lamotrigine or carbamazepine can be useful therapies for trigeminal neuralgia in multiple sclerosis. *Eur. Neurol.* 2000; 44(1):45-8

[19] Lossignal DA, Plehiers B, Body JJ. Gabapentin and cancer pain: a pilot study. *Rev. Med. Brux.* 2004 Oct; 25(5): 429-35.

[20] Caraceni A, Zecca E, Bonezzi C, et al. gabapentin for neuropathic cancer pain: a randomized controlled trial from the gabapentin cancer pain study group. *J. Clin. Oncol.* 2004 Jul 15;22(14): 2909-17.

[21] D'Aleo G, Rifici C, Sessa E, et al. R3 norciceptive reflex in multiple sclerosis patients with paraoxymal symptoms treated with gabapentin. *Fuc. Neurol.* 2000 Oct-Dec; 15(4): 205-9.

[22] Houtchens MK, Richert JR, Sami A, Rose JW. Open label gabapentin treatment for pain in multiple sclerosis. *Mult. Scler.* 1997 Aug; 3(4): 250-3.

[23] Levendoglu F, Ogun CO, Ozerbil O, et al. Gabapentin is a first line drug for the treatment of neuropathic pain in spinal cord injury. *Spine* 2004 Apr 16; 29(7):743-51.

[24] Ahn SH, Park HW, Lee RS, et al. Gabapentin effects on neuropathic pain compared among patients with spinal cord injury and different durations of symptoms. *Spine* 2003 Feb 15; 28(4): 341-6.

[25] Putzke JD, Richards JS, Kezar L, et al. Long-term use of gabapentin treatment of pain after traumatic spinal cord injury. *Clin. J. Pain* 2002 Mar-Apr; 18(2): 116-21.

[26] Ness TJ, San Pedro EC, Richards JS. A case of spinal cord injury-related pain with baseline rCBF brain SPECT imagine and beneficial response to gabapentin. *Pain* 1998 Nov;78 (2): 139-43.

[27] Hahn K, Arendt G, Brain JS, et al. A placebo-controlled trial of gabapentin for painful HIV-associated sensory neuropathies. *J. Neurol.* 2004 Oct; 251(10): 1260-6.

[28] La Spina I, Porazzi D, Maggiolo F, et al. Gabapentin in painful HIV related neuropathy: a report of 19 patients' preliminary observations. *Eur. J. Neurol.* 2001 Jan; 8(1): 71-5.

[29] Garcia-Callejo FJ, Velert-Vila MM, Talamantes-Escib F, et al. Clinical response of gabapentin for glossopharyngeal neuralgia. *Rev. Neural.* 1999 Feb 16-18; 28(4): 380-4.

[30] Chen H, Deshpande AD, Jiang R, et al. An epidemiological investigation of off-label anticonvulsant drug use in Georgia Medicaid population. *Phamacoepidemiol Drug Safe* 2004 Dec14.

[31] Covinton EC. Anticonvulsants for neuropathic pain and detoxification. *Cleve. Clin. J. Med.* 1998; 65 Suppl 1: SI 21-9.

[32] Albertazzi P, Bottazzi M, Purdie DW. Gabapentin for management of hot flashes, a case series. *Menopause* 2003 May-Jun; 10(3): 214-7.

[33] Kuma p, Jain MK. Gabapentin in management of pentazocine dependence: a potent analgesic- anticraving agent. *J. Assoc. Physicians India* 2003 Jul; 51: 672-6.

[34] Spira PJ, Beran PG. Gabapentin in the prophylaxis of chronic daily headache: a randomized placebo controlled study. *Neurology* 2003 Dec 23; 61(12): 1753-9.

[35] Freye E, Levy JV, Partecke L. Use of gabapentin for attenuation of symptoms following rapid opiate detoxication (ROD)-correlation with neurophyiological parameters. *Neuro. Physiol. Clin.* 2004 Apri; 34 (2): 81-9.

[36] Zapp JJ, Gabapentin for the treatment of tinnitus: A case report. *Ear. Nose Throat J.* 2001 Feb; 80 (2): 114-6.

[37] Menigaux C, Adam F, Guignard B, et al. Preoperative gabapentin decrease anxiety and improves early functional recovery from knee surgery. *Anesth. Analg.* 2005, 100 (5): 1394-9.

[38] Pandey CK, Navka DV, Giri PJ, et al. Evaluation of the optional preemptive dose of Gabapentin for postoperative pain relief after lumber diskectomy: a randomized double blind placebo-controlled study. *J. Neurosurg. Anesiol.* 2005 April; 17 (2):65-8.

[39] Pandey CK, Sahay S, Gupta D, et al. Preemptive gabapentin decrease postoperative pain after lumber discoidectomy. *Can. J. Anesth.* 2004 Dec; 51 (10): 986-9.

[40] Turan A, Karamanlioglu B, Memis D, et al. Analgesic effects of gabapentin after spinal surgery. *Anesthesiology* 2004 Apri; 100(4): 935-8.

[41] Pararius MG, Mennander S, Suominen P, et al. Gabapentin for the prevention of postoperative pain after vaginal hysrectomy. *Pain* 2004 Jul; 110(1-2): 175-81.

[42] Turan A, Karamanlioglu B, Memis D, et al. The analgesic effect of gabapentin after total abdominal hysterectomy. *Anesth. Analg.* 2004 May; (5): 1370-3.

[43] Dierking G, Duedahl TH, Rasmnsen ML, et al. Effects of gabapentin on postoperative morphine consumption and pain after abdominal hysterectomy: a randomized double blind trial. *Acta Anesthiol. Scand.* 2004 Mar; 48(3); 322-7.

[44] Turan A, Memis D, Karamanlioglu B, et al. The analgesic effects of Gabapentin in monitored anesthesia care for ear-nose-throat surgery. *Anesth. Analg.* 2004 Aug; 99(2): 375-8.

[45] Gilron I, Orr E, Tu D, et al. A placebo-controlled randomized clinical trial of perioperative administration of gabapentin, rofecox b and their combination for spontaneous and movement-evoked pain after abdominal hysterectomy. *Pain* 2005 Jan; 113(1-2):191-200.

[46] Eckhardt K, Ammon S, Hofmann U, et al. Gabapentin enhances the analgesic effects of morphine in healthy volunteers. *Anesth. Analg.* 2000 July; 91(1): 185-91.

[47] Werner MU, Perkins FM, Holte K, et al. Effects of gabapentin in acute inflammatory pain in humans. *Reg. Anesth. Pain Med.* 2001 Jul-Aug; 26(4): 322-8.

[48] Lesser H, Sharma U, LaMoreaux L, Poole RM. Pregablin relieves symptoms of painful diabetic neuropathy. *Neurology* 2004; 63; 2104-2110.

[49] Frampton JE, Scott LJ. Pregablin in the treatment of painful diabetic peripheral neurapathy. *Drugs* 2004; 64(24): 2813-20.

[50] Frampton JE, Foster RH, Pregablin: in the treatment of postherpetic neuralgia. *Drugs* 2005; 65(1): 111-8.

[51] Crofford LJ, Rowbatham MC, Mease PJ, et al. Pregablin for the treatment of fibromyalgia syndrome: Result of a randomized double-blind placebo controlled trial. *Arthritis Rheum.* 2005 Apr; 52(4): 1264-73.

[52] Atli A, Dodra S. Zonisamide in the treatment of painful diabetic neuropathy: a randomized, double blind, placebo-controlled pilot study. *Pain Med.* 2005 May-Jun;6(3): 225-34.

[53] Sobieszek G, Borowicz KK, Kimber-trojiar Z et al. Zonisamide: A new antiepileptic drug. *Pol. J. Pharmacol.* 2003 Sep-Oct; 55(5): 683-9.

[54] Drake ME Jr. Greathouse NJ, Renner JB, et al. Open-label Zonisamide for refractory migraine. *Clin. Neuropharmacol.* 2004 Nov-Dec; 27(6): 278-80.

[55] Takahashi Y, Hashimoton K, Tsuji S. Successful use of zonisamide for central poststroke pain. *J. Pain* 2004 Apr; 5(3): 192-4.

[56] Wermeling DP. Ziconotide: an intrathecally administered N type calcium channel antagonist for the treatment of chronic pain. *Phamacotherapy* 2005 Aug; 25(8): 1084-94.

[57] Staats PS, Yearwood T, Charapata SG. Et al. Intrathecal ziconotide in the treatment of refractory pain in patients with cancer or AIDS: a randomized controlled trial. *JAMA* 2004 Jan 7:291(1): 63-70.

[58] Wermeling D, Drass M, Ellis D, et al. Pharmacokinetics and pharmacodynamics of intrathecal ziconotide in chronic pain patients. *J. Clin. Pharmacol.* 2003 Jun; 43(6):624-36.

[59] Alanassoff PG, Hartmamsgruber MW, Thrasher J, et al. Ziconotide, a new N-type calcium Channel blocker, administed intrathecally for acute postoperative pain. *Reg. Anesth. Pain. Med.* 2000 May-June; 25(3): 274-8.

[60] LuKyanetz EA, Shkryl VM, Lostyuk PG. Selective blockade of N-type calcium channels by levetiracetam. *Epilepsia* 2002; 43:9.

[61] Enggaard TP, Klitgeard NA, Sindrnp SH. Specific effect of levetiracetam in experimental human pain models. *Eur. J. Pain.* 2006 Apr; 10(3): 193-8.

[62] Price MJ. Levetiracetam in the treatment of neuropathic pain: three case studies. *Clinical J. Pain.* 2004 Jan-Feb; 20(1): 33-6.

[63] Dunteman ED. Levetiracetam as an adjunctive analgesic in neuroplastic plexopathies: case series and commentary. *J. Pain Palliat. Care Pharmacother.* 2005; 19(1):35-43.

[64] Rowbotham MC, Manville NS, Ren J. Pilot tolerability and effectiveness study of levetiracetam for postherpetic neuralgia. *Neurology* 2003; 61:866-867.

[65] Cochran JW. Levetiracetam as migraine prophylaxis. *Clin. J. Pain.* 2004 May-Jun 20(3):198-9.

[66] Yaksh TL. Calcium channels as therapeutic targets in neuropathic pain. *The J. of Pain* 2006 Jan;7 ( 1 suppl 1):S13-S30.

[67] Waxman SG, Cummins TR, Dib-Hajj S, et al. Sodium Channels, excitability of primary sensory neurons, and molecular basis of pain. *Muscle Nerve.* 1999 Sep; 22(9): 1177-87.

[68] Quashoff S, Grosskreutz J, Schroder JM, et al. Calcium potentials and tetrodotoxin-resistant sodium potentials in unmyeliated C-fibers of biopsied human sural nerve. *Neuroscience* 1995; 69:955-965.

[69] Stebbing MJ, Eschenfelder S, Habler HJ, et al. Changes in the action potential in sensory neurons after axotomy in vivo. *Neuro Report* 1999; 10:201-206.

[70] Mao JR, Chen L. Systemic lidocaine for neuropathic pain relief. *Pain Jul*; 87(1): 7-17.

[71] Peterson P, Kastrup J, Zeeberg I, Boysen G. Chronic pain with intravenous lidocaine. *Neurol. Res.* 1986 Sep; 8(3): 189-90.

[72] Attal N, Gaude V, Brasseur L, et al. Intravenous lidocaine in central pain: a double blind placebo-controlled psychophysical study. *Neurology* 2000 Feb. 8; 54(3): 564-74.

[73] Cahana A, Shvelzon V, Dolbug O, et al. Intravenous lidocaine for chronic pain: an 18 month experience. *Harefuah* 1998 May 1; 134(9): 692-4, 751, 750

[74] Cahana A, Carota A, Montadon ML, et al. The long-term effect of repeated intravenous lidocaine on central pain and possible correlation in positron emission tomography measurements. *Anesth. Anal.* 2004 Jun; 98(6): 1581-4.

[75] Scrivani SJ, Chandry A, Maeiewicz RJ,et al. Chronic neurologic facial pain: lack of response to intravenous lidocaine infusion- a new treatment o chronic painful diabetic neuropathy. *J. Orofac. Pain.* 1999 spring 13(2)89-96.

[76] Kamanli A, Kaya A Ardicoglu O, et al. Comparision of lidocaine injection, botulinum toxin injection and dry needling to trigger points in myofascial pain syndrome. *Pheumatol. Int.* 2005 Oct;25 (8): 604-11.

[77] Kastrup J, Petersen P, Dejgard A, et al. Intravenous lidocain infusion – a new treatment of chronic painful diabetic neuropathy. *Pain* 1987 Jan 28(1): 69-75.

[78] Ackerman WE 3rd, Colclough GW, Juneja MM. Bellinger K.. The management of oral mexiletine and intravenous lidocaine to treat chronic painful symmetrical diabetic neuropathy. *J. Ky. Med. Assoc.* 1991 Oct; 89(10): 500-1.

[79] Dejgard A, Petersen P, Kastrup J. Mexiletine for treatment of chronic diabetic neuropathy. *Lancet* 1998 Jan2-9; 1(8575-6): 9-11.

[80] Attal N, Bouhassira D. Translating basic research on sodium channels in human neuropathic pain. *The J. of Pain.* 2006 Jan; (1 suppl 1) S31-37.

[81] Davis RW. Successful treatment for phantom pain. *Orthopedics* 1993 Jun; 16(6): 691-5.

[82] Finnerup NB, Biering-Sorensen F, Johannesen IL, et al. Intravenous lidocaine relieves spinal cord injury pain: a randomized control trial. *Anesthesiology* 2005 May; 102(5): 1023-30.

[83] Kvarnstrom A, Karlsten R, Quiding H, Gordh T. The analgesic effect of intravenous ketamine and lidocaine on pain after spinal cord injury. *Acta Anesthesiol. Scand.* 2004 Apr; 48(4):498-506.

[84] Nathan A, Rose JB, Guite JW, et al. Primary erythromelalgia in a child responding to intravenous lidocaine and oral mexiletine treatment. *Pediatrics.* 2005 Apr; 115(4) e504-7.

[85] Cohen SP, Lubin E, Stojanovic M. Intravenous lidocaine in the treatment of hiccup. *South. Med. J.* 2001 Nov; 94(11):1124-5

[86] Sjogren P, Banning AM, Hebsgaard K, et al. Intravenous lidocaine in the treatment of chronic pain caused by bone metastases. *Ugeskr. Laeger.* 1989 Aug 21;151(34): 2144-6.

[87] Williams DR, Stark RJ. Intravenous lidocaine infusion for the treatment of chronic daily headache with substantial medication overdose. *Cephalagia* 2003 Dec; 23(10): 963-71.

[88] Argoff CE, Galer BS, Jensen MP, et al. Effectiveness of the lidocaine patch 5% on pain qualities in three chronic pain states: assessment with the neuropathic pain scale. *Curr. Med. Res. Opin.* 2004;20 suppl 2:S21-8.

[89] Galer BS, Gamnaitoni AR, Oleka N, et al. Use of the lidocaine patch 5% in reducing intensity of various pain qualities responded by patients with low back pain. *Curr. Med. Res. Opin.* 2004; 20. suppl 2: S5-12.

[90] Meier T, Faust M, Huppe M, et al. Reduction of chronic pain for non-postherpetic peripheral neuropathyes after topical treatment with a lidocaine patch. *Schmerz* 2004 Jun; 18(3): 172-8.

[91] Davies PS, Galer BS. Review of lidocaine patch 5% studies in the treatment of postherpetic neuralgia. *Drugs* 2004; 64(9): 937-47.

[92] Hines R, Keaney D, Moskowitz MH, et al. Use of lidocaine patch 5% for chronic low back pain: a report of four case. *Pain Med.* 2002 Dec; 3(4):361-5.

[93] White WT, Patel N, Drass M, Dalamachu S. Lidocaine patch 5% with systemic analgesics such as gabapentin: a rational polyphamacy approach for the treatment of chronic pain. *Pain Med.* 2003 Dec; 4(4);321-30.

[94] Killian JM, Fromm GH. Carbamazepine in the treatment of neuralgia. *Arch. Neurol.* 1968 Aug; 19(2):129-36.

[95] Rockliff BW, Davis EH. Controlled sequential trials of carbamazrpine in trigeminal neuralgia. *Arch. Neuro.* 1966 Aug; 15(2):129-36.

[96] Campbell FG, Graham JG, Zikha KJ. Clinical trial of cabamazepine in trigeminal neuralgia. *J. Neurosurg. Neurol. Psych.* 1966 June; 29(3): 265-7.

[97] Nicol CF. A four year double blind, randomized study of tegretol in facial pain. *Headache* 1969 Apr; 9(1): 54-7.

[98] McQuay H, Carrol D, Jadad AR, et al. Anticonvulsant drugs for management of pain: a systemic review. *BMJ* 1995 Oct 21; 311(7012): 1047-52.

[99] Zakrzecoska JM, Patsalos PN. Oxacarbazepine: a new drug in the management of intractable trigeminal neuralgia. *J. Nerol. Surg. Psychiatry.* 1989 Apr; 52(4):472-6.

[100] Beydoun A, Schimidt D, D'Souza J. Metaanalysis of comparative trials of oxacarbazepine versus carbamazepine in trigeminal neuralgia. *J. Pain.* 2002;3(suppl 1);38.

[101] Beydoun A, Kobertz SA, Carrazana EJ. Efficacy of oxacarbazepine in the treatment of painful diabetic neuropathy. *Clin. J. Pain.* 2005 May-jun; 20(3):174-8.

[102] Dogra S, Beydoun A, Mazzola J, et al. Oxacarbazepine in painful neurapathy: a randomized placebo-controlled study. *Eur. J. Pain.* 2005 Oct; 9(5): 543-54.

[103] Criscuolo S, Auletta C, Lippi S, et al. Oxacarbazepine monotherapy in postherpetic neuralgia unresponsive to carbamazepine and gabapentin. *Acta Neuro. Scand.* 2005 Apr; 111(4): 229-32.

[104] Lalwanik K, Schoham A, Kol JL, McGraw T. Use of oxacarbazepine to treat a pediatric patient with resistant CRPS. *J. Pain.* 2005 Oct; 6(10): 704-6.

[105] Magenta P, Arghetti S, Dipalma F, et al. Oxacarbazepine is effective and safe in the treatment of neuropathic pain: pooled analysis of seven clinical studies. *Neurol. Sci.* 2005 Oct; 26(4):218-26.

[106] Solaro C, Messmer Uccelli M, Uccelli A, et al. Low dose of gabapentin combined with either lamotrigine or carbamazepine can be useful therapies for trigeminal neuralgia in multiple sclerosis. *Eur. Neurol.* 2000; 44 (1): 45-8.

[107] Sander-Kiesling A, Rumpold SG, Dorn C, et al. Lamotrigine monotherapy for control of neuralgia after nerve section. *Acta Anesthesiol. Scand.* 2002 Nov; 46(10):1261-4.

[108] Finnerup NB, Sindrup SH, Bach FW, et al. Lamotrigine in spinal cord injury pain: a randomized controlled trial. *Pain* 2003 Apr; 96(3): 375-83.

[109] Devulder J, Deleat M. Lamotrigine in the treatment of chronic refractory neuropathic pain. *J. Pain Symptom. Manage.* 2000 May; 19(5):398-403.

[110] Simpson DM, McArthur JC, Olney R, et al. Lamotrigine for HIV-associated painful sensory neuropathies: a placebo-controlled trial. *Neurology* 2003 May13;60(9): 1508-14.

[111] Markman JD, Dworkin RH. Ion channel targets and treatment efficacy in neuropathic pain. *The J. of Pain* 2006 Jan (7) 1s: S38-47.

[112] Raskin P, Donofrio PD, Rosenthal NR, et al. Topiramate VS placebo in painful diabetic neuropathy: analgesic and metabolic effects. *Neurology* 2004 Sep 14; 63(5): 865-73.

[113] Donofrio PD, Raskin P, Rosenthal NR, et al. Safety and effectiveness of topiramate for the management of painful diabetic peripheral neuropathy in an open-label extension study. *Clin. Ther.* 2005 Sep; 27(9):1420-31.

[114] Thienel U, Neto W, Schwabe SK, et al. Topiramate in painful diabetic polyneuropathy: findings from three double blind placebo-controlled trials. *Acta Neurol. Scand.* 2004 Oct; 110(4): 221-31.

[115] Khoromi S, Patsalides A, Parada S, et al. Topiramate in chronic lumber radicular pain. *J. Pain.* 2005 Dec;6(12):829-36.

[116] Borzy JC, Koch TK, Schimschock JR. Effectiveness of topiramate in the treatment of pediatric chronic daily headache. *Pediatr. Neurol.* 2005 Nov; 33(5): 314-6.

[117] Campistol J, Campos J, Casas C, Herranz JL. Topiramate in the prophylactic treatment of migraine in children, *J. Child. Neurol.* 2005 Mar; 20(3): 251-3.

[118] Hershey AD, Powers SW, Vockell AL, et al. Effectiveness of topiramate in the prevention of childhood headaches. *Headache* 2002 Sep;42(8): 810-8.

[119] Mathew NT, Kailasam J, Meadors L. Prophylaxis of migraine, transformed migraine and cluster headache with topiramate. *Headache* 2002 Sep; 42(8): 796-803.

*Chapter III*

# Spinal N-Methyl-D-Aspartate Receptor Mechanisms of Central Sensitization and Persistent Pain Following Tissue Injury

*Wei Guo, Ronald Dubner and Ke Ren*[*]

Department of Biomedical Sciences, Dental School; Program in Neuroscience, University of Maryland, Baltimore, MD 21201, USA

## Abstract

Studies in recent years have shed light on the cellular and molecular mechanisms underlying persistent pain. We now know that the increased nociceptor activity after injury leads to hyperexcitability in the central nervous system (CNS) and subsequent hyperalgesia and spontaneous pain. Convincing evidence demonstrates that the development of persistent pain involves activation of N-methyl-D-aspartate (NMDA) receptors, a subtype of the ionotropic glutamate receptor family. NMDA receptors are involved in activity-dependent neuronal plasticity and play a key role in response to tissue injury and inflammation. The NMDA receptor is a receptor-ion channel complex and characterized by a voltage-dependent block by $Mg^{2+}$, significant $Ca^{2+}$ inflow upon activation, and slow kinetics. At least seven subunits contribute to the formation of the NMDA receptor, NR1, NR2A-D and NR3A/B. The functional NMDA receptor channel comprises two heterodimers each formed by one NR1 and one NR2 subunits. Studies indicate that NMDA receptors contribute to the initiation and maintenance of central sensitization or spinal dorsal horn hyperexcitability and the development of persistent pain. The injury-induced increase in NMDA receptor function involves posttranslational modulation. The NR1 and NR2B subunits in the spinal cord are phosphorylated after peripheral inflammation with a temporal profile corresponding to the development of

---

[*] Correspond to: K. Ren, Ph.D. Dept. BMS Rm. 5A12, 666 W. Baltimore St., Baltimore, MD 21201-1510. Ph: (410) 706-3250. Fax: (410) 706-0865. E-mail: kren@umaryland.edu

behavioral hyperalgesia. The phosphorylation of the NMDA receptors requires activation of protein kinases such as PKA, PKC and protein tyrosine kinase Src. The signal transduction upstream to NR2B tyrosine phosphorylation also involves G-protein coupled receptors and IP$_3$-mediated intracellular calcium release. The findings of the role of NMDA receptors in central sensitization have significant impact on the search for novel approaches for the treatment of persistent pain. The efficacy of the NMDA receptor antagonists in persistent pain has been assessed in animal models as well as in clinical studies. Antagonism of the NMDA receptor may add a new dimension to the management of persistent pain. Although the psychotomimetic side effects produced by most NMDA receptor antagonists have hampered the use of NMDA receptor antagonists in chronic pain, the basic research in this area should help to develop new directions in the antagonism of the NMDA receptor activation for pain control. These include manipulation of the components of the signal transduction pathways upstream to NMDA receptor phosphorylation, including scaffold proteins in the postsynaptic density, protein kinases and phosphatases and co-factors, searching for optimal combination of NMDA receptor antagonists with other agents, and the development of subunit specific NMDA receptor antagonists with a reduced aversive profile.

# Introduction

Chronic pain conditions often develop after tissue or nerve injury and persist for months or years, even when the injury has healed. Different from transient or acute pain, chronic pain is non-protective and difficult to treat, thus representing a major health problem. Studies in recent years have shed light on the cellular and molecular mechanisms underlying persistent pain. We now know that the increased nociceptor activity after injury leads to hyperexcitability in the central nervous system (CNS) including spinal and medullary dorsal horns and subsequent hyperalgesia and spontaneous pain [1-3]. Among the multiple receptor mechanisms, convincing evidence demonstrates that the development of persistent pain involves activation of N-methyl-D-aspartate (NMDA) receptors, a subtype of the ionotropic glutamate receptor family [4,5]. This line of research has been generating novel targets of drug development for the control of persistent pain.

# The Structure, Function and Pharmacology of the NMDA Receptor

L-glutamate and possibly several other excitatory amino acids (EAA) function as major excitatory neurotransmitters in the mammalian CNS. The receptors that mediate EAAs' action consist of two groups of ionotropic and metabotropic receptors [5,6]. The ionotropic glutamate receptors are further divided into the three subtypes that are preferably activated by NMDA, alpha-animno-3-hydroxy-5-methyl-4-isoxazole propionic acid (AMPA), and kainate, and are named after these agonists, respectively [7-10]. The metabotropic glutamate receptors (mGluRs) consist of three subgroups (I-III). Ample evidence indicates that NMDA receptors are involved in activity-dependent neuronal plasticity, expressed as changes in synaptic strength and neuronal activity during development and learning [11]. This NMDA receptor-dependent CNS plasticity is also a key phenomenon in response to tissue injury and inflammation [1].

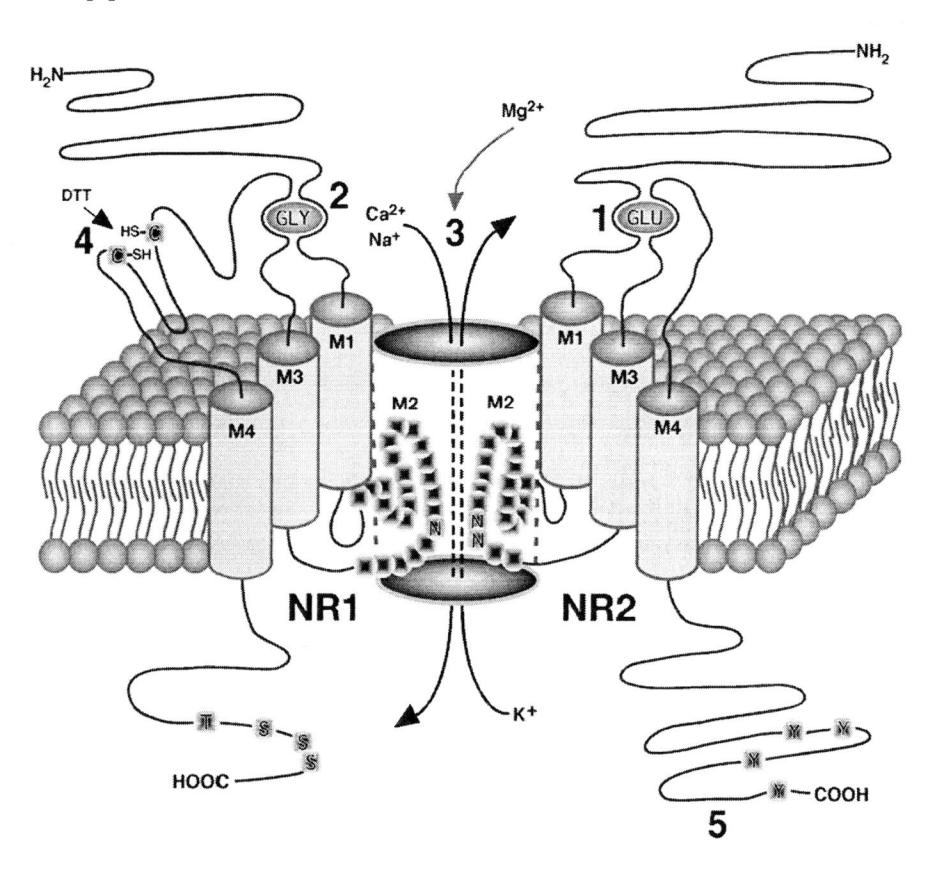

Figure 1. The molecular and functional model of the NMDA receptor ion channel complex. See text for details

The NMDA receptor is a receptor-ion channel complex [5,12] (Fig. 1). The NMDA receptor channel is characterized by a voltage-dependent $Mg^{2+}$ block, significant $Ca^{2+}$ inflow upon activation, and slow kinetics. The activation of the NMDA receptor requires the removal of the $Mg^{2+}$ block by depolarization. The current knowledge of the molecular basis of the function of the NMDA receptor channel complex is summarized in figure 1 and briefly discussed below.

At least seven subunits contribute to the formation of the NMDA receptor, NR1 (or GluRzeta1), NR2A-D (or GluRepsilon 1-4) and NR3A/B. Further, there are three regions (exon 5, 21 and 22 of the NR1 gene) of alternative splicing, named N1, C1, and C2 cassettes, on the NR1 protein [13-15]. The functional NMDA receptor channel comprises two heterodimers each formed by one of the NR1 splice variants and one NR2 subunit (NR2A-D) [16]. Each NR1 or NR2 subunit has 1) four hydrophobic membrane domains (M1-M4) in which M1 and M3-4 are transmembrane-spanning domains and M2 is thought to make a hairpin turn within the membrane; 2) a large extracellular N-terminus domain and an extracellular loop between M3 and M4; 3) an intracellular carboxy-terminus domain which involves about 100 aa' for NR1 and 400-600 aa' for NR2 subunits. The contribution of the NR3 subunit to the NMDA receptor is less certain [5].

Activation of the NMDA receptor requires binding of an EAA ligand and a co-agonist. Glutamate (GLU) binds to the agonist site on the NR2 subunit and glycine (GLY) acts through a strychnine-insensitive site on the NR1 subunit as a co-agonist of the NMDA receptor. The putative binding sites for GLU and GLY are formed in a region preceding M1 and the loop domain separating M3 and M4 on NR2 and NR1 subunits, respectively (bi-lobed formation) [17].

The NMDA receptor channel is highly permeable to $Ca^{2+}$ and subject to the $Mg^{2+}$ block under resting conditions. The pore of the NMDA channel is formed in a region consisting of the M2 segments of both NR1 and NR2 subunits, although parts of the M1 and M3 segments may also contribute [18]. The analysis by site-directed mutagenesis has revealed that the asparagine (N) sites in the M2 segment of the NR1 and NR2 subunits govern both $Ca^{2+}$ permeability and $Mg^{2+}$ block in the NMDA receptor channel [19-21]. Mutation of the N sites by glutamine markedly reduces the $Mg^{2+}$ block and $Ca^{2+}$ permeability.

A number of endogenous compounds, including zinc, protons, polymines spermine and spermidine, and sulfhydryl (SH) redox reagents, act at multiple modulatory sites on the NMDA receptor assembly to either facilitate or inhibit the receptor activation. Zinc inhibits NMDA receptor function through both voltage-dependent and voltage-independent mechanisms [22,23]. Protons inhibit NMDA receptor function through interactions with the NR1 subunit [24]. Polyamines increase the binding of [$^3$H] MK-801 [25], suggesting that they could facilitate activation of the NMDA receptor by glutamate. Polyamines may also suppress the NMDA receptor function under certain conditions. The N1 insert (including Lys211) from exon 5 of the NR1 gene is involved in regulation of pH sensitivity, and the effects of zinc and polyamines on NMDA receptor [23]. Dithiothreitol (DTT), an SH group reducing agent, enhances NMDA receptor responses via two cysteine residues (C744 and C798) of the NR1 subunit [21] (Fig. 1). Mutation of these two cysteine residues eliminates potentiation of the receptor by DTT and spermine, and inhibition by protons, suggesting an interaction between modulatory sites of the NMDA receptor channel complex.

Phosphorylation is an important mode of regulation of NMDA receptor activity [27,28]. There are multiple sites on the NR1 and NR2 subunits that are targets of several protein kinases and phosphatases, including protein kinase A (PKA), protein kinase C (PKC), $Ca^{2+}$/calmodulin-dependent protein kinase II (CaMKII), tyrosine kinases, and protein tyrosine phosphatases. For example, some putative phosphorylation sites are identified at the C1 insert from the exon 21 of the NR1 gene (Threonine879, Serine890, 896, 897) [29]. Some tyrosine residues (Y837, 842 of NR2A, Y1472 of NR2B) of the NR2 subunits are phosphorylated to modulate NMDA receptor channel opening and receptor internalization [30-32]. The activity of protein tyrosine phosphatases controls the gain of the NMDA receptor [33,34].

Based on molecular structure and function of the NMDA receptor, multiple classes of agents or drugs can be used to affect the activity of the NMDA receptor, thus achieving a variety of therapeutic goals, including control of chronic pain conditions (Fig. 1). These agents are 1) agonist recognition site antagonists, usually the phosphonoamino acid antagonists, that compete for the recognition sites of L-GLU [e.g. (±)-2-amino-5-phosphonopentanoic acid (AP-5), and (±)-3-(2-carboxypiperazin-4-yl)-propyl-1-phosphonic acid (CPP)]; 2) strychnine-insensitive GLY site antagonists that block the binding of the co-agonist glycine [e.g. HA-966, and 7-chlorokynurenic acid (7-Cl kynurenic acid)]; 3) channel blockers that act at the intra-ion channel sites to inhibit receptor associated channels [e.g. $Mg^{2+}$, dizocilpine maleate (MK-801), and ketamine]; 4) A variety of agents that act on the different modulatory sites such as the sulfhydryl redox site [35]; and 5) kinase inhibitors that affect the C-terminal phosphorylation. According to studies using recombinant NMDA receptors, the pharmacological properties of NMDA receptors vary with their subunit composition [36]. The NR1/NR2C receptor is much less sensitive to $Mg^{2+}$ and MK-801 block than that of NR1/NR2A and NR1/NR2B receptors. The sensitivity of the ligand recognition site to AP-5 is in the order of NR1/NR2A > NR1/NR2B > NR1/NR2C ≥ NR1/NR2D. The sensitivity to the GLY site antagonist 7-Cl kynurenic acid is in the order of NR1/NR2C > NR1/NR2B > NR1/NR2A ≈ NR1/NR2D. The atypical NMDA receptor antagonist ifenprodil may be a selective antagonist at the NR2B subunit.

## NMDA Receptors in Spinal Nociceptive Processing and Dorsal Horn Hyperexcitability

A number of earlier studies suggest that the NMDA receptor plays a role in processing nociceptive input to the spinal dorsal horn. Injection of NMDA into the spinal subarachnoid space of mice produces a behavioral hyperalgesic effect [37]. In contrast, intrathecal injection of the NMDA receptor antagonist suppresses aversive nocifensive responses in rats [38]. This is consistent with the observations that glutamate exists in primary afferent terminals in the superficial spinal dorsal horn [39] and the NMDA-sensitive binding site is present in the dorsal horn [40]. Nagy et al. [41] have further shown differential synaptic distribution of the NMDA receptor subunits in the rat spinal cord. Glutamate is released upon C-fiber intensity dorsal root stimulation in spinal cord slices [42]. *In vivo* studies confirm that noxious stimulation induces an increase in glutamate and aspartate in the dorsal lumbar spinal cord of freely moving rats [43]. Knee joint arthritis induces aspartate and glutamate release into the rat spinal dorsal horn [44].

Dorsal horn nociceptive neurons exhibit the wind-up phenomenon in response to repeated stimulation of peripheral nerves [45]. When stimulation intensity is strong enough to activate C-fibers and stimulation frequencies are greater than once per two to three seconds, the responses of such neurons will increase with each subsequent stimulus. As a result, the responses to latter stimuli will be much greater than the original response and are often followed by a significant afterdischarge. Wind-up may trigger central hyperexcitability and result in prolonged nociceptive states [46]. This phenomenon has been related to a centrally mediated temporal summation and used to explain pain summation with repetitive or persistent stimulation. The wind-up of dorsal horn neurons is sensitive to NMDA receptor antagonists. Dickenson and Sullivan [47], and Davies and Lodge [48] observed simultaneously in rats that wind-up of dorsal horn nociceptive neurons is selectively reduced by a competitive NMDA receptor antagonist, AP-5, and a non-competitive NMDA receptor antagonist, ketamine. Thus, NMDA receptor activation is coupled to the functional plasticity of the spinal cord associated with repetitive stimulation.

Dorsal horn hyperexcitability after tissue injury is often referred to as central sensitization [46,49], which is evidenced by a reduced threshold, an increased responsiveness and an expansion of the receptive fields of dorsal horn nociceptive neurons [1,3,50,51]. The enlargement of the receptive fields size is a measure of neuronal hyperexcitability. In the normal rat, the receptive fields of dorsal horn nociceptive neurons innervating the hind paw are typically small and restricted to one or more toes or toe pads [50,52]. After injection of the inflammatory agent CFA into one hind paw, the receptive fields of these neurons are greatly enlarged and more complex [52,53]. There is an appearance of discontinuous fields, fields with areas of differing sensitivity, and additional responses to joint movement. The receptive fields from the CFA-inflamed paw are over 2 fold larger than those in control animals [52]. The alteration of the receptive fields is a reflection of the activity-dependent plasticity of the spinal and medullary dorsal horns in response to changes in stimulus input, which has been observed under a variety of experiment conditions including adjuvant-induced polyarthritis [54,55] and temporomandibular joint inflammation [56], chemical irritation of the cutaneous [57] or deep masseter muscle tissue [58], surgical incision of the skin [59], electrical stimulation [50,60], noxious pinch [61] and ischemia [62].

The expanded receptive fields of nociceptive neurons in the superficial laminae or the neck of the dorsal horn following complete Freund's adjuvant-induced inflammation are sensitive to the NMDA receptor antagonist. We have examined the effects of MK-801, an NMDA receptor channel blocker, on the receptive fields of dorsal horn neurons [53]. Extracellular recordings were made from dorsal horn neurons at 24 h after injection of CFA into one hind paw. Both edema and behavioral hyperalgesia had reached their maximal magnitude at this time [52]. As shown in Fig. 2, 5 of the 8 neurons recorded from the rat superficial dorsal horn had receptive fields that extended over nearly the entire plantar surface of the paw. The receptive fields of the 3 other neurons occupied approximately half of the ventral surface of the hind paw. After administration of MK-801 (cumulative dose of 7 mg/kg, i.v.), there was a dose-dependent and statistically significant reduction in the receptive field size of these nociceptive neurons in CFA-treated rats [53]. MK-801 also prevented the dynamic expansion of the receptive fields produced by inflammation or electrical stimulation [53]. In contrast, MK-801 did not produce significant changes in the receptive field size in normal rats. The NMDA receptor antagonists also reduce the facilitation of the flexor reflex produced by C-fiber strength electrical stimulation of the sural nerve or by the cutaneous application of mustard oil [63] and suppress background and mechanically evoked activity of spinal neurons in cats with knee joint inflammation [64].

The antagonism of the receptive field expansion by the NMDA receptor antagonist has important implications for understanding central sensitization or activity-dependent plasticity in the spinal dorsal horn. The cutaneous receptive fields of dorsal horn neurons in normal individuals are surrounded by an excitatory subliminal fringe [57,65,66]. The area of the fringe can extend from a small area adjacent to the center of the receptive fields to almost the entire hindlimb [57]. Stimulation applied to this fringe usually only induces low amplitude EPSPs without action potentials. Functionally, ineffective synapses may also surround the edge of the receptive fields [67,68]. The presence of the receptive field fringe and the ineffective synapses forms a physiological basis for understanding receptive field plasticity under different conditions. It is likely that in rats with CFA-induced inflammation the subliminal fringe of the receptive fields becomes suprathreshold and an additional part of the receptive fields.

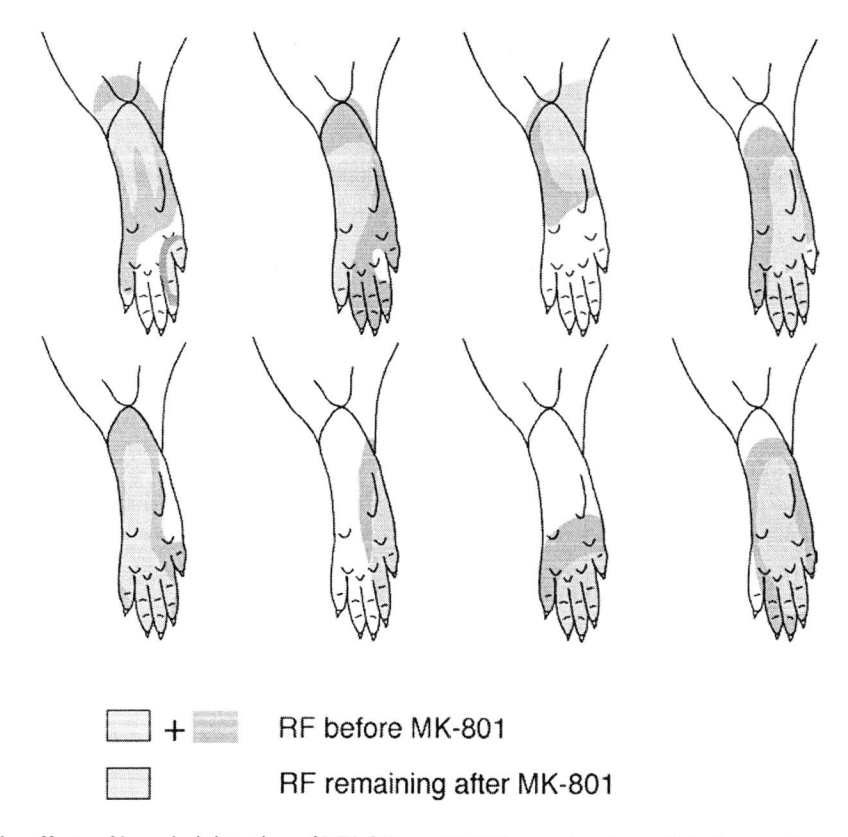

☐ + ▨  RF before MK-801
☐  RF remaining after MK-801

Figure 2. The effects of i.v. administration of MK-801, an NMDA receptor channel blocker, on the receptive field (RF) size of nociceptive specific neurons recorded from the superficial dorsal horn ipsilateral to the injection of CFA. The extent of the RFs of these neurons before (gray plus hatched areas) and after (hatched area) the administration of MK-801 is shown. The experiments were performed at 24 h after the injection of CFA into a hind paw (From [53], with permission from IASP)

We have hypothesized that expanded receptive fields will result in greater overlap of receptive fields and lead to a greater number of neurons activated by a stimulus than the number activated by the same stimulus applied in the absence of receptive field expansion. Such a mechanism correlates increased neuronal activity with more intense pain and may at least partially explain mechanical allodynia [69,70]. Importantly, the NMDA receptor is involved in this plastic change of receptive fields. A sequence of events may occur following peripheral tissue or nerve injury. As proposed by Dubner [70], an increased nociceptive neuronal barrage from the periphery would lead to increased depolarization at NMDA receptor sites, facilitated by neuropeptide release (substance P, CGRP and dynorphin). The activation of NMDA receptors contributes to the increased excitability of dorsal horn neurons and central sensitization. With over-excitation, excessive depolarization could result in EAA excitotoxicity, cell dysfunction and a loss of inhibitory mechanisms. There would be a further enlargement of receptive fields of dorsal horn neurons and hyperexcitability, leading to persistent hyperalgesia.

# Cellular and Molecular Mechanisms of NMDA Receptor Activation in Inflammatory Pain

Recent molecular and biochemical analyses further establish the role of NMDA receptors in central sensitization and persistent hyperalgesia. After a conditional deletion of the NR1 subunit of the NMDA receptor in the lumbar spinal cord of adult mice by the localized injection of an adenoassociated virus expressing Cre recombinase into floxed NR1 mice, the formalin-induced nocifensive behavior is reduced by 70% [71]. Intrathecal injection of small interfering RNAs (siRNAs) targeting the NR2B subunit of the NMDA receptor suppresses the expression of NR2B mRNAs and proteins and abolishes formalin-induced nocifensive behavior in rats [72]. The properties of NMDA receptor channels are altered by inflammation. Rat dorsal horn neurons that receive inputs from the inflamed hind paw exhibit a reduced $Mg^{2+}$ block and enhanced NMDA responses at negative potentials [73].

## NMDA Receptor Subunit Phosphorylation

The injury-induced increase in NMDA receptor function involves posttranslational modulation. The NR1 subunit is phosphorylated by PKA on serine 890 and 897 and by PKC on serine 896. These phosphorylation events can be monitored with phosphorylation site-specific antibodies [28,74]. A time-dependent and lasting NR1 phosphorylation at serine 896 and 897 after CFA-induced inflammation has been observed [75]. Carrageenan also induces an increase in NR1 serine phosphorylation in the rat spinal cord [76]. There is an enhanced phosphorylation of NR1 on serine 897 in dorsal horn spinothalamic tract neurons after intradermal injection of capsaicin in rats [77]. The NR1 serine 897 phosphorylation of superficial dorsal horn spinothalamic cells after capsaicin is mediated by PKA, and the phosphorylation of spinothalamic cells in the deep dorsal horn involves both PKA and PKC [78]. Noxious heat stimulation induces phosphorylation of NR1 on serine 896 in dorsal horn neurons [79]. Excitotoxic injury of the rat spinal cord induces excessive grooming behavior that is associated with an increase in NR1 serine phosphorylation [80]. The increased NR1 serine phosphorylation in dorsal horn neurons is correlated with the maintenance of allodynia in neuropathic rats [81]. All these findings support the idea that the phosphorylation of NR1 subunits is related to the increased synaptic efficacy and the development of central sensitization after injury. Brenner et al. [79] showed that NR1 serine 896 phosphorylation occurred in the endoplasmic reticulum, suggesting a role for NR1 subunit phosphorylation in trafficking of the NR1 subunit to the cell membrane.

Studies on hippocampal, forebrain and other disease systems have indicated importance of the NR2 subunit to NMDA receptor function and synaptic plasticity. The NR2 subunit can determine synaptic localization and function of the NMDA receptor. Deletion of the C-terminal tail of the NR2 subunit impairs NMDA receptor mediated synaptic activity [12,82,83]. Phosphorylation of multiple sites in the cytoplasmic C termini of the NR2 subunits is known to modulate NMDA receptor activity and affect synaptic transmission [74,84]. Tyrosine phosphorylation of the NR2 subunits plays a key role in signal transduction pathways for NMDA receptor activation [85-87]. NMDA receptor gating is closely regulated by tyrosine kinase Src that phosphorylates tyrosine residues on the NR2 subunits [30,87,88]. Intracellular application of Src leads to an increase in NMDA receptor channel current [89].

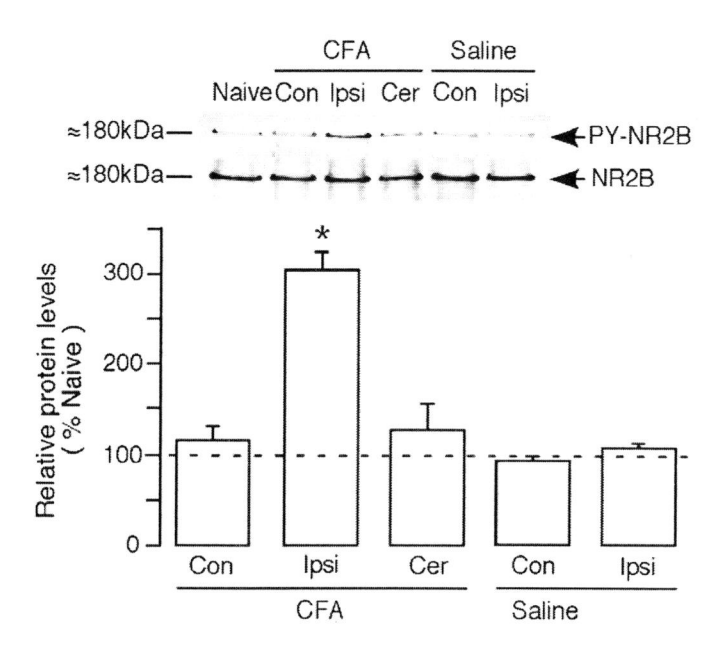

Figure 3. Selective increases in NR2B tyrosine phosphorylation after inflammation. Proteins were extracted from L4,5 spinal cord of non-inflamed naïve (N) rats and rats at 24h after complete Freund's adjuvant or saline injection into one hind paw. The spinal dorsal horn was divided at the midline into the ipsilateral (ipsi) and contralateral (Con) halves. Cervical spinal cord (Cer) was used as a control. The upper blot shows the immunoreactive bands against anti-phosphotyrosine 4G-10 (PY-NR2B) after immunoprecipitation of extracted proteins with anti-NR2B antibodies. The lower blot shows immunobands against NR2B antibodies after stripping and reprobing the same membrane previously probed with 4G-10 antibodies. The levels of tyrosine phosphorylation are normalized to the respective NR2B immunoreactive bands. The relative phosphotyrosine protein levels (mean ± S.E.M.) are expressed as a percentage of the naïve controls for the purpose of illustration. Raw data were used for statistical comparisons. Asterisks indicate significant differences ($p<0.05$) from the naïve controls. N = 5 per time point. Dashed line indicates the control levels in non-inflamed rats. (From [99], with permission from Society for Neuroscience)

It has been shown that the major tyrosine phosphorylated protein in the postsynaptic density (PSD) is the NR2B subunit of the NMDA receptor [85]. Tyrosine phosphorylation of the NR2 subunits, particularly the NR2B subunit, has been associated with long-term potentiation (LTP) [90,91], as well as neuropathological conditions [92,93].

NR2B mRNAs and proteins are expressed in dorsal horn neurons [94-96] and protein tyrosine kinases are expressed in the spinal cord [97]. We have produced inflammation and hyperalgesia in rats and examined the tyrosine phosphorylation of the spinal NR2 subunits in relation to the development and maintenance of hyperalgesia. Compared to control samples from naive and saline-injected rats and contralateral dorsal horn, the levels of NR2B tyrosine phosphorylation in the ipsilateral spinal dorsal horn are selectively increased after peripheral inflammation (Fig. 3) [98,99]. Formalin injection in the hind paw also induces an increase in NR2B tyrosine phosphorylation in rats [100]. Kovacs et al. [101] show that an NR2B subunit specific NMDA receptor antagonist CI-1041 blocks wind-up of dorsal horn neurons, further supporting a role of the NR2B subunit in spinal hyperexcitability. Hind paw inflammation did not induce a change in NR2A tyrosine phosphorylation in the spinal cord of the rat [98], which appears consistent with a report that deletion of the GluRepsilon 1 (NR2A) gene did not alter CFA-induced pain behavior in mice [102]. However, hind paw inflammation induces an enhanced NR2A tyrosine phosphorylation in the rostral ventromedial medulla, an important supraspinal structure involved in descending pain modulation [103], suggesting a differential functional involvement of the NR2 subunits at spinal and supraspinal levels in response to injury. The NR2 tyrosine phosphorylation was apparently not observed after carrageenan-induced inflammation [76]. These correlative findings support the hypothesis that NR2B tyrosine phosphorylation is involved in the development of spinal plasticity and hyperalgesia after inflammation. Recent studies have identified seven specific tyrosine residues on the C-terminus of the NR2B subunit that are phosphorylated by Fyn, a Src family tyrosine kinase, *in vitro* [104]. Among those tyrosine residues, tyr-1472 appears to be the major Fyn-mediated phosphorylation site and tyr-1472 phosphorylation is enhanced after induction of LTP in mouse hippocampal slices [104]. Phosphorylation of tyr-1472 by Fyn helps to retain NR2B in the postsynaptic density and facilitate synaptic responses [32]. Using a phosphorylation site-specific antibody, Abe et al. [105] show that Fyn kinase-mediated NR2B tyrosine phosphorylation at tyr1472 is essential for the maintenance of neuropathic pain. It would be very interesting to determine whether a deletion of the specific tyrosine site on the NR2B subunit affect the development of CFA-induced hyperalgesia.

## Temporal Profile and Input Dependency of NMDA Receptor Phosphorylation

The time course of the increased phosphorylation of the NMDA receptor after inflammation is very similar for the NR1 and NR2B subunit [75,98]. A key phenomenon common to serine and tyrosine sites of the NMDA receptor is that the changes in phosphorylation occur almost immediately after peripheral insult. In animals receiving intradermal capsaicin that activates small-diameter nociceptors, serine residues on the NR1 subunit are phosphorylated within 30 min of the stimulation [77,78]. The extracellular signal-regulated protein kinases (ERK) in spinal and dorsal root ganglion neurons are phosphorylated within a minute of an intense noxious peripheral or C-fiber electrical stimulus [106,107]. Importantly, thermal hyperalgesia and mechanical allodynia can be detected within minutes after inflammation [98,108]. These correlated behavioral and biochemical findings indicate that NMDA receptor phosphorylation plays a key role in the *initiation* of central sensitization and subsequently, pain hypersensitivity. It is noted that serine phosphorylation of the NR1 subunit waned around day 7 and no significant increase in phosphorylation was found at day 14 after inflammation [103]. The inflammation-induced NR2B tyrosine phosphorylation shows a similar time course [98]. However, CFA-induced hyperalgesia and allodynia produced by thermal and mechanical stimuli do not fully recover at two weeks after inflammation, although they are significantly attenuated [109,110]. Thus, the NMDA receptor phosphorylation may play less of a role in maintaining the late persistent phase of inflammatory hyperalgesia. Further studies should address the contribution of other receptors and kinases and related cellular pathways and central nervous system circuitry to the later phases of hyperalgesia.

The inflammation-induced increase in NR1 serine 896 and NR2B tyrosine phosphorylation depends on primary afferent drive. After pretreatment of the hind paw with 2% lidocaine before the injection of CFA, the increase in phosphoserine 896 NR1 was attenuated or abolished at 10-30 min, and recovered after 2 h post-CFA [75,98], when compared to rats pre-treated with saline. This blockage corresponds to a period when behavioral signs of hyperalgesia also disappeared, suggesting that the phosphorylation is dependent upon primary afferent input [98]. The reappearance of phosphorylation after local anesthesia block further indicates that NR1 serine 896 and NR2B tyrosine phosphorylation are not only initiated, but also maintained by primary afferent input. These observations strengthen the view that altered central nociceptive processing is initiated and dynamically maintained by input from the site of injury [98,111].

It was unexpected that the increased NR1 serine 897 phosphorylation was not affected by local anesthetic block [75]. An incomplete anesthesia of the injected paw was unlikely since the same procedure was followed as in other experiments that verify effective anesthesia. It appears that factors other than activation of nociceptors at the site of injury may have contributed to the maintenance of phosphorylation. Many chemical mediators are known to be released from the site of inflammation. Intraplantar injection of carrageenan, lipopolysaccharide or bacterial endotoxin produces mechanical hyperalgesia associated with an upregulation of proinflammatory cytokines such as tumor necrosis factor-alpha, interleukin (IL)-1beta, IL-6 and nerve growth factor in the injected skin [112-114]. Endothelins and prostaglandins are also released after injury and the phospholipase-cyclooxygenase-prostanoid cascade is activated [115,116]. Some of these factors may reach the central target via the circulation. A unilateral hind paw inflammation induces an increased cyclooxygenase-2 expression in both sides of the lumbar spinal cord as well as the cervical cord [117], suggesting a non-somatotopically related activation. More interestingly, complete blockage of the sciatic nerve for more than 24 h is unable to completely eliminate cyclooxygenase-2 mRNA induction in the spinal cord or the increased prostaglandin $E_2$ levels in the cerebrospinal fluid after peripheral inflammation [117]. These observations support the hypothesis that chemical mediators released during inflammatory reactions not only directly activate nociceptors on site but also produce an effect on central neurons via other unknown pathways [118]. Future studies on the underlying mechanisms of dorsal horn hyperexcitability and protein phosphorylation that outlast, or are independent of the primary afferent nociceptive drive will be important for our understanding of some forms of persistent pain.

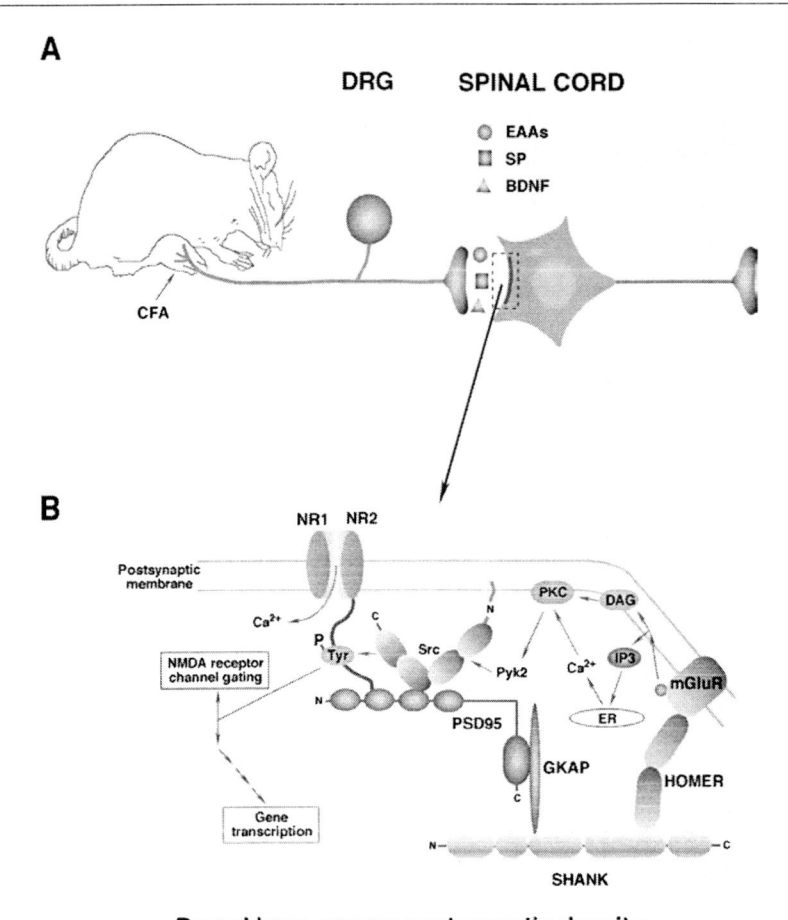

**Dorsal horn neuron postsynaptic density**

Figure 4. Proposed mGluR-NMDA receptor coupling and related protein tyrosine kinase pathways in dorsal horn neurons after inflammation. A. After injection of complete Freund's adjuvant (CFA) into the hind paw, tissue injury and inflammation occur, which activate peripheral nociceptors. There is a reduction of excitation threshold, increased expression of sodium channels, and release of inflammatory cytokines and mediators, all leading to peripheral sensitization. The injury initiates primary afferent barrage that goes into the spinal dorsal horn, release neurotransmitters including excitatory amino acids (EAAs) transmitters, substance P (SP), brain-derived neurotrophic factor (BDNF) and calcitonin gene-related peptide (CGRP, not illustrated). A cascade of events will follow the activation of EAA and other receptors, eventually leading to sensitization of dorsal horn neurons, so called dorsal horn hyperexcitability or central sensitization. The signaling events that would occur in the postsynaptic density (dashed rectangle) in postsynaptic dorsal horn neurons after peripheral inflammation are detailed in B. B. The NMDA receptor and group I mGluRs-HOMER are linked through the binding of PSD95 (postsynaptic density-95 protein) and SHANK with GKAP (guanylate kinase-associated protein). Src, a protein tyrosine kinase, is associated with NMDA receptor via interaction with PSD95. After primary afferent activation, tyrosine (Tyr) residues in the C-termini of the NR2B subunits are phosphorylated through Pyk2-Src pathways. The upstream events to Src-tyrosine signaling likely involve activation of group I mGluRs, an increase in intracellular $Ca^{2+}$ through $IP_3$-endoplastic reticulum (ER) pathways, and protein kinase C activation through the diacylglycerol (DAG) pathway. Tyrosine phosphorylation of the NMDA receptor will potentiate the NMDA receptor channel gating and trigger a cascade leading to increased gene transcription of the target genes. These events contribute to amplification of synaptic input, central sensitization and the development of hyperalgesia

## Postsynaptic Density and mGLuR-NMDA Receptor Coupling

The NMDA receptor forms multiprotein complexes with postsynaptic density proteins including receptors, adaptor proteins, and protein kinases [119]. This super protein complex also includes Src family protein tyrosine kinases [33,99,120,121] that are important modulators of NMDA receptor channels [30]. The protein scaffold in the postsynaptic density allows for efficient intracellular signaling. The NMDA receptor subunits can be phosphorylated by kinases intrinsic to the postsynaptic density. The functional integrity of the PSD is necessary for the expression of persistent pain behaviors. Inhibiting the expression of PSD-95 (postsynaptic density-95 protein) in spinal neurons significantly attenuates nocifensive facilitation by NMDA [122]. Mice with a mutated PSD-95 gene did not develop NMDA receptor-dependent hyperalgesia and allodynia after neuropathy [123]. Targeted disruption of the PSD-93 gene attenuates NMDA receptor-dependent persistent pain after CFA or nerve injury [124].

In CNS neurons, NMDARs are physically linked to mGluRs in the postsynaptic density (Fig. 4). The group I mGluRs bind Homer protein, and the latter binds Shank, a family of postsynaptic proteins [125]. Shank also is linked to PSD-95 via binding with GKAP (guanylate kinase-associated protein) [126]. Postsynaptic density-95 protein is known to interact with NR2A/B subunits of the NMDA receptor in spinal neurons [122]. Our co-immunoprecipitation and double immunofluorescent labeling experiments indicate that, in the spinal dorsal horn, mGluR-Homer-Shank complex and NMDA receptors are biochemically linked through related postsynaptic density proteins PSD-95 and Shank [99] (Fig. 4).

The interaction between the mGluRs and NMDA receptors has received increased attention as a mechanism of modulation of neuronal plasticity. Group I mGluRs have been implicated in a variety of pain conditions associated with inflammation, neuropathy, and spinal injury [127-134]. The application of group I mGluR antagonists have been shown to reduce spinothalamic neuronal activity and mechanical allodynia [128,135]. Antisense ablation of $mGluR_1$ inhibits spinal nociceptive transmission [136]. The mGluR agonist evoked response is enhanced in the spinal cord from hyperalgesic but not naive animals, which is reversed by an NMDA receptor antagonist [137]. Activation of mGluR potentiates NMDA current in dissociated rat spinal dorsal horn neurons [138], *Xenopus* oocytes [139-141], CA3 pyramidal cells [142], and NMDAR-mediated synaptic transmission in the rat dentate gyrus [143], and is necessary for NMDA-induced long term potentiation [144]. Selective activation of mGluR1 increases NR2 subunit tyrosine phosphorylation in cortical neurons *in vitro* from mouse [145].

After receiving strong primary afferent drive generated from peripheral nociceptors by inflammation, a cascade of events in the postsynaptic density of dorsal horn neurons may lead to NMDA receptor phosphorylation (Fig. 4). One important signaling pathway for NR2B tyrosine phosphorylation involves the coupling between group I mGluRs and NMDA receptors [99]. We have provided evidence that intrathecal administration of the group I mGluR antagonists blocks inflammation-induced NR2B tyrosine phosphorylation [98,99]. This effect should be attributed to the blockage of postsynaptic mGluRs and its interaction with NMDA receptors but not presynaptic modulation. Although mGluRs are present in presynaptic terminals, the activation of presynaptic mGluRs functions to reduce presynaptic glutamate release [146]. In a dorsal horn slice preparation, the group I (DHPG), but not group II (APDC) and III (L-AP4), mGluR agonists, induces NR2B tyrosine phosphorylation similar to that seen *in vivo* after inflammation [99]. These results demonstrate a role for interactions or coupling between metabotropic and ionotropic glutamate receptors in the development of spinal plasticity.

The coupling with mGluRs may not be the sole upstream pathway leading to NR2B tyrosine phosphorylation. In addition, intrathecal administration of an NK1 receptor antagonist also attenuated NR2B tyrosine phosphorylation [98]. Previous studies have also suggested an interaction between spinal NMDA and NK1 tachykinin receptor systems in the processing of nociceptive information [147-151]. The wind-up phenomenon also involves the NK1 receptor. Mice lacking the NK1 receptor do not exhibit wind-up of the hind paw withdrawal responses that is shown in the wild-type control animals [152]. This raises the possibility that the coupling through G-protein-linked receptors may be a common mechanism for regulating the function of the NMDA receptor. An interaction with NMDA receptors has been implicated in the mechanisms of opioid tolerance and opioid-induced abnormal pain sensitivity [153,154]. Additional G-protein-linked receptors including muscarinic acetylcholine [155], bradykinin [156] and somatostatin [157] receptors have been shown to mediate upregulation of NMDA receptor function, suggesting the presence of abundant signaling pathways. In light of the recent findings, the hypothesis that the induction of spinal dorsal horn sensitization after inflammation is related primarily to activity of NMDA, AMPA, NK1 and Trk B receptors [3,158] needs to be revised to include the coupling between ionotropic and G-protein-linked receptors as a mechanism underlying the initiation and facilitation of central sensitization.

## Protein Kinases and Signaling Cascade Related to NMDA Receptor Phosphorylation

Using intrathecal administration of selective PKC and PKA inhibitors, we have verified some of the upstream protein kinases that mediate serine phosphorylation of the NR1 subunit in the spinal dorsal horn [75]. The results are consistent with previous characterization in other cellular systems that NR1 serine 896 is phosphorylated by PKC activation and NR1 serine 897 is phosphorylated by PKA [74,159]. On the other hand, a protein phosphatase inhibitor further enhances the capsaicin-induced NMDA receptor phosphorylation [160]. The NR1 serine 897 phosphorylation in the spinal cord is also blocked by a PKC inhibitor chelerythrine [75]. A similar phenomenon is the increase in phosphoserine 897 NR1 in spinothalamic tract neurons after capsaicin treatment involving both PKA and PKC activation [78]. Since PKC cannot directly phosphorylate serine 897 of the NR1 subunit as shown in NR1 fusion proteins, human embryonic kidney 293 cells, and hippocampal neurons [74], these results suggest an interaction between the PKC and PKA pathways in producing NR1 serine 897 phosphorylation after inflammation. The activation of PKC may facilitate PKA activity to phosphorylate NR1 serine 897 in the spinal cord.

The upstream kinases that phosphorylate the NR2B subunit of the NMDA receptor belong to the family of Src protein tyrosine kinases [88,161,162]. The direct evidence that

Src participate in NR2B phosphorylation after activity-dependent plasticity in the spinal cord comes from the findings that the inflammation-induced increase in NR2B tyrosine phosphorylation is abolished by intrathecal administration of genistein, a tyrosine kinase inhibitor, and PP2 and CGP77675, two selective Src family protein tyrosine kinases inhibitors [98,99]. Importantly, intrathecal administration of PP2 prior to injection of CFA delays the onset of mechanical hyperalgesia and allodynia [98]. Post-treatment of PP2 also blocked NR2B tyrosine phosphorylation and inflammatory hyperalgesia, suggesting that NR2B phosphorylation plays a role in maintaining central hyperexcitability. Intravenous or intrathecal administration of Src40-49, a 10 amino acid peptide that inhibits upregulation of the NMDA receptor function by Src [163], suppresses phase 2, but not phase 1 formalin response [100]. Protein kinase C is known to potentiate NMDA receptor activation [139,164,165]. Phosphorylation of the NMDA receptor by PKC helps to remove $Mg^{2+}$ block of the NMDA receptor channel, leading to an increased sensitivity of the receptor to glutamate [164]. The $mGluR_1$-mediated potentiation of NMDA receptors involves intracellular calcium release and PKC [141] and PKC activation induces NR2 tyrosine phosphorylation in the rat hippocampus [166].

We have examined the involvement of PKC in inflammation-induced NR2B tyrosine phosphorylation. Using an intrathecal protocol, the increase in NR2B tyrosine phosphorylation was blocked by pretreatment with chelerythrine, a selective PKC inhibitor [98]. Direct activation of PKC by PMA (phorbol-12-myristate-13-acetate, PKC activator) in spinal dorsal horn slices also mimics CFA-induced NR2B tyrosine phosphorylation [99]. The PMA-induced NR2B tyr-P was blocked by pretreatment of the slice with CGP 77675, a Src inhibitor, and chelerythrine.

The Src family protein tyrosine kinases are activated by the proline-rich tyrosine kinase 2 (PYK2)/cell-adhesion kinase beta (CAKbeta) pathway [167,168] that is sensitive to an increase in intracellular calcium [169]. PKC may stimulate Src through the PYK2/CAKbeta pathway [88] and induce NR2 tyrosine phosphorylation [166]. The major forms of PKC (alpha, beta, gamma) have a calcium-binding site and require $Ca^{2+}$ together with diacylglycerol (DAG) for activation (Fig. 4B). Thus, both PYK2 and PKC activation require an increase in intracellular calcium. One potential source of the increase in intracellular $Ca^{2+}$ in spinal neurons after inflammation is through activation of G-protein-linked receptors since they have been shown to be involved in inflammation-induced NR2B tyrosine phosphorylation [98,99]. A logical hypothesis is that calcium is mobilized from intracellular stores through the activation of the inositol 1,4,5-triphosphate ($IP_3$) pathway following mGluR activation. We have directly tested this hypothesis with the administration of $IP_3$ receptor antagonists. Intrathecal pretreatment of 2APB, a membrane permeable $IP_3$ receptor antagonist that does not affect $Ca^{2+}$ release from the ryanodine-sensitive $Ca^{2+}$ stores [170] blocked NR2B tyrosine phosphorylation after inflammation. The basal levels of NR2B tyrosine phosphorylation were not affected by the same doses of 2APB. In contrast, the NR2B tyrosine phosphorylation was not affected by the agents that block the inflow of extracellular calcium through calcium permeable channels. Such agents include NMDA receptor channel blockers, AMPA/KA receptor antagonists, and inhibitors of the voltage-dependent calcium channels [99]. Further, direct application of the $IP_3$ receptor agonist (D-$IP_3$) to the spinal slice preparation induces a significant increase in NR2B tyrosine phosphorylation [99]. The IP$_3$-induced increase in tyrosine phosphorylation is blocked by pretreatment with a Src inhibitor. These results establish that activation of the IP$_3$-PKC pathway is sufficient to induce spinal dorsal horn NR2B tyrosine phosphorylation. Consistently, the group I mGluR agonist-induced NR2B tyrosine phosphorylation also requires PKC, intracellular calcium release, and Src activation [98,99].

Taken together, these findings suggest that the signal transduction upstream to NR2B tyrosine phosphorylation involves G-protein coupled receptors and subsequent phospholipase C activation, IP$_3$-mediated intracellular calcium release, PKC, and Src family protein tyrosine kinases. Interestingly, PD98059, a mitogen-activated protein kinase kinase (MAPKK/MEK) inhibitor, did not block inflammation-induced NR2B tyrosine phosphorylation, although PD98059 has been shown to inhibit spinal ERK activation and nociception [106,171]. The activity of MAP kinase may represent a down stream, or a parallel signaling pathway to inflammation-induced dorsal horn NR2B tyrosine phosphorylation.

# Antihyperalgesic Effect of the NMDA Receptor Antagonists

The findings of the role of NMDA receptors in central sensitization have significant impact on the search for novel approaches for the treatment of persistent pain [2,70,172-177]. The efficacy of the NMDA receptor antagonists in persistent pain has been assessed in animal models as well as in clinical studies.

## Animal Studies

The formalin response, a model of chemical nociception, is inhibited by NMDA receptor antagonists [178-180]. Carrageenan-induced hyperalgesia is attenuated by MK-801 [181]. The behavioral hyperalgesia in nerve-injured rats is attenuated or blocked by MK-801 [180,182-184]. The autotomy behavior and neuronal responses to noxious hindlimb ischemia are also mediated by NMDA receptors [62,185].

One promising aspect of the use of the NMDA receptor antagonist for persistent pain is that antagonists acting at any constituent of the NMDA receptor should be able to interrupt normal function of the receptor since functional integrity of all components of the receptor complex is essential for the activation of the receptor (Fig. 1). This hypothesis has been tested in animal pain models. We have injected NMDA receptor antagonists with different mechanisms of action into the lumbar subarachnoid space of the rat with hind paw inflammation and hyperalgesia [53,98,186,187]. The results show that inflammatory hyperalgesia is significantly attenuated by AP-5 and CPP, the two competitive antagonists acting at the glutamate binding site (Site #1 in Fig. 1); 7-Cl kynurenic acid, an antagonist against the glycine co-agonist binding (Site #2 in Fig. 1); MK-801 and ketamine, two NMDA receptor channel blockers (Site #3 in Fig. 1); and PP2 {4-amino-5-(4-chlorophenyl)-7-(*t*-butyl)pyrazolo[3,4-d]pyrimidine}, a Src family tyrosine kinase inhibitor (Site #5 in Fig. 1). Yashpal et al. [188] show that intrathecal administration of a PKC inhibitor, GF 109203X or chelerythrine, significantly attenuated formalin responses and secondary mechanical hyperalgesia in rats. Laughlin et al. [189] also demonstrate that DTT, a sulfhydryl reducing agent that potentiates NMDA receptor responses (Site #4 in Fig. 1), enhances NMDA-induced thermal hyperalgesia and formalin-induced nocifensive behavior, as well as the long lasting allodynia induced by intrathecal administration of dynorphin. The potentiation of nocifensive behaviors by DTT is blocked by DTNB [5,5'-dithio-bis-(2-nitrobenzoic acid)], an oxidizing agent. Interestingly, magnesium deficiency in rats is associated with a behavioral hyperalgesia, which can be reversed by $MgSO_4$ and the inhibitors of NMDA receptors, PKC, nitric oxide synthase, and neurokinin receptors [190].

When tested on rats without injury, NMDA receptor antagonists do not produce significant analgesia until the doses used produce visible motor dysfunction [37,182,184,186,191]. The basal responses of spinal neurons to C-fiber input also are not affected by the NMDA receptor antagonists [48,63,178] and the receptive field size of dorsal horn nociceptive neurons of normal rats is not affected by MK-801 [53]. It appears that NMDA receptor antagonists selectively produce antinociceptive effects under conditions where noxious inputs are tonically active and produce altered processing and hyperexcitability at the level of the spinal dorsal horn. These situations include injection of inflammatory agents to produce tissue injury [53,186,192-194], chronic constriction of the sciatic nerve to develop neuropathic pain [184], intradermal injection of formalin to activate nociceptive neurons [178], occlusion of blood vessels to induce post-exercise ischemic pain [195] or excitation of dorsal horn neurons [62], and neurectomy of peripheral nerves that leads to autotomy [185].

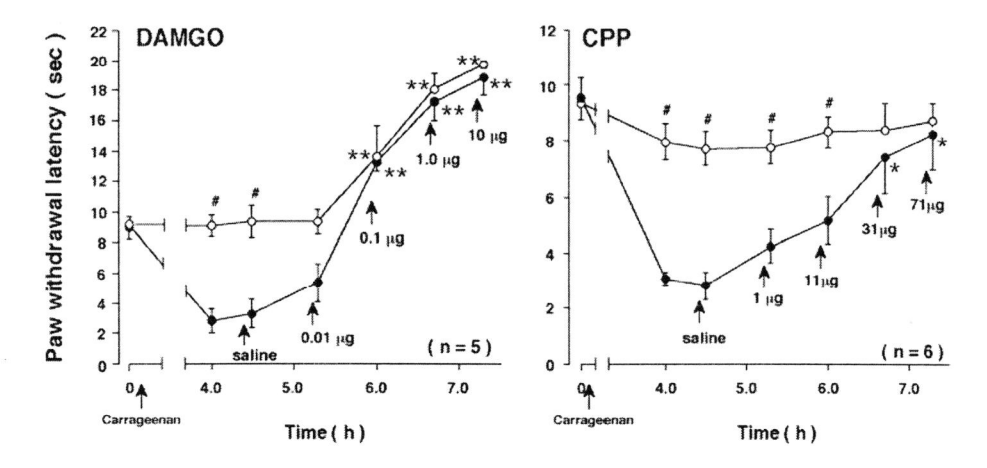

Figure 5. Comparison of the effects of the opioid receptor agonist and NMDA receptor antagonist on paw withdrawal latencies of rats after tissue injury. Cumulative doses of a mu-opioid receptor agonist DAMGO [(D-Ala$^2$,MePhe$^4$,Gly-ol$^5$) enkephalin] (Left) and a competitive NMDA receptor antagonist CPP [(±)-3-(2-carboxypiperazin-4-yl)-propyl-1-phosphonic acid] (Right) were administered intrathecally at times indicated by arrows. Saline was injected as a control. Rats received an injection of carrageenan into one hind paw. Withdrawal latencies (sec) of both injected (filled circles) and non-injected (open circles) paws from a noxious thermal stimulus are plotted against time course (h) of the experiments. *, p < 0.05, **, p < 0.01: Post-drug latencies vs. prior to drug (post-carrageenan). #, p<0.05: significant differences from that prior to carrageenan injection. (From [186], with permission from Elsevier)

By comparing their effects with those of opioid receptor agonists, it is clear that NMDA receptor antagonists are antihyperalgesic, but not analgesic (Fig. 5). Although both classes of agents produce antinociception in the rat inflammation model, opioid agonists differ from the NMDA receptor antagonists in that they increase the paw withdrawal latency of the non-inflamed paw [186,192]. Intrathecal DAMGO, a mu-opioid receptor agonist, significantly increases the withdrawal latency of both inflamed and non-inflamed paws (Fig. 5). The NMDA receptor antagonist CPP, however, only prolongs the withdrawal latency of the inflamed paw and did not affect the contralateral non-inflamed paw (Fig. 5). Hypersensitivity states in flexor motoneurons due to repetitive C-fiber strength stimulation or application of a chemical irritant to the skin were also reduced by MK-801 and CPP at doses that did not modify baseline reflexes [63]. NMDA receptor antagonists do not affect normal synaptic transmission but block wind-up of dorsal horn neurons [101]. Thus, the evidence supports the view that changes in central pain processing have occurred in response to prolonged noxious stimulation or tissue injury and NMDA receptors are actively involved in this process. Distinct from opioid agonists, which produce antinociception in non-inflamed as well as inflamed conditions, selective attenuation of the behavioral hyperalgesia by NMDA receptor antagonists suggests that this group of agents may be helpful in controlling pain where activation of the NMDA receptor is a major source of excessive depolarization and hyperexcitability.

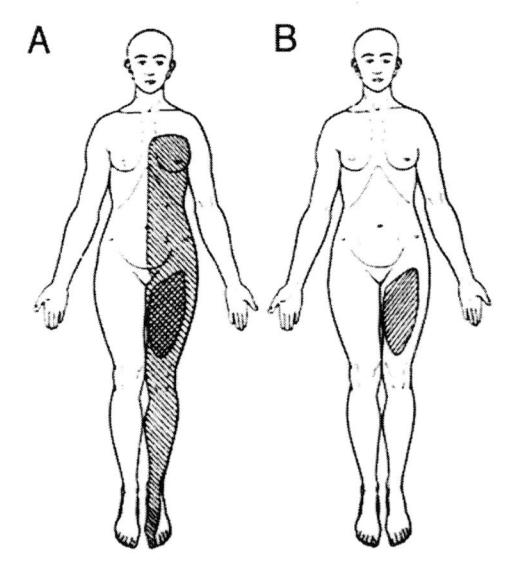

Figure 6. Effect of the NMDA receptor antagonist CPP on neurogenic pain in humans. The patient had developed severe and intractable pain in the left leg (cross-hatched area in A and hatched area in B) due to the injury of the anterior cutaneous branches of the femoral nerve after repeated surgery on left leg for varicose veins. The pain includes continuous deep pain, and allodynia; and spread outside of the territory of the injured nerve (hatched area in A). Intrathecal administration of one dose of CPP (200 nmol) abolished spread of pain. However, pain in the injured territory still existed (hatched area in B). Another 500 nmol of CPP did not produce further pain relief. CPP produced psychotomimetic effects include anxiety, uneasiness, hyperacusis, which was controlled by diazepam. In a 2-week follow-up, pain was still reduced. (Adapted form [199], with permission from IASP)

## Human Studies

Human pain sensation also shows temporal summation, a situation similar to wind-up as seen in animal studies [196,197]. The temporal summation of human pain sensation, particularly the second pain, parallels the long latency C-fiber input-evoked response of dorsal horn nociceptive neurons and thus appears to be a good correlate of wind-up. NMDA receptor antagonists have been tested on humans in clinical settings. Price et al. [198] show that the temporal summation of second pain is selectively attenuated by an NMDA receptor antagonist, dextromethorphan. A case report by Kristensen, Svensson and Gordh [199] shows that the wind-up-like component of an intractable neurogenic pain is eliminated after intrathecal administration of a competitive NMDA receptor antagonist CPP (Fig. 6). Interestingly, CPP only inhibited the spread of pain outside of the territory of the injured nerve and left the thermal pain threshold unchanged. Dextromethorphan has shown certain efficacy against postoperative hyperalgesia [200,201] and painful diabetic neuropathy [202], although it lacks an analgesic effect [203-205]. Ketamine, a non-competitive NMDA receptor antagonist, reduces ischemic pain and allodynia [195]. The NMDA receptor also contributes to the development and maintenance of human visceral pain hypersensitivity [206]. These clinical observations are consistent with findings from the animal studies and indicate the involvement of NMDA receptors in pain hypersensitivity.

Based on information gathered from animal studies, antagonism of the NMDA receptor at the spinal level may add a new dimension to the management of persistent pain. However, the psychotomimetic side effects produced by most NMDA receptor antagonists have hampered the use of NMDA receptor antagonists in chronic pain [e.g. 199]. The basic research in this area should help point to new directions in the use of the NMDA receptor antagonist for pain control. Manipulation of the components of the signal transduction pathways upstream to NMDA receptor phosphorylation, including scaffold proteins in the postsynaptic density, protein kinases and phosphatases and co-factors, may be an alternative and efficient approach for inhibiting pain hypersensitivity. This requires thorough understanding of the cellular and molecular mechanisms of NMDA receptor activation and modulation under persistent pain conditions.

Since the NMDA receptor interacts with multiple receptor systems, searching for optimal combination of NMDA receptor agents with other agents is another way to overcome side effects associated with higher doses. Amantadine, a clinically available NMDA receptor antagonist, has been shown to have a synergistic interaction with morphine in the second phase of the formalin test in rats [207]. Intrathecal co-administration of AP-5 and morphine is maximally effective in a rat experimental pancreatitis model [208]. Electroacupuncture combined with MK-801 prolongs anti-hyperalgesia in rats with peripheral inflammation [209]. Blocking central NMDA receptors appears necessary for enhancing analgesia induced through peripheral opioid mechanisms in the formalin model [210]. The development of subunit specific NMDA receptor antagonists with a reduced aversive profile is also promising [175,211-216]. Animal studies have pointed to a significant contribution of NR2B subunits in persistent pain conditions [98,217,218]. New NR2B-selective antagonists have been shown to produce antihyperalgesia with minimal or no side effects [95,219,220].

## Acknowledgement

The authors' work is supported by NIH grants DA10275, NS41384, DE11964, DE15374.

## References

[1] Dubner R; Ruda MA. Activity-dependent neuronal plasticity following tissue injury and inflammation. *Trends Neurosci.* 1992, 15:96-103.

[2] Coderre TJ; Katz J; Vaccarino AL; Melzack R. Contribution of central neuroplasticity to pathological pain: review of clinical and experimental evidence. *Pain.* 1993, 52:259-285.

[3] Woolf CJ; Salter MW. Neuronal plasticity: increasing the gain in pain. *Science.* 2000 288:1765-1769.

[4] Monaghan, DT; Wenthold, RJ. *The ionotropic glutamate receptors.* Totowa, N.J.: Humana Press Inc. 1996.

[5] Kew JN; Kemp JA. Ionotropic and metabotropic glutamate receptor structure and pharmacology. *Psychopharmacology* (Berl). 2005, 179:4-29.

[6] Masu M; Nakajima Y; Moriyoshi K; Ishii T; Akazawa C; Nakanashi S. Molecular characterization of NMDA and metabotropic glutamate receptors. *Ann. N. Y. Acad. Sci.* 1993, 707:153-164.

[7] Collingridge GL; Lester RA. Excitatory amino acid receptors in the vertebrate central nervous system. *Pharmacol. Rev.* 1989, 41:143-210.

[8] Monaghan DT; Bridges RJ; Cotman CW. The excitatory amino acid receptors: their classes, pharmacology, and distinct properties in the function of the central nervous system. *Annu. Rev. Pharmacol. Toxicol.* 1989, 29:365-402.

[9] Ozawa S; Kamiya H; Tsuzuki K. Glutamate receptors in the mammalian central nervous system. *Prog. Neurobiol.* 1998, 54:581-618.

[10] Dingledine R; Borges K; Bowie D; Traynelis SF. The glutamate receptor ion channels. *Pharmacol. Rev.* 1999, 51:7-61.

[11] Perez-Otano I; Ehlers MD. Homeostatic plasticity and NMDA receptor trafficking. *Trends Neurosci.* 2005, 28:229-238.

[12] Mori H; Mishina M. Structure and function of the NMDA receptor channel. *Neuropharmacology.* 1995, 34:1219-1237.

[13] Sugihara H; Moriyoshi K; Ishii T; Masu M; Nakanishi S. Structures and properties of seven isoforms of the NMDA receptor generated by alternative splicing. *Biochem. Biophys. Res. Commun.* 1992, 185:826-832.

[14] Laurie DJ; Putzke J; Zieglgansberger W; Seeburg PH; Tolle TR. The distribution of splice variants of the NMDAR1 subunit mRNA in adult rat brain. *Brain Res. Mol. Brain Res.* 1995, 32:94-108.

[15] Zukin RS; Bennett MV. Alternatively spliced isoforms of the NMDARI receptor subunit. *Trends Neurosci.* 1995, 18:306-313.

[16] Furukawa H, Singh SK, Mancusso R, Gouaux E. Subunit arrangement and function in NMDA receptors. *Nature.* 2005 Nov 10;438(7065):185-92.

[17] Laube B; Hirai H; Sturgess M; Betz H; Kuhse J. Molecular determinants of agonist discrimination by NMDA receptor subunits: analysis of the glutamate binding site on the NR2B subunit. *Neuron.* 1997, 18:493-503.

[18] Kashiwagi K; Pahk AJ; Masuko T; Igarashi K; Williams K. Block and modulation of N-methyl-D-aspartate receptors by polyamines and protons: role of amino acid residues in the transmembrane and pore-forming regions of NR1 and NR2 subunits. *Mol. Pharmacol.* 1997, 52:701-713.

[19] Burnashev N; Schoepfer R; Monyer H; Ruppersberg JP; Gunther W; Seeburg PH; Sakmann B. Control by asparagine residues of calcium permeability and magnesium blockade in the NMDA receptor. *Science.* 1992, 257:1415-1419.

[20] Mori H; Masaki H; Yamakura T; Mishina M. Identification by mutagenesis of a Mg(2+)-block site of the NMDA receptor channel. *Nature.* 1992, 358:673-675.

[21] Sakurada K; Masu M; Nakanishi S. Alteration of Ca2+ permeability and sensitivity to Mg2+ and channel blockers by a single amino acid substitution in the N-methyl-D-aspartate receptor. *J. Biol. Chem.* 1993, 268:410-415.

[22] Paoletti P; Ascher P; Neyton J. High-affinity zinc inhibition of NMDA NR1-NR2A receptors. J Neurosci. 1997, 17:5711-25. Erratum in: *J. Neurosci.* 1997, 17(20):following

[23] Traynelis SF; Burgess MF; Zheng F; Lyuboslavsky P; Powers JL. Control of voltage-independent zinc inhibition of NMDA receptors by the NR1 subunit. *J. Neurosci.* 1998, 18:6163-6175.

[24] Traynelis SF; Hartley M; Heinemann SF. Control of proton sensitivity of the NMDA receptor by RNA splicing and polyamines. *Science.* 1995, 268:873-876.

[25] Ransom RW; Stec NL. Cooperative modulation of [3H]MK-801 binding to the N-methyl-D-aspartate receptor-ion channel complex by L-glutamate, glycine, and polyamines. *J. Neurochem.* 1988, 51:830-836.

[26] Sullivan JM; Traynelis SF; Chen HS; Escobar W; Heinemann SF; Lipton SA. Identification of two cysteine residues that are required for redox modulation of the NMDA subtype of glutamate receptor. *Neuron.* 1994, 13:929-936.

[27] Raymond LA; Tingley WG; Blackstone CD; Roche KW; Huganir RL. Glutamate receptor modulation by protein phosphorylation. *J. Physiol. Paris.* 1994, 88:181-192.

[28] Hatt H. Modification of glutamate receptor channels: molecular mechanisms and functional consequences. *Naturwissenschaften.* 1999, 86:177-186.

[29] Tingley WG; Roche KW; Thompson AK; Huganir RL. Regulation of NMDA receptor phosphorylation by alternative splicing of the C-terminal domain. *Nature.* 1993, 364:70-73.

[30] Yu XM; Askalan R; Keil GJ 2nd; Salter MW. NMDA channel regulation by channel-associated protein tyrosine kinase Src. *Science.* 1997, 275:674-678.

[31] Wenthold RJ; Prybylowski K; Standley S; Sans N; Petralia RS. Trafficking of NMDA receptors. *Annu. Rev. Pharmacol. Toxicol.* 2003, 43:335-358.

[32] Prybylowski K; Chang K; Sans N; Kan L; Vicini S; Wenthold RJ. The synaptic localization of NR2B-containing NMDA receptors is controlled by interactions with PDZ proteins and AP-2. *Neuron.* 2005, 47:845-857.

[33] Lei G; Xue S; Chery N; Liu Q; Xu J; Kwan CL; Fu YP; Lu YM; Liu M; Harder KW; Yu XM. Gain control of N-methyl-D-aspartate receptor activity by receptor-like protein tyrosine phosphatase alpha. *EMBO J.* 2002, 21:2977-2989.

[34] Pelkey KA; Askalan R; Paul S; Kalia LV; Nguyen TH; Pitcher GM; Salter MW; Lombroso PJ. Tyrosine phosphatase STEP is a tonic brake on induction of long-term potentiation. *Neuron.* 2002, 34:127-138.

[35] Lipton SA; Stamler JS. Actions of redox-related congeners of nitric oxide at the NMDA receptor. *Neuropharmacology.* 1994, 33:1229-1233.

[36] Sucher NJ; Awobuluyi M; Choi YB; Lipton SA. NMDA receptors: from genes to channels. *Trends Pharmacol. Sci.* 1996 17:348-355.

[37] Aanonsen LM; Wilcox GL. Nociceptive action of excitatory amino acids in the mouse: effects of spinally administered opioids, phencyclidine and sigma agonists. *J. Pharmacol. Exp. Ther.* 1987, 243:9-19.

[38] Cahusac PM; Evans RH; Hill RG; Rodriquez RE; Smith DA. The behavioural effects of an N-methylaspartate receptor antagonist following application to the lumbar spinal cord of conscious rats. *Neuropharmacology.* 1984, 23:719-724.

[39] De Biasi S; Rustioni A. Glutamate and substance P coexist in primary afferent terminals in the superficial laminae of spinal cord. *Proc. Natl. Acad. Sci. U S A.* 1988, 85:7820-7824.

[40] Monaghan DT; Cotman CW. Distribution of N-methyl-D-aspartate-sensitive L-[3H]glutamate-binding sites in rat brain. *J. Neurosci.* 1985, 5:2909-2919.

[41] Nagy GG; Watanabe M; Fukaya M; Todd AJ. Synaptic distribution of the NR1, NR2A and NR2B subunits of the N-methyl-d-aspartate receptor in the rat lumbar spinal cord revealed with an antigen-unmasking technique. *Eur. J. Neurosci.* 2004, 20:3301-3312.

[42] Kangrga I; Randic M. Tachykinins and calcitonin gene-related peptide enhance release of endogenous glutamate and aspartate from the rat spinal dorsal horn slice. *J. Neurosci.* 1990, 10:2026-2038.

[43] Skilling SR; Smullin DH; Beitz AJ; Larson AA. Extracellular amino acid concentrations in the dorsal spinal cord of freely moving rats following veratridine and nociceptive stimulation. *J. Neurochem.* 1988, 51:127-132.

[44] Sluka KA; Jordan HH; Willis WD; Westlund KN. Differential effects of N-methyl-D-aspartate (NMDA) and non-NMDA receptor antagonists on spinal release of amino acids after development of acute arthritis in rats. *Brain Res.* 1994, 664:77-84.

[45] Mendell LM. Physiological properties of unmyelinated fiber projection to the spinal cord, *Exp. Neurol.* 1966, 16:316-332.

[46] Woolf CJ. Windup and central sensitization are not equivalent. *Pain.* 1996, 66:105-108.

[47] Dickenson AH; Sullivan AF. Evidence for a role of the NMDA receptor in the frequency dependent potentiation of deep rat dorsal horn nociceptive neurones following C fibre stimulation. *Neuropharmacology.* 1987, 26:1235-1238.

[48] Davies SN; Lodge D. Evidence for involvement of N-methylaspartate receptors in 'wind-up' of class 2 neurones in the dorsal horn of the rat. *Brain Res.* 1987, 424:402-406.

[49] Woolf CJ. Evidence for a central component of post-injury pain hypersensitivity. *Nature*. 1983, 306:686-688.

[50] Cook AJ; Woolf CJ; Wall PD; McMahon SB. Dynamic receptive field plasticity in rat spinal cord dorsal horn following C-primary afferent input. *Nature*. 1987, 325:151-153.

[51] Ren K; Dubner R. Central Nervous System Plasticity and Persistent Pain. *J. Orofacial. Pain.* 1999, 13:155-163.

[52] Hylden JL; Nahin RL; Traub RJ; Dubner R. Expansion of receptive fields of spinal lamina I projection neurons in rats with unilateral adjuvant-induced inflammation: the contribution of dorsal horn mechanisms. *Pain*. 1989, 37:229-243.

[53] Ren K; Hylden JLK; Williams GM; Ruda MA; Dubner R. The effects of a non-competitive NMDA receptor antagonist, MK-801, on behavioral hyperalgesia and dorsal horn neuronal activity in rats with unilateral inflammation. *Pain*. 1992, 50:331-344.

[54] Menetrey D; Besson JM. Electrophysiological characteristics of dorsal horn cells in rats with cutaneous inflammation resulting from chronic arthritis. *Pain*. 1982, 13:343-364.

[55] Calvino B; Villanueva L; Le Bars D. Dorsal horn (convergent) neurones in the intact anaesthetized arthritic rat. I. Segmental excitatory influences. *Pain*. 1987, 28:81-98.

[56] Iwata K; Tashiro A; Tsuboi Y; Imai T; Sumino R; Morimoto T; Dubner R; Ren K. Medullary dorsal horn neuronal activity in rats with persistent temporomandibular joint and perioral inflammation. *J. Neurophysiol*. 1999, 82:1244-1253.

[57] Woolf CJ; King AE. Dynamic alterations in the cutaneous mechanoreceptive fields of dorsal horn neurons in the rat spinal cord. *J. Neurosci*. 1990, 10:2717-2726.

[58] Hu JW; Sessle BJ; Raboisson P; Dallel R; Woda A. Stimulation of craniofacial muscle afferents induces prolonged facilitatory effects in trigeminal nociceptive brain-stem neurones. *Pain*. 1992, 48:53-60.

[59] Kawamata M; Koshizaki M; Shimada SG; Narimatsu E; Kozuka Y; Takahashi T; Namiki A; Collins JG. Changes in response properties and receptive fields of spinal dorsal horn neurons in rats after surgical incision in hairy skin. *Anesthesiology*. 2005, 102:141-151.

[60] Cervero F; Shouenborg J; Sjolund BH; Waddell PJ. Cutaneous inputs to dorsal horn neurones in adult rats treated at birth with capsaicin. *Brain Res*. 1984, 301:47-57.

[61] Laird JM; Cervero F. A comparative study of the changes in receptive-field properties of multireceptive and nocireceptive rat dorsal horn neurons following noxious mechanical stimulation. *J. Neurophysiol*. 1989, 62:854-863.

[62] Sher GD; Mitchell D. N-methyl-D-aspartate receptors mediate responses of rat dorsal horn neurones to hindlimb ischemia. *Brain Res*. 1990, 522:55-62.

[63] Woolf CJ; Thompson SW. The induction and maintenance of central sensitization is dependent on N-methyl-D-aspartic acid receptor activation; implications for the treatment of post-injury pain hypersensitivity states. *Pain*. 1991, 44:293-299.

[64] Schaible HG; Grubb BD; Neugebauer V; Oppmann M. The Effects of NMDA Antagonists on Neuronal Activity in Cat Spinal Cord Evoked by Acute Inflammation in the Knee Joint. *Eur. J. Neurosci*. 1991, 3:981-991.

[65] Brown AG; Fyffe RE. Form and function of dorsal horn neurones with axons ascending the dorsal columns in cat. *J. Physiol*. 1981, 321:31-47.

[66] Saadé N; Jabbur SJ; Wall PD. Effects of 4-aminopyridine, GABA and bicuculline on cutaneous receptive fields of cat dorsal horn neurons. *Brain Res.* 1985, 344:356-359.

[67] Merrill EG; Wall PD. Factors forming the edge of a receptive field: the presence of relatively ineffective afferent terminals. *J. Physiol.* 1972, 226:825-846.

[68] Markus H; Pomeranz B. Saphenous has weak ineffective synapses in sciatic territory of rat spinal cord: electrical stimulation of the saphenous or application of drugs reveal these somatotopically inappropriate synapses. *Brain Res.* 1987, 416:315-321.

[69] Dubner R; Sharav Y; Gracely RH; Price DD. Idiopathic trigeminal neuralgia: sensory features and pain mechanisms. *Pain.* 1987, 31:23-33.

[70] Dubner R. Neuronal plasticity and pain following peripheral tissue inflammation or nerve injury. In: Bond MR; Charlton JE; Woolf CJ, editors. *Proceedings of the VIth World Congress on Pain*, Amsterdam: Elsevier; 1991; pp. 263-276.

[71] South SM; Kohno T; Kaspar BK; Hegarty D; Vissel B; Drake CT; Ohata M; Jenab S; Sailer AW; Malkmus S; Masuyama T; Horner P; Bogulavsky J; Gage FH; Yaksh TL; Woolf CJ; Heinemann SF; Inturrisi CE. A conditional deletion of the NR1 subunit of the NMDA receptor in adult spinal cord dorsal horn reduces NMDA currents and injury-induced pain. *J. Neurosci.* 2003, 23:5031-5040.

[72] Tan PH; Yang LC; Shih HC; Lan KC; Cheng JT. Gene knockdown with intrathecal siRNA of NMDA receptor NR2B subunit reduces formalin-induced nociception in the rat. *Gene Ther.* 2005, 12:59-66.

[73] Guo H; Huang LY. Alteration in the voltage dependence of NMDA receptor channels in rat dorsal horn neurones following peripheral inflammation. *J. Physiol.* 2001, 537(Pt 1):115-123.

[74] Tingley WG; Ehlers MD; Kameyama K; Doherty C; Ptak JB; Riley CT; Huganir RL. Characterization of protein kinase A and protein kinase C phosphorylation of the N-methyl-D-aspartate receptor NR1 subunit using phosphorylation site-specific antibodies. *J. Biol. Chem.* 1997, 272:5157-5166.

[75] Guo W; Zou S-P; Ikeda T; Dubner R; Ren K. Rapid and lasting increase in serine phosphorylation of rat spinal cord NMDAR1 and GluR1 subunits after peripheral inflammation. *Thalamus and Related Systems* 2005, (in press).

[76] Caudle RM, Perez FM, Del Valle-Pinero AY, Iadarola MJ. Spinal cord NR1 serine phosphorylation and NR2B subunit suppression following peripheral inflammation. *Mol. Pain.* 2005 Sep 2;1:25.

[77] Zou X; Lin Q; Willis WD. Enhanced phosphorylation of NMDA receptor 1 subunits in spinal cord dorsal horn and spinothalamic tract neurons after intradermal injection of capsaicin in rats. *J. Neurosci.* 2000, 20:6989-6997.

[78] Zou X; Lin Q; Willis WD. Role of protein kinase A in phosphorylation of NMDA receptor 1 subunits in dorsal horn and spinothalamic tract neurons after intradermal injection of capsaicin in rats. *Neuroscience.* 2002, 115:775-786.

[79] Brenner GJ; Ji RR; Shaffer S; Woolf CJ. Peripheral noxious stimulation induces phosphorylation of the NMDA receptor NR1 subunit at the PKC-dependent site, serine-896, in spinal cord dorsal horn neurons. *Eur. J. Neurosci.* 2004, 20:375-384.

[80] Caudle RM; Perez FM; King C; Yu CG; Yezierski RP. N-methyl-D-aspartate receptor subunit expression and phosphorylation following excitotoxic spinal cord injury in rats. *Neurosci. Lett.* 2003, 349:37-40.

[81] Gao X; Kim HK; Chung JM; Chung K. Enhancement of NMDA receptor phosphorylation of the spinal dorsal horn and nucleus gracilis neurons in neuropathic rats. *Pain.* 2005, 116:62-72.

[82] Sprengel R; Suchanek B; Amico C; Brusa R; Burnashev N; Rozov A; Hvalby O; Jensen V; Paulsen O; Andersen P; Kim JJ; Thompson RF; Sun W; Webster LC; Grant SG; Eilers J; Konnerth A; Li J; McNamara JO; Seeburg PH. Importance of the intracellular domain of NR2 subunits for NMDA receptor function in vivo. *Cell.* 1998, 92:279-289.

[83] Cull-Candy S; Brickley S; Farrant M. NMDA receptor subunits: diversity, development and disease. *Curr. Opin. Neurobiol.* 2001, 11:327-335.

[84] Lu WY; Jackson MF; Bai D; Orser BA; MacDonald JF. In CA1 pyramidal neurons of the hippocampus protein kinase C regulates calcium-dependent inactivation of NMDA receptors. *J. Neurosci.* 2000, 20:4452-4461.

[85] Moon IS; Apperson ML; Kennedy MB. The major tyrosine-phosphorylated protein in the postsynaptic density fraction is N-methyl-D-aspartate receptor subunit 2B. *Proc. Natl. Acad. Sci. U S A* 1994, 91:3954-3958.

[86] Lau LF; Huganir RL. Differential tyrosine phosphorylation of N-methyl-D-aspartate receptor subunits. *J. Biol. Chem.* 1995, 270:20036-20041.

[87] Xiong ZG; Pelkey KA; Lu WY; Lu YM; Roder JC; MacDonald JF; Salter MW. Src potentiation of NMDA receptors in hippocampal and spinal neurons is not mediated by reducing zinc inhibition. *J. Neurosci.* 1999, 19:RC37(1-6).

[88] Ali DW; Salter MW. NMDA receptor regulation by Src kinase signalling in excitatory synaptic transmission and plasticity. *Curr. Opin. Neurobiol.* 2001, 11:336-342.

[89] Wang YT; Salter MW. Regulation of NMDA receptors by tyrosine kinases and phosphatases. *Nature.* 1994, 369:233-235.

[90] Rosenblum K; Dudai Y; Richter-Levin G. Long-term potentiation increases tyrosine phosphorylation of the N-methyl-D-aspartate receptor subunit 2B in rat dentate gyrus in vivo. *Proc. Natl. Acad. Sci. U S A* 1996, 93:10457-10460.

[91] Rostas JA; Brent VA; Voss K; Errington ML; Bliss TV; Gurd JW. Enhanced tyrosine phosphorylation of the 2B subunit of the N-methyl-D-aspartate receptor in long-term potentiation. *Proc. Natl. Acad. Sci. U S A* 1996, 93:10452-10456.

[92] Menegoz M; Lau LF; Herve D; Huganir RL; Girault JA. Tyrosine phosphorylation of NMDA receptor in rat striatum: effects of 6-OH-dopamine lesions. *Neuroreport* 1995, 7:125-128.

[93] Dunah AW; Wang Y; Yasuda RP; Kameyama K; Huganir RL; Wolfe BB; Standaert DG. Alterations in subunit expression, composition, and phosphorylation of striatal N-methyl-D-aspartate glutamate receptors in a rat 6-hydroxydopamine model of Parkinson's disease. *Mol. Pharmacol.* 2000, 57:342-352.

[94] Yung KK. Localization of glutamate receptors in dorsal horn of rat spinal cord. *Neuroreport* 1998, 9:1639-1644.

[95] Boyce S; Wyatt A; Webb JK; O'Donnell R; Mason G; Rigby M; Sirinathsinghji D; Hill RG; Rupniak NM. Selective NMDA NR2B antagonists induce antinociception without motor dysfunction: correlation with restricted localisation of NR2B subunit in dorsal horn. *Neuropharmacology* 1999, 38:611-623.

[96] Karlsson U; Sjodin J; Angeby Moller K; Johansson S; Wikstrom L; Nasstrom J. Glutamate-induced currents reveal three functionally distinct NMDA receptor populations in rat dorsal horn - effects of peripheral nerve lesion and inflammation. *Neuroscience.* 2002, 112:861-868.

[97] Ross CA; Wright GE; Resh MD; Pearson RC; Snyder SH. Brain-specific src oncogene mRNA mapped in rat brain by in situ hybridization. *Proc. Natl. Acad. Sci. U S A* 1988, 85:9831-9835.

[98] Guo W; Zou S; Guan Y; Ikeda T; Tal M; Dubner R; Ren K. Tyrosine phosphorylation of the NR2B subunit of the NMDA receptor in the spinal cord during the development and maintenance of inflammatory hyperalgesia. *J. Neurosci.* 2002, 22:6208-6217.

[99] Guo W; Wei F; Zou S; Robbins MT; Sugiyo S; Ikeda T; Tu JC; Worley PF; Dubner R; Ren K. Group I metabotropic glutamate receptor NMDA receptor coupling and signaling cascade mediate spinal dorsal horn NMDA receptor 2B tyrosine phosphorylation associated with inflammatory hyperalgesia. *J. Neurosci.* 2004, 24:9161-9173.

[100] Liu XJ; Gingrich JR; Salter MW. A role for non-receptor tyrosine kinase Src in pain hypersensitivity. 11th World Congress on Pain Abstr. Seattle, IASP Press, 2005, p. 285.

[101] Kovacs G; Kocsis P; Tarnawa I; Horvath C; Szombathelyi Z; Farkas S. NR2B containing NMDA receptor dependent windup of single spinal neurons. *Neuropharmacology* 2004, 46:23-30.

[102] Petrenko AB; Yamakura T; Baba H; Sakimura K. Unaltered pain-related behavior in mice lacking NMDA receptor GluRepsilon 1 subunit. *Neurosci. Res.* 2003, 46:199-204.

[103] Guo W; Robbins MT; Wei F; Zou S; Dubner R; Ren K. Supraspinal brain-derived neurotrophic factor signaling: a novel mechanism for descending pain facilitation. *J. Neurosci.* 2006, 26:126-137.

[104] Nakazawa T; Komai S; Tezuka T; Hisatsune C; Umemori H; Semba K; Mishina M; Manabe T; Yamamoto T. Characterization of Fyn-mediated tyrosine phosphorylation sites on GluR epsilon 2 (NR2B) subunit of the N-methyl-D-aspartate receptor. *J. Biol. Chem.* 2001, 276:693-699.

[105] Abe T; Matsumura S; Katano T; Mabuchi T; Takagi K; Xu L; Yamamoto A; Hattori K; Yagi T; Watanabe M; Nakazawa T; Yamamoto T; Mishina M; Nakai Y; Ito S. Fyn kinase-mediated phosphorylation of NMDA receptor NR2B subunit at Tyr1472 is essential for maintenance of neuropathic pain. *Eur. J. Neurosci.* 2005, 22:1445-1454.

[106] Ji RR; Baba H; Brenner GJ; Woolf CJ. Nociceptive-specific activation of ERK in spinal neurons contributes to pain hypersensitivity. *Nat. Neurosci.* 1999, 2:1114-1119.

[107] Dai Y; Iwata K; Fukuoka T; Kondo E; Tokunaga A; Yamanaka H; Tachibana T; Liu Y; Noguchi K. Phosphorylation of extracellular signal-regulated kinase in primary afferent neurons by noxious stimuli and its involvement in peripheral sensitization. *J. Neurosci.* 2002, 22:7737-7745.

[108] Ji RR; Befort K; Brenner GJ; Woolf CJ. ERK MAP kinase activation in superficial spinal cord neurons induces prodynorphin and NK-1 upregulation and contributes to persistent inflammatory pain hypersensitivity. *J. Neurosci.* 2002, 22:478-485.

[109] Iadarola MJ; Douglass J; Civelli O; Naranjo JR. Differential activation of spinal cord dynorphin and enkephalin neurons during hyperalgesia: evidence using cDNA hybridization. *Brain Res.* 1988, 455:205-212.

[110] Ren K. An improved method for assessing mechanical allodynia in the rat. *Physiol. Behav.* 1999, 67:711-716.

[111] Gracely RH; Lynch SA; Bennett GJ. Painful neuropathy: altered central processing maintained dynamically by peripheral input. Pain. 1992, 51:175-194. Erratum in: *Pain* 1993, 52:251-253.

[112] Woolf CJ; Allchorne A; Safieh-Garabedian B; Poole S. Cytokines, nerve growth factor and inflammatory hyperalgesia: the contribution of tumour necrosis factor alpha. *Br. J. Pharmacol.* 1997, 121:417-424.

[113] Cunha JM; Cunha FQ; Poole S; Ferreira SH. Cytokine-mediated inflammatory hyperalgesia limited by interleukin-1 receptor antagonist. *Br. J. Pharmacol.* 2000, 130:1418-1424.

[114] Safieh-Garabedian B; Poole S; Haddad JJ; Massaad CA; Jabbur SJ; Saade NE. The role of the sympathetic efferents in endotoxin-induced localized inflammatory hyperalgesia and cytokine upregulation. *Neuropharmacology.* 2002, 42:864-872.

[115] Svensson CI; Yaksh TL. The spinal phospholipase-cyclooxygenase-prostanoid cascade in nociceptive processing. *Annu. Rev. Pharmacol. Toxicol.* 2002; 42:553-583.

[116] Khodorova A; Navarro B; Jouaville LS; Murphy JE; Rice FL, Mazurkiewicz JE; Long-Woodward D; Stoffel M; Strichartz GR; Yukhananov R; Davar G. Endothelin-B receptor activation triggers an endogenous analgesic cascade at sites of peripheral injury. *Nat. Med.* 2003, 9:1055-1061.

[117] Samad TA; Moore KA; Sapirstein A; Billet S; Allchorne A; Poole S; Bonventre JV; Woolf CJ. Interleukin-1beta-mediated induction of Cox-2 in the CNS contributes to inflammatory pain hypersensitivity. *Nature.* 2001, 410:471-475.

[118] Watkins LR; Maier SF. Immune regulation of central nervous system functions: from sickness responses to pathological pain. *J. Intern. Med.* 2005, 257:139-155.

[119] Fujita A; Kurachi Y. SAP family proteins. *Biochem. Biophys. Res. Commun.* 2000, 269:1-6.

[120] Tezuka T; Umemori H; Akiyama T; Nakanishi S; Yamamoto T. PSD-95 promotes Fyn-mediated tyrosine phosphorylation of the N-methyl-D-aspartate receptor subunit NR2A. *Proc. Natl. Acad. Sci. U S A.* 1999, 96:435-440.

[121] Kalia LV; Salter MW. Interactions between Src family protein tyrosine kinases and PSD-95. *Neuropharmacology.* 2003, 45:720-728.

[122] Tao YX; Huang YZ; Mei L; Johns RA. Expression of PSD-95/SAP90 is critical for N-methyl-D-aspartate receptor-mediated thermal hyperalgesia in the spinal cord. *Neuroscience.* 2000, 98:201-206.

[123] Garry EM; Moss A; Delaney A; O'Neill F; Blakemore J; Bowen J; Husi H; Mitchell R; Grant SG; Fleetwood-Walker SM. Neuropathic sensitization of behavioral reflexes and

spinal NMDA receptor/CaM kinase II interactions are disrupted in PSD-95 mutant mice. *Curr. Biol.* 2003, 13:321-328.

[124] Tao YX; Rumbaugh G; Wang GD; Petralia RS; Zhao C; Kauer FW; Tao F; Zhuo M; Wenthold RJ; Raja SN; Huganir RL; Bredt DS; Johns RA. Impaired NMDA receptor-mediated postsynaptic function and blunted NMDA receptor-dependent persistent pain in mice lacking postsynaptic density-93 protein. *J. Neurosci.* 2003, 23:6703-6712.

[125] Tu JC; Xiao B; Naisbitt S; Yuan JP; Petralia RS; Brakeman P; Doan A; Aakalu VK; Lanahan AA; Sheng M; Worley PF. Coupling of mGluR/Homer and PSD-95 complexes by the Shank family of postsynaptic density proteins. *Neuron.* 1999, 23:583-592.

[126] Naisbitt S; Kim E; Tu JC; Xiao B; Sala C; Valtschanoff J; Weinberg RJ; Worley PF; Sheng M. Shank, a novel family of postsynaptic density proteins that binds to the NMDA receptor/PSD-95/GKAP complex and cortactin. *Neuron.* 1999, 23:569-582.

[127] Meller ST; Dykstra CL; Gebhart GF. Acute mechanical hyperalgesia is produced by coactivation of AMPA and metabotropic glutamate receptors. *Neuroreport.* 1993, 4:879-882.

[128] Mills CD; Xu GY; Johnson KM; McAdoo DJ; Hulsebosch CE. AIDA reduces glutamate release and attenuates mechanical allodynia after spinal cord injury. *Neuroreport.* 2000, 11:3067-3070.

[129] Karim F; Wang CC; Gereau RW 4th. Metabotropic glutamate receptor subtypes 1 and 5 are activators of extracellular signal-regulated kinase signaling required for inflammatory pain in mice. *J. Neurosci.* 2001, 21:3771-3779.

[130] Walker K; Bowes M; Panesar M; Davis A; Gentry C; Kesingland A; Gasparini F; Spooren W; Stoehr N; Pagano A; Flor PJ; Vranesic I; Lingenhoehl K; Johnson EC; Varney M; Urban L; Kuhn R. Metabotropic glutamate receptor subtype 5 (mGlu5) and nociceptive function. I. Selective blockade of mGlu5 receptors in models of acute, persistent and chronic pain. *Neuropharmacology.* 2001, 40:1-9.

[131] Dolan S; Nolan AM. Behavioral evidence supporting a differential role for spinal group I and II metabotropic glutamate receptors in inflammatory hyperalgesia in sheep. *Neuropharmacology.* 2002, 43:319-326.

[132] Hudson LJ; Bevan S; McNair K; Gentry C; Fox A; Kuhn R; Winter J. Metabotropic glutamate receptor 5 upregulation in A-fibers after spinal nerve injury: 2-methyl-6-(phenylethynyl)-pyridine (MPEP) reverses the induced thermal hyperalgesia. *J. Neurosci.* 2002, 22:2660-2668.

[133] Neugebauer V. Metabotropic glutamate receptors--important modulators of nociception and pain behavior. *Pain.* 2002, 98:1-8.

[134] Zhang L; Lu Y; Chen Y; Westlund KN. Group I metabotropic glutamate receptor antagonists block secondary thermal hyperalgesia in rats with knee joint inflammation. *J. Pharmacol. Exp. Ther.* 2002, 300:149-156.

[135] Neugebauer V; Chen PS; Willis WD. Role of metabotropic glutamate receptor subtype mGluR1 in brief nociception and central sensitization of primate STT cells. *J. Neurophysiol.* 1999, 82:272-282.

[136] Young MR; Blackburn-Munro G; Dickinson T; Johnson MJ; Anderson H; Nakalembe I; Fleetwood-Walker SM. Antisense ablation of type I metabotropic glutamate receptor mGluR1 inhibits spinal nociceptive transmission. *J. Neurosci.* 1998, 18:10180-10188.

[137] Boxall SJ; Berthele A; Tolle TR; Zieglgansberger W; Urban L. mGluR activation reveals a tonic NMDA component in inflammatory hyperalgesia. *Neuroreport.* 1998, 9:1201-1203.

[138] Cerne R; Randic M. Modulation of AMPA and NMDA responses in rat spinal dorsal horn neurons by trans-1-aminocyclopentane-1,3-dicarboxylic acid. *Neurosci. Lett.* 1992,144:180-184.

[139] Kelso SR; Nelson TE; Leonard JP. Protein kinase C-mediated enhancement of NMDA currents by metabotropic glutamate receptors in Xenopus oocytes. *J. Physiol.* 1992, 449:705-718.

[140] Lan JY; Skeberdis VA; Jover T; Zheng X; Bennett MV; Zukin RS. Activation of metabotropic glutamate receptor 1 accelerates NMDA receptor trafficking. *J. Neurosci.* 2001, 21:6058-6068.

[141] Skeberdis VA; Lan J; Opitz T; Zheng X; Bennett MV; Zukin RS. mGluR1-mediated potentiation of NMDA receptors involves a rise in intracellular calcium and activation of protein kinase C. *Neuropharmacology.* 2001, 40:856-865.

[142] Benquet P; Gee CE; Gerber U. Two distinct signaling pathways upregulate NMDA receptor responses via two distinct metabotropic glutamate receptor subtypes. *J. Neurosci.* 2002, 22:9679-9686.

[143] O'Connor JJ; Rowan MJ; Anwyl R. Long-lasting enhancement of NMDA receptor-mediated synaptic transmission by metabotropic glutamate receptor activation. *Nature.* 1994, 367:557-559.

[144] O'Connor JJ; Rowan MJ; Anwyl R. Tetanically induced LTP involves a similar increase in the AMPA and NMDA receptor components of the excitatory postsynaptic current: investigations of the involvement of mGlu receptors. *J. Neurosci.* 1995, 15(3 Pt 1):2013-2020.

[145] Heidinger V; Manzerra P; Wang XQ; Strasser U; Yu SP; Choi DW; Behrens MM. Metabotropic glutamate receptor 1-induced upregulation of NMDA receptor current: mediation through the Pyk2/Src-family kinase pathway in cortical neurons. *J. Neurosci.* 2002, 22:5452-5461.

[146] Pin JP; Duvoisin R. The metabotropic glutamate receptors: structure and functions. *Neuropharmacology.* 1995, 34:1-26.

[147] Dougherty PM; Willis WD. Enhancement of spinothalamic neuron responses to chemical and mechanical stimuli following combined micro-iontophoretic application of N-methyl-D-aspartic acid and substance P. *Pain.* 1991, 47:85-93.

[148] Rusin KI; Jiang MC; Cerne R; Randic M. Interactions between excitatory amino acids and tachykinins in the rat spinal dorsal horn. *Brain Res. Bull.* 1993, 30:329-338.

[149] Seguin L; Millan MJ. The glycine B receptor partial agonist, (+)-HA966, enhances induction of antinociception by RP 67580 and CP-99,994. *Eur. J. Pharmacol.* 1994, 253:R1-3.

[150] Marvizon JC; Martinez V; Grady EF; Bunnett NW; Mayer EA. Neurokinin 1 receptor internalization in spinal cord slices induced by dorsal root stimulation is mediated by NMDA receptors. *J. Neurosci.* 1997, 17:8129-8136.

[151] Wu ZZ; Guan BC; Li ZW; Yang Q; Liu CJ; Chen JG. Sustained potentiation by substance P of NMDA-activated current in rat primary sensory neurons. *Brain Res.* 2004, 1010:117-126.

[152] De Felipe C; Herrero JF; O'Brien JA; Palmer JA; Doyle CA; Smith AJ; Laird JM; Belmonte C; Cervero F; Hunt SP. Altered nociception, analgesia and aggression in mice lacking the receptor for substance P. *Nature.* 1998, 392:394-397.

[153] Trujillo KA; Akil H. Inhibition of morphine tolerance and dependence by the NMDA receptor antagonist MK-801. *Science.* 1991, 251:85-87.

[154] Mao J. Opioid-induced abnormal pain sensitivity: implications in clinical opioid therapy. *Pain.* 2002, 100:213-217.

[155] Lu WY; Xiong ZG; Lei S; Orser BA; Dudek E; Browning MD; MacDonald JF. G-protein-coupled receptors act via protein kinase C and Src to regulate NMDA receptors. *Nat. Neurosci.* 1999, 2:331-338.

[156] Wang H; Kohno T; Amaya F; Brenner GJ; Ito N; Allchorne A; Ji RR; Woolf CJ. Bradykinin produces pain hypersensitivity by potentiating spinal cord glutamatergic synaptic transmission. *J. Neurosci.* 2005, 25:7986-7992.

[157] Pittaluga A; Feligioni M; Longordo F; Arvigo M; Raiteri M. Somatostatin-induced activation and up-regulation of N-methyl-D-aspartate receptor function: mediation through calmodulin-dependent protein kinase II, phospholipase C, protein kinase C, and tyrosine kinase in hippocampal noradrenergic nerve endings. *J. Pharmacol. Exp. Ther.* 2005, 313:242-249.

[158] Hunt SP; Mantyh PW. The molecular dynamics of pain control. *Nat. Rev. Neurosci.* 2001, 2:83-91.

[159] Mammen AL; Kameyama K; Roche KW; Huganir RL. Phosphorylation of the alpha-amino-3-hydroxy-5-methylisoxazole4-propionic acid receptor GluR1 subunit by calcium/calmodulin-dependent kinase II. *J. Biol. Chem.* 1997, 272:32528-32533.

[160] Zhang X; Wu J; Lei Y; Fang L; Willis WD. Protein phosphatase modulates the phosphorylation of spinal cord NMDA receptors in rats following intradermal injection of capsaicin. *Brain Res. Mol. Brain Res.* 2005, 138:264-272.

[161] Chen C; Leonard JP. Protein tyrosine kinase-mediated potentiation of currents from cloned NMDA receptors. *J. Neurochem.* 1996, 67:194-200.

[162] Salter MW; Kalia LV. Src kinases: a hub for NMDA receptor regulation. *Nat. Rev. Neurosci.* 2004, 5:317-328.

[163] Gingrich JR; Pelkey KA; Fam SR; Huang Y; Petralia RS; Wenthold RJ; Salter MW. Unique domain anchoring of Src to synaptic NMDA receptors via the mitochondrial protein NADH dehydrogenase subunit 2. *Proc. Natl. Acad. Sci. U S A.* 2004, 101:6237-6242.

[164] Chen L; Huang LY. Protein kinase C reduces Mg2+ block of NMDA-receptor channels as a mechanism of modulation. *Nature.* 1992, 356:521-523.

[165] Zheng X; Zhang L; Wang AP; Bennett MV; Zukin RS. Protein kinase C potentiation of N-methyl-D-aspartate receptor activity is not mediated by phosphorylation of N-

methyl-D-aspartate receptor subunits. *Proc. Natl. Acad. Sci. U S A.* 1999, 96:15262-15267.

[166] Grosshans DR; Browning MD. Protein kinase C activation induces tyrosine phosphorylation of the NR2A and NR2B subunits of the NMDA receptor. *J. Neurochem.* 2001, 76:737-744.

[167] Dikic I; Tokiwa G; Lev S; Courtneidge SA; Schlessinger J. A role for Pyk2 and Src in linking G-protein-coupled receptors with MAP kinase activation. *Nature.* 1996, 383:547-550.

[168] Huang Y; Lu W; Ali DW; Pelkey KA; Pitcher GM; Lu YM; Aoto H; Roder JC; Sasaki T; Salter MW; MacDonald JF. CAKbeta/Pyk2 kinase is a signaling link for induction of long-term potentiation in CA1 hippocampus. *Neuron.* 2001, 29:485-496.

[169] Girault JA; Costa A; Derkinderen P; Studler JM; Toutant M. FAK and PYK2/CAKbeta in the nervous system: a link between neuronal activity, plasticity and survival? *Trends Neurosci.* 1999, 22:257-263.

[170] Maruyama T; Kanaji T; Nakade S; Kanno T; Mikoshiba K. 2APB, 2-aminoethoxydiphenyl borate, a membrane-penetrable modulator of Ins(1,4,5)P3-induced Ca2+ release. *J. Biochem.* (Tokyo). 1997, 122:498-505.

[171] Kawasaki Y; Kohno T; Zhuang ZY; Brenner GJ; Wang H; Van Der Meer C; Befort K; Woolf CJ; Ji RR. Ionotropic and metabotropic receptors, protein kinase A, protein kinase C, and Src contribute to C-fiber-induced ERK activation and cAMP response element-binding protein phosphorylation in dorsal horn neurons, leading to central sensitization. *J. Neurosci.* 2004, 24:8310-8321.

[172] Dickenson AH. A cure for wind up: NMDA receptor antagonists as potential analgesics. *Trends Pharmacol. Sci.* 1990, 11:307-309.

[173] Parsons CG; Danysz W; Quack G. Glutamate in CNS disorders as a target for drug development: an update. *Drug News Perspect.* 1998, 11:523-569.

[174] Szekely JI; Torok K; Mate G. The role of ionotropic glutamate receptors in nociception with special regard to the AMPA binding sites. *Curr. Pharm. Des.* 2002, 8:887-912.

[175] Zhuo M. Glutamate receptors and persistent pain: targeting forebrain NR2B subunits. *Drug Discov. Today.* 2002, 7:259-267.

[176] Smith PF. Therapeutic N-methyl-D-aspartate receptor antagonists: will reality meet expectation? *Curr. Opin. Investig. Drugs.* 2003, 4:826-832.

[177] Chazot PL. The NMDA receptor NR2B subunit: a valid therapeutic target for multiple CNS pathologies. *Curr. Med. Chem.* 2004, 11:389-396.

[178] Haley JE; Sullivan AF; Dickenson AH. Evidence for spinal N-methyl-D-aspartate receptor involvement in prolonged chemical nociception in the rat. *Brain Res.* 1990, 518:218-226.

[179] Nasstrom J; Karlsson U; Post C. Antinociceptive actions of different classes of excitatory amino acid receptor antagonists in mice. *Eur. J. Pharmacol.* 1992, 212:21-29.

[180] Chaplan SR; Malmberg AB; Yaksh TL. Efficacy of spinal NMDA receptor antagonism in formalin hyperalgesia and nerve injury evoked allodynia in the rat. *J. Pharmacol. Exp. Ther.* 1997, 280:829-838.

[181] Yamamoto T; Shimoyama N; Mizuguchi T. The effects of morphine, MK-801, an NMDA antagonist, and CP-96,345, an NK1 antagonist, on the hyperesthesia evoked by carageenan injection in the rat paw. *Anesthesiology*. 1993, 78:124-133.

[182] Davar G; Hama A; Deykin A; Vos B; Maciewicz R. MK-801 blocks the development of thermal hyperalgesia in a rat model of experimental painful neuropathy. *Brain Res*. 1991, 553:327-330.

[183] Mao J; Price DD; Mayer DJ; Lu J; Hayes RL. Intrathecal MK-801 and local nerve anesthesia synergistically reduce nociceptive behaviors in rats with experimental peripheral mononeuropathy. *Brain Res*. 1992, 576:254-262.

[184] Yamamoto T; Yaksh TL. Spinal pharmacology of thermal hyperesthesia induced by constriction injury of sciatic nerve. Excitatory amino acid antagonists. *Pain*. 1992, 49:121-128.

[185] Seltzer Z; Cohn S; Ginzburg R; Beilin B. Modulation of neuropathic pain behavior in rats by spinal disinhibition and NMDA receptor blockade of injury discharge. *Pain*. 1991, 45:69-75.

[186] Ren K; Williams GM; Hylden JL; Ruda MA; Dubner R. The intrathecal administration of excitatory amino acid receptor antagonists selectively attenuated carrageenan-induced behavioral hyperalgesia in rats. *Eur. J. Pharmacol*. 1992, 219:235-243.

[187] Ren K; Dubner R. NMDA receptor antagonists attenuate mechanical hyperalgesia in rats with unilateral inflammation of the hindpaw. *Neurosci. Lett*. 1993, 163:22-26.

[188] Yashpal K; Pitcher GM; Parent A; Quirion R; Coderre TJ. Noxious thermal and chemical stimulation induce increases in 3H-phorbol 12,13-dibutyrate binding in spinal cord dorsal horn as well as persistent pain and hyperalgesia, which is reduced by inhibition of protein kinase C. *J. Neurosci*. 1995, 15(5 Pt 1):3263-3272.

[189] Laughlin TM; Kitto KF; Wilcox GL. Redox manipulation of NMDA receptors in vivo: alteration of acute pain transmission and dynorphin-induced allodynia. *Pain*. 1998, 80:37-43.

[190] Begon S; Pickering G; Eschalier A; Mazur A; Rayssiguier Y; Dubray C. Role of spinal NMDA receptors, protein kinase C and nitric oxide synthase in the hyperalgesia induced by magnesium deficiency in rats. *Br. J. Pharmacol*. 2001, 134:1227-1236.

[191] Yaksh TL. Behavioral and autonomic correlates of the tactile evoked allodynia produced by spinal glycine inhibition: effects of modulatory receptor systems and excitatory amino acid antagonists. *Pain*. 1989, 37:111-123.

[192] Hylden JL; Thomas DA; Iadarola MJ; Nahin RL; Dubner R. Spinal opioid analgesic effects are enhanced in a model of unilateral inflammation/hyperalgesia: possible involvement of noradrenergic mechanisms. *Eur. J. Pharmacol*. 1991, 194:135-143.

[193] Ma QP; Allchorne AJ; Woolf CJ. Morphine, the NMDA receptor antagonist MK801 and the tachykinin NK1 receptor antagonist RP67580 attenuate the development of inflammation-induced progressive tactile hypersensitivity. *Pain*. 1998, 77:49-57.

[194] Kawamata T; Omote K; Sonoda H; Kawamata M; Namiki A. Analgesic mechanisms of ketamine in the presence and absence of peripheral inflammation. *Anesthesiology*. 2000, 93:520-528.

[195] Klepstad P; Maurset A; Moberg ER; Oye I. Evidence of a role for NMDA receptors in pain perception. *Eur. J. Pharmacol*. 1990, 187:513-518.

[196] Price DD. Characteristics of second pain and flexion reflexes indicative of prolonged central summation. *Exp. Neurol.* 1972, 37:371-387.
[197] Ren K. Wind-up and the NMDA receptor: from animal studies to humans. *Pain.* 1994, 59:157-158.
[198] Price DD; Mao J; Frenk H; Mayer DJ. The N-methyl-D-aspartate receptor antagonist dextromethorphan selectively reduces temporal summation of second pain in man. *Pain.* 1994, 59:165-174.
[199] Kristensen JD; Svensson B; Gordh T Jr. The NMDA-receptor antagonist CPP abolishes neurogenic 'wind-up pain' after intrathecal administration in humans. *Pain.* 1992, 51:249-253.
[200] Kawamata T; Omote K; Kawamata M; Namiki A. Premedication with oral dextromethorphan reduces postoperative pain after tonsillectomy. *Anesth. Analg.* 1998, 86:594-597.
[201] Gordon SM; Dubner R; Dionne RA. Antihyperalgesic effect of the N-methyl-D-aspartate receptor antagonist dextromethorphan in the oral surgery model. *J. Clin. Pharmacol.* 1999, 39:139-146.
[202] Sang CN; Booher S; Gilron I; Parada S; Max MB. Dextromethorphan and memantine in painful diabetic neuropathy and postherpetic neuralgia: efficacy and dose-response trials. *Anesthesiology.* 2002, 96:1053-1061.
[203] Ilkjaer S; Nielsen PA; Bach LF; Wernberg M; Dahl JB. The effect of dextromethorphan, alone or in combination with ibuprofen, on postoperative pain after minor gynaecological surgery. *Acta Anaesthesiol. Scand.* 2000, 44:873-877.
[204] Plesan A; Sollevi A; Segerdahl M. The N-methyl-D-aspartate-receptor antagonist dextromethorphan lacks analgesic effect in a human experimental ischemic pain model. *Acta Anaesthesiol. Scand.* 2000, 44:924-928.
[205] Weinbroum AA; Rudick V; Paret G; Ben-Abraham R. The role of dextromethorphan in pain control. *Can. J. Anaesth.* 2000, 47:585-596.
[206] Willert RP; Woolf CJ; Hobson AR; Delaney C; Thompson DG; Aziz Q. The development and maintenance of human visceral pain hypersensitivity is dependent on the N-methyl-D-aspartate receptor. *Gastroenterology.* 2004, 126:683-692.
[207] Snijdelaar DG; van Rijn CM; Vinken P; Meert TF. Effects of pre-treatment with amantadine on morphine induced antinociception during second phase formalin responses in rats. *Pain.* 2005 Nov 15; [Epub ahead of print]
[208] Lu Y; Vera-Portocarrero LP; Westlund KN. Intrathecal coadministration of D-APV and morphine is maximally effective in a rat experimental pancreatitis model. *Anesthesiology.* 2003, 98:734-740.
[209] Zhang RX; Wang L; Wang X; Ren K; Berman BM; Lao L. Electroacupuncture combined with MK-801 prolongs anti-hyperalgesia in rats with peripheral inflammation. *Pharmacol. Biochem. Behav.* 2005, 81:146-151.
[210] Sevostianova N; Danysz W; Bespalov AY. Analgesic effects of morphine and loperamide in the rat formalin test: Interactions with NMDA receptor antagonists. *Eur. J. Pharmacol.* 2005 Nov 16; [Epub ahead of print]

[211] Kew JN; Trube G; Kemp JA. State-dependent NMDA receptor antagonism by Ro 8-4304, a novel NR2B selective, non-competitive, voltage-independent antagonist. *Br. J. Pharmacol.* 1998, 123:463-472.

[212] During MJ; Symes CW; Lawlor PA; Lin J; Dunning J; Fitzsimons HL; Poulsen D; Leone P; Xu R; Dicker BL; Lipski J; Young D. An oral vaccine against NMDAR1 with efficacy in experimental stroke and epilepsy. *Science.* 2000, 287:1453-1460.

[213] Chizh BA; Headley PM; Tzschentke TM. NMDA receptor antagonists as analgesics: focus on the NR2B subtype. *Trends Pharmacol. Sci.* 2001, 22:636-642.

[214] Malmberg AB; Gilbert H; McCabe RT; Basbaum AI. Powerful antinociceptive effects of the cone snail venom-derived subtype-selective NMDA receptor antagonists conantokins G and T. *Pain.* 2003, 101:109-116.

[215] Layer RT; Wagstaff JD; White HS. Conantokins: peptide antagonists of NMDA receptors. *Curr. Med. Chem.* 2004, 11:3073-3084.

[216] Borza I; Kolok S; Ignacz-Szendrei G; Greiner I; Tarkanyi G; Galgoczy K; Horvath C; Farkas S; Domany G. Indole-2-carboxamidines as novel NR2B selective NMDA receptor antagonists. *Bioorg. Med. Chem. Lett.* 2005, 15:5439-5441.

[217] Wei F; Wang GD; Kerchner GA; Kim SJ; Xu HM; Chen ZF; Zhuo M. Genetic enhancement of inflammatory pain by forebrain NR2B overexpression. *Nat. Neurosci.* 2001, 4:164-169.

[218] Wilson JA; Garry EM; Anderson HA; Rosie R; Colvin LA; Mitchell R; Fleetwood-Walker SM. NMDA receptor antagonist treatment at the time of nerve injury prevents injury-induced changes in spinal NR1 and NR2B subunit expression and increases the sensitivity of residual pain behaviours to subsequently administered NMDA receptor antagonists. *Pain.* 2005, 117:421-432.

[219] Taniguchi K; Shinjo K; Mizutani M; Shimada K;, Ishikawa T; Menniti FS;, Nagahisa A. Antinociceptive activity of CP-101,606, an NMDA receptor NR2B subunit antagonist. *Br. J. Pharmacol.* 1997, 122:809-812.

[220] Claiborne CF; McCauley JA; Libby BE;, Curtis NR; Diggle HJ; Kulagowski JJ; Michelson SR; Anderson KD; Claremon DA; Freidinger RM; Bednar RA; Mosser SD; Gaul SL; Connolly TM; Condra CL; Bednar B; Stump GL; Lynch JJ; Macaulay A; Wafford KA; Koblan KS; Liverton NJ. Orally efficacious NR2B-selective NMDA receptor antagonists. *Bioorg. Med. Chem. Lett.* 2003, 13:697-700.

*Chapter IV*

# NMDA Receptor Antagonists and Clinical Pain Management

*Jianren Mao*[*]

Pain Research Group, MGH Pain Center
Department of Anesthesia and Critical Care, Massachusetts General Hospital
Harvard Medical School, Boston, MA 02114

## Abstract

Among several major glutamate receptor subtypes, the N-methyl-D-aspartate (NMDA) receptor is perhaps the most extensively studied over the last two decades. There is compelling preclinical evidence indicating a critical role for NMDA receptors in the central mechanisms of pathological pain, which has led to the proposed use of NMDA receptor antagonists in the clinical pain management. In this chapter, a small sample of clinical trials using clinically available NMDA receptor antagonists will be discussed. Comparisons will be made between preclinical and clinical findings regarding the role of NMDA receptor antagonists in animal pain behaviors and clinical pain conditions. Disparities between preclinical and clinical findings using NMDA receptor antagonists will be discussed in light of the important role of translational pain research in bridging the gap between preclinical and clinical studies.

## Introduction

Over the last two decades, the role of the central glutamatergic system in general, and the N-methyl-D-aspartate (NMDA) receptor in particular, in the neural mechanisms of pathological pain has been extensively investigated in preclinical studies. As extensively discussed in a separate chapter in this volume, these preclinical studies have provided

---

[*] Phone: 6177262338. Fax: 6177242719. E-mail: jmao@partners.org

compelling evidence for a critical role of NMDA receptors in the induction and maintenance of pain behaviors induced by pathological conditions such as inflammation and nerve injury. The cellular mechanisms underlying the NMDA receptor function also have been well examined. These preclinical studies suggest that NMDA receptor antagonists could be used as a promising pharmacological tool for the clinical management of chronic pathological pain. Indeed, a large number of clinical trials have been carried out to evaluate the potential application of NMDA receptor antagonists in the clinical setting. As discussed in this chapter, the effects of clinically available NMDA receptor antagonists vary with different trial and clinical pain conditions. Since there are a large volume of clinical data and have been extensive reviews on this topic, only representative samples of such clinical trials will be cited in this chapter to facilitate the discussion on the importance of translational pain research as a tool to improve preclinical and clinical pain research.

# Effect of NMDA Receptor Antagonists in Preclinical Studies

The NMDA receptor is a major glutamate receptor subtype. Glutamate and aspartate are endogenous ligands of NMDA receptors. As discussed in detail in a separate chapter in this volume, the NMDA receptor consists of subunits including NR1 and one of NR2 or NR3 subunits [1; more references can be found in another chapter in this volume]. Various combinations of NR1 and other NR subunits thus determine the property of NMDA receptor activity. The NMDA receptor is both voltage- and ligand-gated. That is, activation of this receptor requires not only an agonist (e.g., glutamate) binding and also cell membrane depolarization to remove a magnesium blockade inside the calcium channel coupled with the NMDA receptor. The NMDA receptor is regulated at multiple sites of its receptor-channel complex including glutamate, glycine, and calcium channel sites. Thus far, clinically available NMDA receptor antagonists such as ketamine and dextromethorphan mainly bind to the calcium channel site and are categorized as non-competitive NMDA receptor antagonists.

NMDA receptors have a large presence in both supraspinal and spinal regions. There appears to be a minimal variation of NMDA receptor distributions within the central nervous system among different species including rats, mice, and human beings. At the supraspinal level, NMDA receptors have been found in the hippocampus, cerebral cortex, thalamus, striatum, cerebellum, and various brainstem nuclei. At the spinal level, NMDA receptors have been demonstrated mainly in the superficial layers of the dorsal horn [1]. Most NMDA receptors are located at the postsynaptic site as revealed using immunocytochemistry. However, presynaptic NMDA receptors have been demonstrated at primary afferent fibers using the combined electron microscopic and immunocytochemical technique [2]. These presynaptic NMDA receptors, among other glutamate receptor subtypes, may have a role in regulating excitatory amino acid release from presynaptic terminals. NMDA receptors play a pivotal role in a number of essential physiological functions including neuroplasticity. However, excessive stimulation of the NMDA receptor could be detrimental to the central nervous system functions leading to neurotoxicity. It is this function of NMDA receptors that has been shown to play a significant role in the development and maintenance of pain behaviors following inflammation (inflammatory pain) and/or nerve injury (neuropathic pain) in a large number of preclinical studies.

In preclinical studies, compelling evidence has emerged indicating a critical role of NMDA receptors in the neural mechanisms of pathological pain behaviors such as hyperalgesia and allodynia associated with neuropathy and inflammation [3–8]. These preclinical studies indicate that 1) NMDA receptors are involved in pathological pain states induced by either partial or complete nerve injury or by persistent inflammation; 2) pain behaviors can be prevented and/or reversed by using either investigational (AP-5, MK-801) or clinically available (ketamine, amantadine, dextrorphan - the active metabolite of dextromethorphan) NMDA receptor antagonists; and 3) both thermal hyperalgesia and mechanical allodynia, as well as spontaneous pain behaviors, can be effectively reduced using an NMDA receptor antagonist.

The data from these preclinical studies regarding the role of NMDA receptors in pain behaviors are reproducible and reliable across different animal models, pathological conditions, and treatment regimens. Thus, preclinical evidence strongly suggests that NMDA receptor antagonists might be useful clinically to prevent the development of pathological pain. More importantly, since NMDA receptor antagonists have been shown to reverse pain behaviors in preclinical studies, a clinically available NMDA receptor antagonist would be expected to have a therapeutic role in treating clinical pain. These are the premises of a large number of clinical trials conducted over the last two decades.

# Effect of NMDA Receptor Antagonists in Clinical Studies

A considerable number of clinical observations (controlled studies and case reports) have been published [9, 10]. Currently, three clinically available NMDA receptor antagonists (ketamine, dextromethorphan, amantadine) with various NMDA receptor antagonist properties have been used for clinical studies. By reviewing these clinical observations, it is rather interesting to note that, unlike almost unequivocal results from preclinical studies, the clinical effects of NMDA receptor antagonists vary considerably among these studies. Both positive and negative outcomes have been reported as shown in small samples of clinical studies summarized in Table 1.

Several observations may be made from these clinical studies. First, in those studies with negative outcomes, postoperative pain such as that following abdominal or knee surgery was generally used as the study pain condition, whereas, in those studies with positive outcomes, neuropathic pain (e.g., complex regional pain syndrome; postherpetic neuralgia) was used as the study condition. Second, an NMDA receptor antagonist often was given preoperatively or intraoperatively as a single dose in these negative outcome studies. In contrast, patients with a positive response to an NMDA receptor antagonist often received either multiple doses or continuous intravenous or subcutaneous infusion over hours, days, or weeks (in some cases). Third, except for few studies in which hyperalgesia was specifically examined using the technique of quantitative sensory testing, visual analog or numerical pain scales were used to report changes in pain intensity in these studies.

### Table 1. Representative Clinical Studies

| Pain Type | Drug | Dose Regimen | Outcome | Ref. |
|---|---|---|---|---|
| Hysterectomy | Ama | 200 mg, iv, pre-op | Negative | [15] |
| Hysterectomy | Dex | 150 mg, po, pre-op | Negative | [16] |
| Knee surgery | Dex | 40 mg, im, pre-op | Negative | [17] |
| Knee surgery | Dex | 200 mg, po, pre-op | Negative | [18] |
| Abd. surgery | Dex | 120 mg, im, pre-op | Negative | [19] |
| Hysterectomy | Dex | 27 mg, po, peri-op | Negative | [20] |
| CNP | Ket | > 100 mg/d, po | Positive | [21] |
| PHN | Dex | 125 mg/d, po | Positive | [22] |
| Hyperalgesia | Ket | 2 µg/kg/min x 72 hr | Positive | [23] |
| PHN | Ket | 0.15 mg/kg/hr x 7 d | Positive | [24] |
| NCP | Ket | 400 mg/day, s.c. | Positive | [25] |
| NCP | Ama | 200 mg/3 hr, i.v. | Positive | [26] |

The tabel includes only a small sample of representative clinical studies. A detailed review can be seen in reference [27].

Legends: Abd: abdominal; CNP: chronic neuropathic pain; PHN: postherpetic neuralgia; NCP: neuropathic (cancer) pain;. Ama: amantadine; Dex: dextromethorphan; Ket: ketamine.; Pre-op: pre-operative; Peri-op: peri-operative; Neg.: Negative result; Pos.: positive result; iv: intravenously; sc: subcutaneously; po: orally; im: intramuscularly.

While the role of NMDA receptors in pain behaviors is strongly supported by a large number of preclinical studies, outcomes from clinical studies using an NMDA receptor antagonist differ dramatically among different study conditions and dose regimens. One obvious limitation in these studies is that clinically available NMDA receptor antagonists are not highly selective and some of these agents are only weak NMDA receptor antagonists. However, even when the same clinically available NMDA receptor antagonist (e.g., ketamine) was used in these studies, clinical outcomes still differ among these studies indicating there may be additional factors contributing to the study outcome.

As discussed below, several factors may have contributed to the discrepancies between preclinical and clinical studies.

*First, there could be a mismatch in study pain conditions.* NMDA receptors are most likely to be involved in pathological pain conditions following nerve injury or persistent inflammation as shown in preclinical studies [5–7] . Importantly, NMDA receptor antagonists have not been shown, in nearly all preclinical studies, to alter baseline nociceptive threshold indicating that an NMDA receptor antagonist itself is unlikely to function as a classic analgesic (e.g., opioid). In many preclinical studies, NMDA receptor antagonists most reliably prevent or reverse hyperalgesia without changing baseline nociceptive threshold. Thus, uncomplicated postoperative pain after either abdominal or knee surgery, which was repeatedly used as a study pain condition in those negative outcome studies, might be less likely to benefit from an NMDA receptor antagonist particularly when an NMDA receptor antagonist is used alone in this setting, because NMDA receptor antagonists are not considered to act as analgesics.

*Second, there could be a mismatch in treatment regimens.* Although a single dose of an NMDA receptor antagonist could transiently reverse pain behaviors, preclinical studies have indicated that repeated doses of an NMDA receptor antagonist often are required to prevent the development of pain behaviors following either nerve injury or inflammation, because a constant or repetitive barrage of peripheral nociceptive input is expected under such conditions [11, 12]. Given that patients who failed to benefit from an NMDA receptor antagonist often received only a single dose regimen, it is likely that an inadequate dosing may have contributed to the lack of treatment benefits in some of these clinical studies.

*Third, there could be a mismatch in the underlying mechanisms.* Preclinical studies have largely focused on the cellular and molecular changes during the early stage following nerve injury or inflammation. While these early responses could indicate neuronal plastic changes in which NMDA receptors play a critical role, they are largely driven by a constant peripheral nociceptive input from nerve injury or inflammation. It remains to be seen whether blocking these early post-injury cellular and molecular changes using an NMDA receptor antagonist would be effective for prevention or reversal of a persistent pain state in the clinical setting. Thus, the effectiveness of an NMDA receptor antagonist could be time-dependent under different clinical conditions.

## NMDA Receptor Antagonists and Preemptive Analgesia

Preemptive analgesia was suggested based on the notion that postoperative pain intensity would be increased if peripheral nociceptive input was not blocked, resulting in central sensitization mediated, at least in part, through the NMDA receptor. Thus, blocking the process of central sensitization perioperatively with a clinically available NMDA receptor antagonist would be expected to prevent or attenuate the development of postoperative pain hypersensitivity. It was expected that the potential preemptive effect using an NMDA receptor antagonist would lead to diminished pain intensity (a lower pain score) and/or reduced consumption of analgesics (such as opioids) during a postoperative period. Nearly every clinical study examining preemptive analgesia was designed along this line of logic. However, the clinical benefit of preemptive analgesia remains largely unclear. Several important issues on this topic are discussed as follows.

*Does central sensitization contribute to postoperative pain?* This question needs to be addressed for two reasons. First, although NMDA receptors play a pivotal role in central sensitization, they are not primarily involved in the processing of nociceptive pain as discussed earlier. Second, because NMDA receptors do not play a major role in the processing of nociceptive pain, an NMDA receptor antagonist by itself could not function as an effective analgesic. Thus, the perioperative use of an NMDA receptor antagonist alone should not be expected to result in significant pain relief since the major component of postoperative pain would be nociceptive pain in nature. On the other hand, certain pain conditions such as that after limb amputation, which is more likely to involve NMDA receptors mechanistically, may respond more effectively to the perioperative use of an NMDA receptor antagonist.

*Can the current clinical study design make a distinction between nociceptive pain and pain hypersensitivity due to central sensitization?* If central sensitization contributes to postoperative pain through increased pain sensitivity, it might be expected that the perioperative use of an NMDA receptor antagonist would lead to a reduced pain score and/or spare of the postoperative analgesic use. However, the current clinical trial design may not be sensitive and specific enough to make the distinction between the drug's effects on pain sensitivity and nociceptive pain itself. In this regard, the clinical endpoints (such as pain score and analgesic consumption) frequently used in most studies are fundamentally insufficient to make such a distinction.

## Conclusion

NMDA receptors are likely to play a significant role in the central mechanisms of pathological pain, which is supported by an overwhelming number of preclinical studies. The fact that clinical study outcomes vary significantly depending on pain condition, dosing regimen, and pain assessment tools suggests that translation between preclinical findings and their clinical application is not a simple one-way (from bench to bedside) process. It is important to recognize both limitations and indications of NMDA receptor antagonists in clinical pain management. While preclinical studies will continue to provide tantalizing results, new concepts, and therapeutic potentials such as new agents targeting NMDA receptor subunits [13, 14], clinical studies need to establish the proper indications, recognize limitations, and compare and contrast various study outcomes. In all of these areas, translational pain research could play a vital role to bridge preclinical and clinical studies and shorten the cycle between basic science research and clinical application.

## References

[1]  Mao J. NMDA and opioid receptors: Their interactions in antinociception, tolerance, and neuroplasticity. *Brain Res. Rev.* 1999; 30:289-304.

[2]  Liu J, Wang H, Sheng M, Jan LY, Jan YN, Basbaum AI. Evidence for presynaptic N-methyl-D-aspartate autoreceptors in the spinal cord dorsal horn. *Proceedings of National Academy of Sciences.* 1994; 91:8383-8387.

[3]  Dickenson AH. A cure for wind-up: NMDA receptor antagonists as potential analgesics. *Trends Pharmacol. Sci.* 1990; 11:307-309.

[4]  Woolf CJ, Thompson SWN. The induction and maintenance of central sensitization is dependent on N-methyl-D-aspartic acid receptor activation: Implications for the treatment of post-injury pain hypersensitivity states. *Pain.* 1991; 44:293-299.

[5]  Woolf CJ, Mannion RJ. Neuropathic pain: Aetiology, symptoms, mechanisms, and management. *Lancet.* 1999; 353: 1959-1964.

[6] Dubner R. Neuronal plasticity and pain following peripheral tissue inflammation or nerve injury. In: Bond M, Charlton E, Woolf CJ, eds. *Proceedings of 5th World Congress on Pain. Pain Research and Clinical Management.* Amsterdam: Elsevier:1991;5:263-276.

[7] Mao J, Price DD, Mayer DJ. Mechanisms of hyperalgesia and opiate tolerance: A current view of their possible interactions. *Pain.* 1995; 62:259-274.

[8] Chaplan SR, Malmberg AB, Yaksh TL. Efficacy of spinal NMDA receptor antagonism in formalin hyperalgesia and nerve injury evoked allodynia in the rat. *J. Pharmacol. Exp. Ther.* 1997; 280: 829-838.

[9] Sindrup SH, Jensen TS. Efficacy of pharmacological treatment of neuropathic pain: An update and effect related to mechanism of drug action. *Pain.* 1999; 83:389-400.

[10] Mao J. Translational pain research: Bridging the gap between basic and clinical pain research. *Pain.* 2002; 97:183-187.

[11] Mao J, Mayer DJ, Hayes RL, Lu J, Price DD. Differential roles of NMDA and non-NMDA receptor activation in induction and maintenance of thermal hyperalgesia in rats with painful peripheral mononeuropathy. *Brain Res.* 1992; 598: 271-278.

[12] Ren K, Williams GM, Hylden JL, Ruda MA, Dubner R. The intrathecal administration of excitatory amino acid receptor antagonists selectively attenuated carrageenan-induced behavioral hyperalgesia in rats. *Eur. J. Pharmacol.* 1992; 219:235-243.

[13] Chazot PL. The NMDA receptor NR2B subunit: a valid therapeutic target for multiple CNS pathologies. *Curr. Med. Chem.* 2004; 389-396.

[14] Tao YX, Raja SN. Are synaptic MAGUK proteins involved in chronic pain. *Trends Phamacol. Sci,* 2004; 25: 397-400.

[15] Gottschalk, A., Schroeder, F., Ufer, M., Oncu, A., Buerkle, H. and Standl, T. Amantadine, a N-methyl-D-aspartate receptor antagonist, does not enhance postoperative analgesia in women undergoing abdominal hysterectomy, *Aneth. Analg.* 2001, 93: 192-196.

[16] Ilkjaer, S., Bach, L.F., Nielsen, P.A., Wernberg, M. and Dahl, J.B. Effect of preoperative oral dextromethorphan on immediate and late postoperative pain and hyperalgesia after total abdominal hysterectomy, *Pain,* 2000; 86:19-24.

[17] Yeh, C.C., Ho, S.T., Kong, S.S., Wu, C.T. and Wong, C.S. Absence of the preemptive analgesic effect of dextromethorphan in total knee replacement under epidural anesthesia, *Acta Anaesthesiol. Sin,* 2000; 38:187-193.

[18] Wadhwa, A., Clarke, D., Goodchild, C.S. and Young, D. Large-dose oral dextromethorphan as an adjunct to patient-controlled analgesia with morphine after knee surgery, *Anesth. Analg,* 2001; 92: 448-454.

[19] Helmy, S.A. and Bali, A. The effect of the preemptive use of the NMDA receptor antagonist dextromethorphan on postoperative analgesic requirements, *Anesth. Analg,* 2001; 92: 739-744.

[20] McConahgy, P.M., McSorley, P., McCaughey, W. and Campbell, W.I. Dextromethorphan and pain after total abdominal hysterectomy, *Br. J. Anaesth,* 1998; 81: 731-736.

[21] Enarson, M.C., Hays, H. and Woodroffe, M.A. Clinical experience with oral ketamine, *J. Pain Symptom Manage*, 1999; 17:384-386.

[22] Klepstad, P. and Borchgrevink, P.C. Four years' treatment with ketamine and a trial of dextromethorphan in a patient with severe post-herpetic neuralgia, *Acta Anaethesiol. Scand,* 1997; 41: 422-426.

[23] Stubhaug, A., Breivik, H., Eide, P.K., Kreunen, M. and Foss, A. Mapping of punctuate hyperalgesia around a surgical incision demonstrates that ketamine is a powerful suppressor of central sensitization to pain following surgery, *Acta Anaesthesiol. Scand*, 1997; 41:1124-1132.

[24] Eide, P.K., Stubhaug, A. and Stenehjem, A.E. Central dysesthesia pain after traumatic spinal cord injury is dependent on N-methyl-D-aspartate receptor activation, *Neurosurgery*, 1995, 37:1080-1087.

[25] Mercadante, S., Lodi, F., Sapio, M., Calligara, M. and Serretta, R. Long-term ketamine subcutaneous continuous infusion in neuropathic cancer pain, *J. Pain Sympt. Manage.* 1995; 10: 564-568.

[26] Pud, D., Eisenberg, E., Spitzer, A., Adler, R., Fried, G. and Yarnisky, D. The NMDA receptor antagonist amantadine reduces surgical neuropathic pain in cancer patients: a double blind, randomized, placebo controlled trial, *Pain*, 1998; 75:349-354.

[27] Sindrup, S.H. and Jensen, T.S. Efficacy of pharmacological treatment of neuropathic pain: an update and effect related to mechanism of drug action, *Pain*, 1999; 83:389-400.

*Chapter V*

# Plasticity of Signaling Molecules and Their Associations after Chronic Morphine: Altered but Not Lost Opioid Receptor-Coupled Functionality

### *Alan R. Gintzler and Sumita Chakrabarti*
Department of Biochemistry, State University of New York,
Downstate Medical Center. 450 Clarkson Ave, Brooklyn, NY

## Abstract

The medicinal usefulness of narcotic analgesics, which remains a preferential treatment for post-surgical and neuropathic pain management, continues to be limited by analgesic tolerance formation. Increased knowledge of the complexity of tolerant mechanisms would help to facilitate the identification of new targets for its pharmacologic amelioration. Opioid tolerance is adaptive, enabling cell survival in the face of the continued perturbing effects of opioids. Consonant with mechanisms that have been shown to underlie desensitization of the β-adrenergic receptor, opioid tolerance was principally thought to involve the loss of opioid receptor function. More recent studies have revealed the greater complexity and multidimensional nature of opioid tolerant-forming mechanisms that occur downstream from the opioid receptor. These are comprised of dynamic processes that make use of the plasticity that is inherent in GPCR signaling mechanisms. Principle among these adaptations is the isoform-specific alteration of the effector enzymes adenylyl cyclase and phospholipase Cβ and augmented phosphorylation of the $G_\beta$ subunit of G proteins. These adaptations profoundly alter, but do not eliminate, the consequences of opioid receptor signaling via Gi/Go, the predominant G proteins that couple to opioid receptors. Recently obtained data also provide direct evidence that chronic morphine markedly enhances the association of the μ-opioid receptor with $G_s$, which would enable a new dimension of opioid receptor signaling to emerge. In the aggregate, these adaptations elicited by chronic morphine permit the continuity of opioid receptor signaling albeit with profoundly altered physiological consequences. They also provide a basis for the well-documented divergence of signaling systems effected by chronic morphine.

# Introduction

The past 30 years have witnessed enormous advances in understanding the biochemistry and molecular biology of opioid receptors and their substrate peptides. However, despite the delineation of many of the physiological, biochemical and molecular biological sequelae of persistent exposure to narcotics, we have a very incomplete understanding of the mechanistic underpinnings of opioid tolerance and it remains a predominant impediment to their medicinal use for chronic pain relief. Nevertheless, the use of morphine and related opiates in the pharmacological management of pain continues unabated, underscoring the need for a more complete understanding of the molecular underpinnings of opioid tolerance. Investigations into tolerance-producing mechanisms are inspired by the conviction that identification of those adaptations that are causally associated with opioid tolerance will facilitate the development of pharmacotherapies that minimize or even eliminate its development. Additionally, it is inspired by the unique perspective such research provides on signal transduction plasticity in the central nervous system.

An impressive array of neurochemical perturbations has been associated with opioid tolerance. Indeed, the plethora of identified biochemical changes elicited by chronic morphine reflects the profound perturbing effects of opioids on CNS equilibria. A major challenge to investigators attempting to elucidate the mechanistic underpinnings of opioid tolerance is to differentiate between those adaptations that are causally associated with opioid tolerance vs. those that are epiphenomena. It is also imperative that unique aspects of acute and chronic opioid receptor pharmacology are incorporated into models of opioid tolerance. Importantly, they should not be predominantly extrapolations of receptor desensitization models that have been extensively developed for other G protein coupled receptors (GPCRs) such as that which has been elegantly formulated by Lefkowitz and co-workers using the $\beta_2$-adrenergic receptor as the GPCR model [1]. These attributes are essential to the medicinal usefulness of any model of opioid tolerance.

# Definition and Categories of Adaptation

Tolerance is always defined relative to specific opioid actions. Notably, analgesia, sedation, respiratory depression, etc., frequently manifest differential tolerance development. This suggests that different opioid functions are mediated via different signaling strategies that could elicit varied adaptational mechanisms. Thus, the general applicability and exclusivity of any model of opioid tolerance should be rigorously assessed and defined relative to the experimental system(s) that was utilized in its development.

The preponderance of adaptations to the persistent presence of morphine that have been postulated to be causally associated with opioid tolerance generally fall into two main categories, those that result in the actual loss of specific opioid receptor-mediated signaling and those that result in the *apparent* loss of this activity via its masking. Examples of adaptations resulting in the loss of opioid action would include the diminution of spare opioid receptors [2], altered opioid receptor density/internalization [3,4] and altered G protein content [5]. Additionally, studies utilizing GTP$\gamma$S$^{35}$ binding, which reflects the exchange of GTP for GDP on the heterotrimeric G protein and thus its activation, have demonstrated decreased opioid receptor G protein coupling following chronic systemic morphine [6].

## Opioid Receptor Phosphorylation

Like all GPCRs, opioid receptors are phosphorylated, which is promoted by agonist binding [7-11]. Phosphorylation of opioid receptors is a prelude to its forming a complex with β-arrestin. Importantly, arrestin binding to GPCRs has dual consequences. It sterically hinders interaction with G proteins resulting in the uncoupling of opioid receptors from their respective G protein(s). This blunts opioid receptor signaling, which is manifest as opioid receptor desensitization. β-arrestin also targets GPCRs to clathrin-coated pits thereby mediating opioid receptor internalization. This can facilitate opioid receptor de-phosphorylation and membrane re-insertion. Alternatively, internalization of opioid receptors can initiate trafficking to other subcellular compartment such as lysozomes where receptor degradation can occur. These events directly parallel those that have been extensively described for the β$_2$-adrenergic receptor [7] and are shared by most, if not all GPCRs.

## Acute Desensitization vs. Sustained Exposure

A critical question, however, is whether or not mechanisms that underlie short-term opioid desensitization that is common among most GRCRs reflect adaptations that are responsible for reductions in opioid agonist potency observed over prolonged time periods, such as occurs clinically. Indeed, numerous considerations suggest that the opioid tolerance that is seen after sustained exposure to opioids requires other modifications of the signal transduction system; it is, unlikely that opioid receptor 'dysfunctionality' can account for the totality of opioid tolerance.

This conclusion is based on multiple observations: (a) profound physiological tolerance to morphine is frequently not accompanied by opioid receptor downregulation [14,15], (b) morphine, which is very tolerant producing, results in little or no opioid receptor internalization [12,16-19], (c) opioid receptor endocytosis has been associated with a *diminution* of receptor desensitization and opioid tolerance [17,20], (d) in some tissue, e.g., the guinea longitudinal muscle myenteric plexus (LMMP) [21], and locus coeruleus [22] the content of G$_{i\alpha}$ is paradoxically increased following chronic morphine, (e) in both the LMMP tissue [23] and periaqueductal gray [24], opioid receptor/effector coupling is increased following chronic morphine and (f) chronic morphine has been shown to *induce* δ-opioid receptor (DOR) function in the midbrain [25]. (g) An important role of receptor internalization/desensitization in tolerance formation is certainly suggested by reports that tolerance formation is markedly blunted in β-arrestin knockout animals [3,26]. This notwithstanding, conclusions drawn from such observations should be tempered by the knowledge that β-arrestin also functions as a scaffolding molecule. For example, membrane recruitment of β-arrestin is not only crucial for intracellular receptor trafficking but also for the activation of a receptor-src kinase complex through which $β_2$-adrenergic receptors activate the MAP kinases Erk1/2 pathway [27]. In fact, components of the c-Jun N-terminal kinase 3 and ERK1/3 MAP kinase cascades as well as the E3 ubiquitin ligase mdm2 and the phosphodiesterase 4D3 and 4D5 isoforms of cAMP are all recruited to GPCRs via β-arrestin. Moreover, there is evidence that the agonist-receptor-arrestin complex can function as an alternative *functional* ternary complex [28], the formation of which could be relevant to tolerant mechanisms. Thus the observed diminution of tolerance formation in β-arrestin knockout animals is consistent with multiple mechanistic inferences and does not unequivocally imply a causal association between opioid receptor internalization and tolerance formation.

Thus, numerous caveats suggest that the receptor desensitization ('dysfunctionality') hypothesis is not sufficient to explain opioid tolerance. Epitomizing this perspective is the massive withdrawal that is precipitated following administration of opioid receptor antagonists to chronic morphine-treated animals. This underscores that the orders of magnitude diminution in opioid analgesic potency following its sustained clinical administration cannot result solely from opioid receptor inactivation.

## Masking Opioid Functionality

An alternative formulation to the 'opioid receptor dysfunctionality' hypothesis is that the loss of opioid action following sustained treatment with opioids is *apparent* and not real. It results from the masking of ongoing opioid receptor signaling. The best-characterized exemplar of adaptations that result in *masking* opioid receptor functionality is adenylyl cyclase (AC) superactivation or AC overshoot [29-32]. This refers to the robust up-regulation of AC activity that is manifest upon the acute withdrawal of an opioid agonist after chronic opioid treatment. This is thought to reflect a compensatory upregulation of AC activity (and not a loss of MOR coupling). Increased AC activity would counter balance the ongoing inhibitory influence of the continued presence of morphine and thereby reestablish 'normal' levels of AC activity. However, AC superactivation is not universally observed. It is not manefest by the LMMP tissue [45], all brain regions [32], or all AC isoforms [54]

Notably, the marked increase in AC activity that ensues following the acute removal of morphine after its prolonged presence underscores the persistence of ongoing morphine inhibition of AC activity. This indicates that opioid receptors continue to signal despite the (apparent) loss of AC inhibitory activity, i.e., the manifestation of opioid tolerance. This inference is supported by the demonstration that re-addition of opioid agonist following its washout from chronic morphine-treated preparations abolishes AC 'superactivation' and reestablishes pre-existing 'tolerant' levels of AC activity. These data further underscore that opioid receptor desensitization and the loss of opioid receptor functionality cannot be the exclusive underpinning of opioid tolerance.

## Downstream Adaptations to Chronic Morphine

The above considerations indicate that while regulatory processes affecting opioid receptors themselves undoubtedly contribute to physiological adaptation to opioids, the complex physiology of adapting to the sustained *in vivo* exposure to opioids cannot be understood solely at this level. The manifestation of opioid tolerance requires additional adaptations downstream from the opioid receptor itself. It is now clear that in addition to adaptations that occur on the level of opioid receptors that 'acutely' reduce effector coupling, long-term adaptations also occur at the cellular, synaptic, and network levels. These contribute to the reestablishment of normal cellular function despite the continued activity of the drug.

A fundamental organizing rubric that permeates formulations of opioid tolerance is that adaptations elicited by chronic opioid administration are protective. Opioids profoundly perturb equilibria in the central nervous system, in response to which compensatory homeostatic process are initiated in an attempt to re-establish initial conditions. Collectively, these adaptations are manifest as the development of opioid tolerance, i.e., higher opioid doses are required to achieve the desired effect. Several recent reviews have cataloged the wide-ranging adaptations that have been associated with chronic opioid treatment, many of which are independent of the opioid receptor itself [33-35]. In the remainder of this chapter, we will confine our discussion of post receptor opioid tolerant-producing strategies to those we have observed on a cellular level.

The perceived deficiencies in prevailing models of opioid tolerance that revolve around hypotheses of opioid receptor 'dysfunctionality' and/or the masking of opioid receptor functionality (i.e., AC superactivation) impelled us to propose complimentary adaptational strategies that would underlie opioid tolerance development. These rely heavily on the duality of intracellular G protein signaling as well as their propensity for pleiotropy.

## Duality and Pleiotropy of G Protein Signaling

The capacity of G proteins for dual intracellular signaling as well as pleiotropy contributes to the richness and diversity of GPCR signaling. G protein duality of signaling derives from their capacity to concomitantly modulate multiple effectors and from the signaling activity of both the $G_\alpha$ as well as $G_{\beta\gamma}$ subunits. For example, $G_i/G_o$, can simultaneously inhibit AC and stimulate phospholipase C$\beta$ via $G_\alpha$ and $G_{\beta\gamma}$, respectively [36]. The ability of both the $G_\alpha$ and $G_{\beta\gamma}$ subunits to modulate the same effector e.g., AC, in a synergistic or antagonistic fashion represents another dimension of dual G protein signaling [37-40]. The ability of GPCRs to simultaneously activate multiple classes of G protein (pleiotropy) further contributes to the flavor and texture of GPCR signaling. For example, many GPCRs exhibit dual coupling to $G_s$ as well as $G_{q11}$ [41] or to $G_i/G_o$ and $G_{q11}$ [42]. Chronic morphine-induced adaptations recently discovered by this laboratory utilize both the duality of intracellular G protein signaling as well as their propensity for pleiotropy.

In contrast to prevailing cellular models of opioid tolerance formation that entail a loss or turning off of opioid receptor signaling, we proposed that chronic morphine elicits the emergence of new opioid receptor-coupled signaling strategies. These results from the altered consequences of opioid receptor G protein coupling that are present in opioid naïve tissue. Altered, but not lost, opioid receptor-coupled signaling following persistent opioid receptor activation was initially deduced from comparisons of the effects of morphine on transmitter release from opioid naïve vs. tolerant/dependent LMMP preparations. In opioid naïve preparations, morphine substantially inhibits the electrically evoked release of methionine enkephalin [43]. Paradoxically, however, in tolerant/dependent preparations, morphine is a prerequisite for such release [44]. In other words, following chronic morphine, the loss of opioid inhibition is accompanied by the manifestation of a facilitative action. This suggested a switch from opioid receptor-coupled inhibitory to excitatory signaling, which was also indicated by the loss of opioid inhibition and the emergence of opioid facilitation of cAMP formation [45,46]. Subsequent research revealed that the latter did not result from a single biochemical perturbation. Instead, it results from a mosaic of changes in the identity and phosphorylation state of (opioid receptor-coupled) AC isoforms as well as the phosphorylation of multiple intervening signaling molecules. This causes changes in dynamic equilibria, offsetting perturbations that result from acute morphine administration.

## Chronic Morphine Induces AC Isoform-Specific Synthesis and Phosphorylation

Chronic morphine qualitatively alters the nature of one of the major effectors that is coupled to opioid receptors. Persistent stimulation of opioid receptors significantly elevates mRNA encoding AC IV [47] and AC VII [48,49]. In contrast, following chronic morphine, levels of AC I mRNA remain unchanged. This, in combination with the specificity of the monoclonal AC antibody used in Western analysis, suggests that the increment in AC protein that is observed following chronic morphine [49] is, most likely, comprised of AC isoforms IV and/or VII.

Changes in the relative preponderance of AC I vs. AC IV and VII protein are functionally very significant since they are differentially dually regulated by the $G_\alpha$ and $G_{\beta\gamma}$ subunits of $G_i/G_o$. Both the $G_\alpha$ and $G_{\beta\gamma}$ subunits of $G_i$ inhibit ACI [37-39]. In contrast, although $G_{i\alpha}$ also inhibits AC IV and VII, they are both conditionally stimulated by $G_{\beta\gamma}$ [37,40,50,51]. Thus, an increment in the relative abundance of AC IV and VII portends a shift in opioid receptor-coupled signaling from AC $G_{i\alpha}$ inhibitory to $G_{\beta\gamma}$ stimulatory.

Importantly, the relevance of AC isoform-specific βγ stimulatory signaling to the directionality (excitatory or inhibitory) of receptor-coupled regulation of AC activity has been directly demonstrated in HEK 293 cells. Coexpression of mutationally active $G_{\beta\gamma}$ with ACII (which is positively modulated by $G_{\beta\gamma}$ [37] converted agonists that act through 'inhibitory' receptors coupled to $G_i$ into stimulators of AC [52,53], as has been reported in the LMMP preparation following chronic morphine [23,44,46]. Analogous findings have been reported for opioid receptor-mediated regulation of AC activity, i.e., morphine dose-dependently inhibits and facilitates dopamine activation of AC type V and AC type VII, respectively [51]. The stimulatory effects of morphine on AC VII are blocked by pertussis toxin as well as the α subunit of transducin suggesting the importance of $G_{\beta\gamma}$ derived from

$G_i$. In COS-7 cells, acute opiate treatment inhibits or stimulates transfected AC activity in an isoform-specific fashion that correlates with the pattern of βγ stimulatory responsiveness [54]. This further underscores the functional significance of the ability of chronic morphine to induce the specific synthesis of those AC isoforms that are stimulated by $G_{\beta\gamma}$.

Paralleling AC isoform-specific synthesis, chronic morphine also markedly enhances the phosphorylation of ACII and/or VII [55]. Notably, $G_{s\alpha}$-independent $G_{\beta\gamma}$ stimulation of ACII and VII is augmented following their phosphorylation [56-58]. Thus, the upregulation of AC isoforms IV and VII concomitant with the enhanced phosphorylation of ACII and VII that ensues following chronic morphine would produce convergent consequences to augment opioid receptor-coupled $G_{\beta\gamma}$ stimulation of AC.

Enhanced opioid receptor-coupled $G_{s\alpha}$-dependent $G_{\beta\gamma}$ stimulation of AC following chronic morphine, predicted from the observed upregulation of ACIV and VII, has in fact been demonstrated [49]. As expected, recombinant $G_{s\alpha}$ ($rG_{s\alpha}$) dose dependently stimulated AC activity in LMMP membranes obtained from opioid naive and tolerant LMMP tissue. Notably, however, the magnitude of the $rG_{s\alpha}$-stimulated increase was significantly greater in LMMP tissue obtained from chronic morphine-treated guinea pigs. Moreover, the observed differential responsiveness to $G_{s\alpha}$ could be abolished by the $G_{\beta\gamma}$ blocking peptide QEHA. Thus, the increased $rG_{s\alpha}$ stimulatory responsiveness of tolerant preparations most likely reflects augmented $G_{\beta\gamma}$ stimulation ($G_{s\alpha}$-dependent) of AC [37]. This would shift opioid receptor-coupled signaling from predominantly $G_{i\alpha}$ inhibitory to $G_{\beta\gamma}$ stimulatory AC signaling. Such a shift would result in the manifestation of opioid tolerance since the persistent opioid inhibition of AC activity via the sustained generation of $G_{i\alpha}$ would be mitigated by the emergence of opioid receptor-coupled stimulation of AC activity that resulted from $G_i$-/$G_o$-derived generation of $G_{\beta\gamma}$.

## GPCR Signaling Complexes

Mounting experimental evidence indicates that GPCRs, G proteins, and effectors are not randomly distributed in the plasma membrane. GPCR signaling mainly occurs within specialized microdomains. The nature and stoichiometry of transducer elements within spatially discrete membrane regions and changes thereof would have a substantial impact on the efficiency and specificity of GPCR signaling [59]. This is another dimension of perturbations that are produced by chronic morphine.

GRK2/3, β-arrestin and the $G_\beta$ subunit of G proteins can be co-immunoprecipitated using either anti-GRK or anti-$G_\beta$ antibodies [48,60]. This suggests that these signaling molecules exist, at least in part, as a multimolecular complex. Strikingly, chronic morphine administration results in the concomitant phosphorylation of all three proteins [48,60]. This is note worthy since phosphorylation of GRK2/3, β-arrestin and $G_\beta$ has varying consequences on their ability to associate. Of particular relevance, phosphorylation of $G_\beta$ decreases interactivity of $G_{\beta\gamma}$ with GRK2/3. This maximizes the availability of $G_{\beta\gamma}$ for interaction with AC (and other effectors), which would further augment $G_{\beta\gamma}$ stimulatory AC signaling. Additionally, phosphorylation of $G_\beta$ enhances (approximately 2-fold) the ability of $G_{\beta\gamma}$ to stimulate AC [61].

Importantly, phosphorylated $G_\beta$, as well as nonphosphorylated $G_\beta$ co-immunoprecipitates with AC. Moreover, the magnitude of $G_\beta$ that co-immunoprecipitates with AC markedly increases following chronic morphine [62]. This indicates that phosphorylated $G_\beta$ ($G_{\beta\gamma}$) associates and thus presumably interacts with AC *in vivo*. It also reveals that AC is a target for the enhanced phosphorylated $G_{\beta\gamma}$ that is generated following chronic morphine treatment, underscoring the physiological relevance of $G_\beta$ phosphorylation to *in vivo* $G_{\beta\gamma}$ stimulatory AC signaling. Thus, increased signaling via $G_{\beta\gamma}$ subunits during opioid tolerance results not only from the ability of chronic morphine to initiate effector modification (AC isoform-specific synthesis) but from chemical modification (phosphorylation) of signaling/transducing molecules as well.

## Importance of PKC to Opioid Tolerance-Producing Mechanisms

The action of PKC has long been considered to be central to opioid tolerance-producing mechanisms. Persistent intrathecal (i.t.) morphine infusion, but not saline, produces a 2-fold increase in dorsal horn PKC phosphorylating activity concomitant with a similar increase in the expression of PKCγ [63]. This strongly suggests that tolerance produced by i.t. morphine infusion is dependent, at least in part, upon an increase in its local phosphorylating activity. Additionally, mice carrying a null mutation in the gene encoding PKCγ manifested approximately half the magnitude of tolerance than did their wild type littermates [64]. Pharmacological manipulation of endogenous PKC activity also indicates the central importance of this signaling enzyme. Intrathecal application of the PKC inhibitors chelerythrine or GF109203X reverses the analgesic tolerance that develops in response to a preceding 5-day i.t. morphine infusion [63] and Go-7874 and sangivamycin, long lasting PKC inhibitors, significantly reversed morphine tolerance for up to 24 h [65].

## PKC and Chronic Morphine-Induced $G_\beta$ Phosphorylation

PKC is intimately involved with the chronic morphine-induced increment in $G_\beta$ phosphorylation; recent work has revealed that $G_\beta$ is one of the substrate proteins that is phosphorylated by PKC in response to chronic morphine. Phosphorylated $G_\beta$ co-immunoprecipitates with PKC. Moreover, following chronic morphine, $^{32}P$ incorporation into the $G_\beta$ that co-immunoprecipitates with PKC significantly increases, which can be abolished by chelerythrine [62]. These data indicate that *in vivo*, $G_\beta$ and PKC not only associate but also functionally interact. Notably, a specific PKC isoform (PKCγ) that co-immunoprecipitates with $G_\beta$, and is increasingly phosphorylated following chronic morphine [62], has been shown to be up-regulated in rat spinal cord following chronic in vivo morphine exposure [66, 67].

The functional significance of the *in vivo* association of PKC (PKCγ) and $G_\beta$ is underscored by the ability of the catalytic subunit of PKC to effectively phosphorylate $G_\beta$ *in vitro* (0.34±0.05 mol of phosphate incorporated/mol of $G_\beta$ [61] and with the markedly superior ability of PKCγ vs. PKCα, PKCζ [61] or PKCβ [68] to *in vitro* phosphorylate $G_\beta$.

Furthermore, the demonstration of the *in vivo* association of PKCγ with G$_\beta$, the augmented phosphorylation of G$_\beta$ following chronic morphine and the increased potency of phosphorylated G$_\beta$ to stimulate AC, in the aggregate, provides a biochemical basis and identifies a substrate for the well-documented relevance of PKC (PKCγ) to opioid tolerance-producing mechanisms.

## PKC Phosphorylates β-Arrestin

Interestingly, PKC can phosphorylate β-arrestin, which also increases following chronic morphine [60]. Chronic morphine-induced phosphorylation of β-arrestin also has important functional consequences. For example, cytoplasmic β-arrestin1 is constitutively phosphorylated and is recruited to the plasma membrane by agonist stimulation of GPCRs. At the plasma membrane, β–arrestin1 is rapidly dephosphorylated. β-arrestin1 dephosphorylation is not required for arrestin binding to receptors, a prelude to rapid desensitization. However, it is a prerequisite for β-arrestin binding to clathrin-coated pits and subsequent receptor endocytosis [69]. Thus, the relative inability of chronic morphine to induce opioid receptor internalization could result from its ability to maintain and even augment the phosphorylation state of β–arrestin. It would also explain the more recent paradoxical observation that chronic morphine treatment also eliminates the capacity of [D-Ala 2, D-Leu 5]enkephalin (DADLE) and etorphine to desensitize opioid-stimulated [$^{35}$S]GTPγS binding and DOR internalization [70].

## Altered Opioid Receptor G Protein Coupling Following Chronic Morphine Exposure

A remaining unresolved issue is whether or not and if so the extent to which chronic morphine induces a change in the relative coupling of opioid receptors to specific G proteins. The μ-opioid receptor (MOR) belongs to the super family of seven transmembrane spanning G protein coupled receptors. Like other members of this receptor family, MOR interacts with multiple G proteins. This is indicated by the observation that MOR activation enhances the photoaffinity labeling of G$_{i\alpha3}$, G$_{i\alpha2}$, and G$_{o\alpha2}$ [71]. Additional evidence that MOR interacts with multiple G proteins is the ability to co-immunoprecipitate MOR with G$_{o\alpha}$, G$_{i\alpha1}$ and G$_{i\alpha3}$ [72]. A shift in the relative coupling of MOR to the members of the G$_i$ and G$_o$ family would not be expected to produce the profound changes in MOR-mediated signaling that has been associated with tolerance formation. However, chronic morphine-induced increased coupling of MOR to G$_s$ would.

## MOR G$_s$ Coupling

The coupling of MOR to G$_s$ has long been controversial. There have been numerous pharmacological observations of excitatory MOR-coupled effects that are resistant to pertussis toxin (PTX; and are thus not mediated via $G_i/G_o$) but are sensitive to cholera toxin (CTX) [23,43,73-75]. Collectively these observations underscore putative coupling of MOR to $G_s$. This not withstanding, in contrast to members of the $G_i$ and $G_o$ families of G proteins, biochemical evidence of MOR coupling to $G_s$ has been difficult to obtain; attempts to demonstrate that $G_s$ co-immunoprecipitates with MOR have not been successful [72,76]. The absence of such data has been largely responsible for excluding formulations of enhanced MOR-$G_s$ coupling from models of tolerance-producing mechanisms.

Prompted by the wealth of pharmacological data suggesting MOR $G_s$ coupling that is enhanced by chronic morphine, we hypothesized that the inability to demonstrate that $G_{s\alpha}$ co-immunoprecipitates with MOR could have resulted from its more predominant coupling to $G_i$ and $G_o$. If this formulation was valid, demonstration that MOR co-immunoprecipitates with $G_s$ should prove to be more feasible; instead of assessing the presence of $G_{s\alpha}$ in MOR IP, we investigated the ability of anti-$G_{s\alpha}$ antibodies to co-IP MOR [77].

## Co-Immunoprecipitation of MOR with $G_{s\alpha}$

Utilizing this approach, we were able to demonstrate that MOR is indeed present in immunoprecipitate obtained with anti-$G_{s\alpha}$ antibodies [77]. Interestingly, the molecular mass of the MOR species that co-immunoprecipitates with $G_{s\alpha}$ is ≈75-80 kDa, which corresponds to the molecular mass of the cloned rat μ-opioid receptor expressed in CHO that is specifically and irreversibly labeled by [$^3$H] β-funaltrexamine [78]. It also corresponds to the molecular mass of MORs that are similarly radiolabeled in brain membranes from several species [79].

## Enhanced MOR $G_{s\alpha}$ Coupling During Opioid Tolerance

As reported previously [80-82], chronic morphine treatment (48 h) produced a substantial decline in the MOR-CHO membrane content of MOR. This notwithstanding and of particular relevance to opioid tolerance producing mechanisms, in both MOR-CHO cells as well as rat spinal cord, chronic morphine treatment substantially increased the magnitude of MOR that was present in the $G_{s\alpha}$ immunoprecipitate. Importantly, this occurred without altering the magnitude of the $G_{s\alpha}$ that was immunoprecipitated [77]. Moreover, while the magnitude of MOR that co-immunoprecipitates with $G_{s\alpha}$ increases following chronic morphine, the opposite pertains to the magnitude of MOR that co-immunoprecipitates with $G_{i\alpha}$; the intensity of the ≈75-80 kDa MOR species that co-immunoprecipitates with $G_{i\alpha}$ from membranes obtained from chronic morphine-treated cells was reduced by ≈39% [77]. A reduction in the magnitude of MOR that co-immunoprecipitates with $G_{i\alpha}$ following chronic morphine is consonant with the documented ability of this treatment to uncouple MOR from inhibitory G protein signaling [83, 84].

It must be borne in mind that although co-immunoprecipitation is a strong indicator of physical association, co-existence in a multimolecular complex does not, necessarily, imply functional interaction. As mentioned above, however, there are numerous indicators that some effects of MOR interaction are mediated via $G_s$. In the guinea pig longitudinal muscle myenteric plexus preparation, CTX (but not PTX) abolishes the facilitation of electrically stimulated transmitter (methionine-enkephalin) release and cAMP formation that is produced by low concentrations of sufentanil [23,43,73]. Analogous observations have been reported in dorsal root ganglion neurons [74] where MOR-mediated prolongation of the $Ca^{2+}$ component of the action potential duration can be abolished by CTX and in F-11 neuroblastoma sensory-neurons in which CTX attenuated opioid stimulation of basal AC activity [85]. More recently, inactivation of $G_i/G_o$ proteins via PTX treatment of Chinese hamster ovary cells stably transfected with MOR was shown to unmask the ability of Tyr-D-Ala-Gly-(NM e)Phe-Gly-ol (DAMGO) to facilitate forskolin activation of AC. The unmasked DAMGO stimulation of AC activity could be abolished by CTX, as was the enhancement of forskolin stimulated AC activity produced by D-Phe-Cys-Tyr-D-Trp-Arg-Thr-Pen-Thr-$NH_2$ (CTAP) [75]. Central analgesic actions of morphine have also shown to be CTX sensitive [86].

## Putative Significance of MOR $G_s$ Coupling

The extent to which enhanced MOR $G_{s\alpha}$ signaling to adaptations that underlie opioid tolerance and dependence remains to be determined. In our formulation, MOR signaling via $G_s$ would occur concomitantly with the adaptations this laboratory has discovered that underlie augmented MOR coupled $G_{\beta\gamma}$ stimulatory AC signaling following chronic morphine, i.e., AC isoform-specific synthesis and phosphorylation, $G_\beta$ phosphorylation, etc. [47,49,55]. Heretofore, the absence of biochemical evidence of MOR $G_s$ coupling has undermined widespread acceptance of $G_s$ mediation of opioid actions and the role of MOR $G_s$ coupling in opioid tolerance-forming mechanisms. Incorporation of MOR $G_s$ coupling into models of acute and chronic opioid actions should now be re-assessed in light of the current demonstration of MOR $G_s$ co-precipitation that is facilitated by chronic morphine exposure.

## Chronic Morphine Alters Phospholipase C Signaling via Isoform-Specific Regulation

Perhaps the most poignant exemplar that chronic morphine elicits adaptations that qualitatively alter, without eliminating, GPCR signaling, is the reciprocal modulation of two isoforms of PLC, PLCβ1 and PLCβ3. PLC is the enzyme responsible for generating two intracellular second messengers via the hydrolysis of phosphatidylinositol 4,5-bisphosphate [87]. Inositol 1,4,5-trisphosphate ($IP_3$) partitions in the cell cytosol and is considered to be a universal $Ca^{2+}$ mobilizing second messenger. Diacylglycerol (DAG) remains in the membrane and is an activator of protein kinase C (PKC).

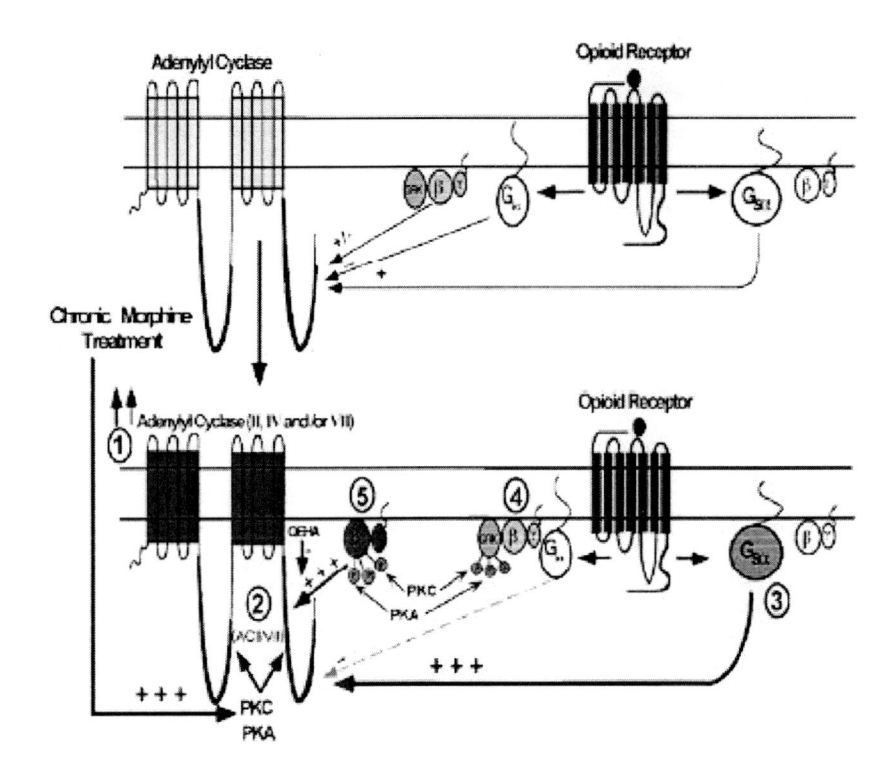

Figure 1. Long-term morphine exposure elicits compensatory adaptations that do not require a loss of MOR G protein coupling. These adaptations involve alterations in the interface between the G protein and its effector molecules. Underlying long-term adaptations to morphine are effector, e.g., adenylyl cyclase (AC) isoform-specific synthesis as well as covalent modification (of effector protein as well as signaling molecules, e.g., G protein receptor kinase (GRK) 2/3, β-arrestin and the $G_\beta$ subunit of G proteins. The cartoon above illustrates that chronic morphine elicits a mosaic of integrated convergent adaptations. These underlie the shift in opioid receptor signaling from $G_{i\alpha}$ inhibitory to $G_{\beta\gamma}$ stimulatory AC signaling that has been associated with tolerance. #1: up-regulation of AC isoforms IV and VII, which are $G_{\beta\gamma}$ stimulated; #2: augmented PKC-mediated phosphorylation of AC. PKC phosphorylation of AC II/VII increases their stimulatory responsiveness to $G_{\beta\gamma}$; #3: Phosphorylation of AC II and VII also increases the stimulatory responsiveness of these isoforms to $G_{s\alpha}$. #4: increased PKA and PKC phosphorylation of GRK/2,3 and $G_\beta$. These signaling molecules are present in a multi-molecular signaling complex as evidenced by their co-immunoprecipitation. Phosphorylation $G_\beta$ decreases the association of $G_{\beta\gamma}$ with GRK, increasing the availability of $G_{\beta\gamma}$ to interact with AC; #5; Phosphorylation of $G_\beta$ by PKC (PKCγ) also increases the potency of $G_{\beta\gamma}$ to stimulate AC. PKCγ, $G_\beta$ and AC can all be co-immunoprecipitated indicating their existence, in part, as a multi-molecular complex. The adaptations described above interact in a multiplicative fashion to augment MOR-coupled $G_{\beta\gamma}$ stimulation of AC activity, which would counteract any ongoing MOR inhibitory AC signaling via $G_{i\alpha}$. #6 Association of MOR with $G_{s\alpha}$ is markedly augmented following chronic morphine suggesting augmented MOR signaling via $G_s$. This would further counteract the inhibitory consequences of MOR signaling via $G_{i\alpha}$ and thus contribute to the manifestation of opioid tolerance.

Molecular cloning and biochemical characterizations have revealed the existence of four types of PLC, β, γ, δ, and ε. These isoforms range in molecular mass (kDa) from 230-260 (ε), 150 (β and γ) to 85 (δ) that are immunologically distinct and products of separate genes. One ε, four β-, two γ and four δ- isoforms have been described in mammalian systems [88].

We focused on PLCβs since they are G protein coupled and are regulated by $G_{\beta\gamma}$ as well as Gαq, which mediate MOR agonist stimulation of PLC activity [89].

Phosphorylation state is also a critical regulatory parameter of PLCβ-isoforms. Phosphorylation of $PLC\beta_1$ and $PLC\beta_3$ via either PKA or PKC, both of which are markedly upregulated following chronic morphine exposure [66,90-94], negatively modulates their activity (see [95,96] and references contained therein). Indeed, following chronic *in vivo* morphine exposure, phosphorylation of PLCβ3 is markedly augmented in both the guinea pig longitudinal muscle myenteric plexus preparation [97] as well as rat spinal cord [98]. Strikingly, however, the phosphorylation of PLCβ1 does not increase after chronic morphine but instead *diminishes*; chronic morphine modulates the phosphorylation (activity) of $PLC\beta_1$ and $PLC\beta_3$ in a *reciprocal* fashion.

Since PLCβ1 and PLCβ3 activities are negatively modulated by phosphorylation, their concomitant reciprocal phosphorylation would alter the relative contribution of these isoforms to $PLC/Ca^{++}$ signaling. Exchange of one isoform for another with comparable regulatory and catalytic properties might not be expected to have notable physiological consequences. However, the chronic morphine-induced shift in the relative predominance of PLCβ1 vs. PLCβ3 should have significant opioid tolerance-associated signaling consequences because of their differential responsiveness to Gαq and $G_{\beta\gamma}$. Gαq/11 subunits (derived from Gq) activate PLCβ1 over a broad concentration range whereas the dose responsiveness for Gαq/11 activation of PLCβ3 is much steeper [99].

## Regulation of PLCβ by G Proteins

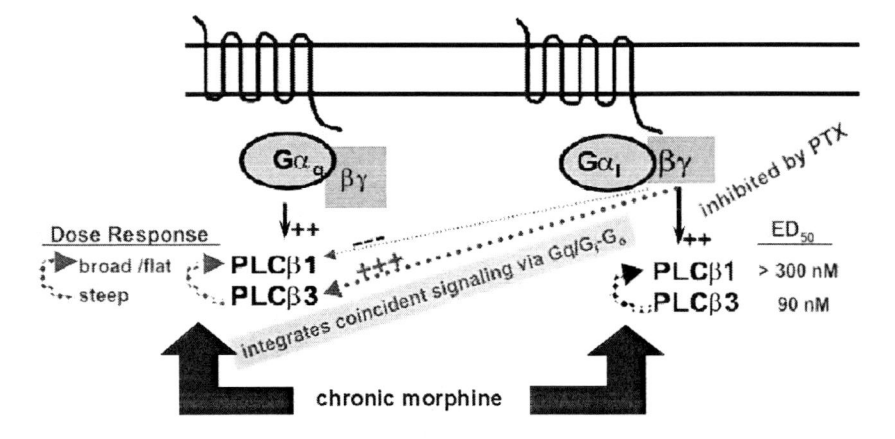

Figure 2. Regulation of PLCββ by G Proteins. The above cartoon illustrates differences in the regulation of PLCβ1 and PLCβ3 by Gαq and $G_{\beta\gamma}$ subunits. PLCβ3 is much more sensitive to Gαq than is PLCβ1. Similarly, Gαq is more effective in stimulating PLCβ3 than PLCβ1. Thus, by increasing the phosphorylation of PLCβ3, which decreases its activity, and decreasing the phosphorylation of PLCβ1, which increases its activity, chronic morphine shifts PLCβ signaling from a 'high gain' Gαq-/$G_{\beta\gamma}$-regulated isoform to one that is more graded in G protein subunit responsiveness. Additionally, $G_{\beta\gamma}$ can synergize with Gαq in stimulating PLCβ3, whereas $G_{\beta\gamma}$ always attenuates Gαq stimulation of PLCβ1. The less than additive regulation of PLCβ3 by Gαq/11 and $G_{\beta\gamma}$ would contribute to the prevalence of a muted, but not lost, PLCβ signaling following chronic morphine.

Efficacy of activation of PLCβ1 and PLCβ3 by $G_{\beta\gamma}$ subunits is also isoform-selective. $G_{\beta\gamma}$ is clearly more effective in stimulating PLCβ3 than PLCβ1 ($ED_{50}$ for $G_{\beta\gamma}$ activation of PLCβ3 and PLCβ1 is 90 nM and >300 nM, respectively [99]. Additionally, PLCβ3, in contrast to PLCβ1, is able to integrate coincident signaling via pathways coupled to Gq and Gi/Go [99]. Thus, the reciprocal modulation PLCβ1 and PLCβ3 following chronic morphine results in the prevalence of PLCβ signaling that is more muted. Chronic morphine shifts PLCβ signaling from a 'high gain' $G\alpha q$-/$G_{\beta\gamma}$-regulated isoform to one that is more graded in G protein subunit responsiveness.

The reciprocal modulation of PLCβ1 and PLCβ3 during the tolerant condition underscores that chronic morphine induces the emergence of alternative signaling strategies via effector modification, and not simply the loss or impairment of MOR G protein coupling. The predominant chronic morphine-induced modification of PLCβ (and AC) isoforms that we have uncovered is phosphorylation, which qualitatively alters the G protein subunit responsiveness of these signaling enzymes. This underscores that the known plasticity in G protein effector interactions is an important substrate for opioid tolerant-producing mechanisms.

## Conclusion

In summary, opioid tolerance formation, long the bane of narcotic medicinal pharmacotherapy, is an active dynamic process that makes use of the plasticity that is inherent in GPCR signaling mechanisms. The mechanisms that subserve opioid tolerance are complex and multifaceted; they involve regulatory parameters in addition to those that have been identified to mediate 'acute desensitization' of the β-adrenergic receptor such as receptor internalization and uncoupling.

Opioid tolerance is adaptive. It enables cell survival in the face of continued exposure to opioids. All cell-based theories of tolerance postulate mechanisms that reinstate initial steady conditions. In the case of AC 'superactivation', up-regulation of the AC system would neutralize the persistent ongoing opioid receptor-coupled inhibition of that system. In the case of the opioid receptor uncoupling/internalization theory, this arrestin-mediated regulation would rapidly desensitize cells to agonist and thereby compensate for the sustained inhibitory action of drugs like morphine that are resistant to proteolytic degradation and thus persist in the extracellular milieu. The chronic morphine-induced augmented AC stimulatory signaling via $G_{\beta\gamma}$ and enhanced $G_s$ coupling that we have demonstrated would neutralize the functional consequences of ongoing opioid receptor-coupled $G_{i\alpha}$ inhibitory signaling, and thereby reinstate naïve steady state cAMP conditions. Increased knowledge of the complexity of tolerant mechanisms would help to understand the spectrum of tolerant-producing strategies that are utilized by different regions of the central nervous system. Such knowledge would also facilitate identifying new targets for its pharmacologic amelioration.

# References

[1] Lefkowitz, RJ, G protein-coupled receptors. III. New roles for receptor kinases and beta-arrestins in receptor signaling and desensitization. *J. Biol. Chem*, 1998, 273: 18677-18680.

[2] Chavkin, C and Goldstein, A, Opioid receptor reserve in normal and morphine-tolerant guinea pig ileum myenteric plexus. *Proc. Natl. Acad. Sci. U.S.A.*, 1984, 81(22): 7253-7257.

[3] Bohn, LM, Gainetdinov, RR, Lin, FT, Lefkowitz, RJ and Caron, MG, Mu-opioid receptor desensitization by beta-arrestin-2 determines morphine tolerance but not dependence. *Nature,* 2000, 408: 720-723.

[4] Chakrabarti, S, Law, P-Y and Loh, HH, Neuroblastoma neuro2A cells stably expressing a cloned m-opioid receptor: a specific cellular model to study acute and chronic effects of morphine. *Mol. Brain Research*, 1995, 30: 269-278.

[5] Ammer, H and Schultz, R, Chronic activation of inhibitory δ-opioid receptors cross-regulates the stimulatory adenylate cyclase-coupled prostaglandin E1 receptor system in neuroblastoma X glioma (NG108-15) hybrid cells. *J.Neurochem.*, 1995, 64(6): 2449-2457.

[6] Sim, LJ, Selley, DE, Dworkin, SI and Childers, SR, Effects of chronic morphine administration on mu opioid receptor-stimulated [$^{35}$S]GTPgammaS autoradiography in rat brain. *J. Neurosci.*, 1996, 16(8): 2684-2692.

[7] Zhang, L, Yu, Y, Mackin, S, Weight, FF, Uhl, GR and Wang, JB, Differential mu opiate receptor phosphorylation and desensitization induced by agonists and phorbol esters. *J. Biol. Chem*, 1996, 271: 11449-11454.

[8] Pei, G, Kieffer, BL, Lefkowitz, RJ and Freedman, NJ, Agonist-dependent phosphorylation of the mouse delta-opioid receptor: involvement of G protein-coupled receptor kinases but not protein kinase C. *Mol. Pharmacol,* 1995, 48: 173-177.

[9] El Kouhen, R, Burd, AL, Erickson-Herbrandson, LJ, Chang, CY, Law, PY and Loh, HH, Phosphorylation of Ser363, Thr370, and Ser375 residues within the carboxyl tail differentially regulates mu-opioid receptor internalization. *J. Biol. Chem*, 2001, 276: 12774-12780.

[10] Appleyard, SM, Celver, J, . Pineda, V, Kovoor, A, Wayman, GA and Chavkin, C, Agonist-dependent desensitization of the kappa opioid receptor by G protein receptor kinase and beta-arrestin. *J. Biol.Chem.*, 1999, 274: 23802-23807.

[11] Appleyard, SM, Patterson, TA, Jin, W and Chavkin, C, Agonist-induced phosphorylation of the k-opioid receptor. *J. Neurochem.*, 1997, 68: 2405-2412.

[12] Kovoor, A, Nappey, V, Kieffer, BL and Chavkin, C, Mu and delta opioid receptors are differentially desensitized by the coexpression of beta-adrenergic receptor kinase 2 and beta-arrestin 2 in xenopus oocytes. *J. Biol. Chem*, 1997, 272: 27605-27611.

[13] McLaughlin, JP, Myers, LC, Zarek, PE, Caron, MG, Lefkowitz, RJ, Czyzyk, TA, Pintar, JE and Chavkin, C, Prolonged kappa opioid receptor phosphorylation mediated by G-protein receptor kinase underlies sustained analgesic tolerance. *J. Biol. Chem*, 2004, 279: 1810-1818.

[14] Simantov, R, Lotem, J and Levy, R, Selectivity in the control of opiate receptor density in the animal and in cultured fetal brain cells. *Neuropeptides*, 1984, 5: 197-200.
[15] Lenoir, D, Barg, J and Simantov, R, Characterization and down-regulation of opiate receptors in aggregating fetal rat brain cells. *Brain Res*, 1984, 304: 285-290.
[16] Sternini, C, Spann, M, Anton, B, Keith, DE, Bunnett, NW, von Zastrow, M, Evans, CJ and Brecha, NC, Agonist-selective endocytosis of μ–opioid receptor by neurons in vivo. *Proc. Natl. Acad. Sci. USA*, 1996, 93: 9241-9246.
[17] Whistler, JL, Chuang, HH, Chu, P, Jan, LY and von Zastrow, M, Functional dissociation of mu opioid receptor signaling and endocytosis: implications for the biology of opiate tolerance and addiction. *Neuron*, 1999, 23: 737-746.
[18] Blanchet, C and Luscher, C, Desensitization of mu-opioid receptor-evoked potassium currents: initiation at the receptor, expression at the effector. *Proc. Natl. Acad. Sci. U S A*, 2002, 99: 4674-4679.
[19] Finn, AK and Whistler, JL, Endocytosis of the mu opioid receptor reduces tolerance and a cellular hallmark of opiate withdrawal. *Neuron*, 2001, 32: 829-839.
[20] Koch, T, Widera, A, Bartzsch, K, Schulz, S, Brandenburg, LO, Wundrack, N, Beyer, A, Grecksch, G and Hollt, V, Receptor endocytosis counteracts the development of opioid tolerance. *Mol. Pharmacol*, 2005, 67: 280-287.
[21] Lang, J and Schulz, R, Chronic opiate receptor activation in vivo alters the level of G-protein subunits in guinea pig myenteric plexus. *Neurosci.*, 1989, 32(2): 503-510.
[22] Nestler, EJ, Erdos, JJ, Terwilliger, R, Duman, RS and Tallman, JF, Regulation of G proteins by chronic morphine in the rat locus coeruleus. *Brain Res*, 1989, 476: 230-239.
[23] Wang, L and Gintzler, AR, Altered μ-opiate receptor-G protein signal transduction following chronic morphine exposure. *J. Neurochem*, 1997, 68: 248-254.
[24] Ingram, SL, Vaughan, CW, Bagley, EE, Connor, M and Christie, MJ, Enhanced opioid efficacy in opioid dependence is caused by an altered signal transduction pathway. *J. Neurosci*, 1998, 18: 10269-10276.
[25] Hack, SP, Bagley, EE, Chieng, BC and Christie, MJ, Induction of delta-opioid receptor function in the midbrain after chronic morphine treatment. *J. Neurosci*, 2005, 25: 3192-3198.
[26] Bohn, LM, Lefkowitz, RJ and Caron, MG, Differential mechanisms of morphine antinociceptive tolerance revealed in (beta)arrestin-2 knock-out mice. *J. Neurosci*, 2002, 22: 10494-10500.
[27] Luttrell, LM, Ferguson, SS, Daaka, Y, Miller, WE, Maudsley, S, Della Rocca, GJ, Lin, F, Kawakatsu, H, Owada, K, Luttrell, DK, Caron, MG and Lefkowitz, RJ, Beta-arrestin-dependent formation of beta2 adrenergic receptor-Src protein kinase complexes. *Science*, 1999, 283: 655-661.
[28] Gurevich, VV, Pals-Rylaarsdam, R, Benovic, JL, Hosey, MM and Onorato, JJ, Agonist-receptor-arrestin, an alternative ternary complex with high agonist affinity. *J. Biol. Chem*, 1997, 272: 28849-28852.
[29] Sharma, SK, Klee, WA and Nirenberg, M, Dual regulation of adenylate cyclase accounts for narcotic dependence and tolerance. *Proc. Natl. Acad. Sci. USA*, 1975, 72: 3092-3096.

[30] Sharma, SK, Nirenberg, M and Klee, WA, Morphine receptors as regulators of adenylate cyclase activity. *Proc. Natl. Acad..Sci. USA.*, 1975, 72: 590-594.

[31] Sharma, SK, Klee, WA and Nirenberg, M, Opiate-dependent modulation of adenylate cyclase. *Proc. Natl. Acad. Sci. USA*, 1977, 74(8): 3365-3369.

[32] Duman, RS, Tallman, JF and Nestler, EJ, Acute and chronic opiate-receptor regulation of adenylate cyclase in brain: specific effects in locus coerulus. *J. Pharmacol. Exp. Ther.*, 1988, 246 No. 3: 1033-1039.

[33] Williams, JT, Christie, MJ and Manzoni, O, Cellular and synaptic adaptations mediating opioid dependence. *Physiol. Rev,* 2001, 81: 299-343.

[34] Vanderah, TW, Ossipov, MH, Lai, J, Malan, TP, Jr. and Porreca, F, Mechanisms of opioid-induced pain and antinociceptive tolerance: descending facilitation and spinal dynorphin. *Pain,* 2001, 92: 5-9.

[35] Nestler, EJ, Molecular basis of long-term plasticity underlying addiction. *Nat. Rev. Neurosci,* 2001, 2: 119-128.

[36] Exton, JH, Regulation of phosphoinositide phospholipases by hormones, neurotransmitters, and other agonists linked to G proteins. *Annu. Rev. Pharmacol. Toxicol*, 1996, 36: 481-509.

[37] Tang, W-J and Gilman, AG, Type-specific regulation of adenylyl cyclase by G protein βγ subunits. *Science*, 1991, 254: 1500-1503.

[38] Taussig, R, Tang, W-J, Hepler, JR and Gilman, AG, Distinct patterns of bidirectional regulation of mammalian adenylyl cyclases. *J.Biol.Chem.,* 1994, 269(8): 6093-6100.

[39] Taussig, R, Quarmby, LM and Gilman, AG, Regulation of purified type I and type II adenylyl cyclases by G protein bg subunits. *J.Biol.Chem.*, 1993, 268(1): 9-12.

[40] Gao, BN and Gilman, AG, Cloning and expression of a widely distributed (type IV) adenylyl cyclase. *Proc.Natl.Acad.Sci.U.S.A.*, 1991, 88: 10178-10182.

[41] Offermanns, S, Wieland, T, Homann, D, Sandmann, J, Bombien, E, Spicher, K, Schultz, G and Jakobs, KH, Transfected muscarinic acetylcholine receptors selectively couple to Gi-type G proteins and Gq/11. *Mol. Pharmacol*, 1994, 45: 890-898.

[42] Jin, LQ, Wang, HY and Friedman, E, Stimulated D(1) dopamine receptors couple to multiple Galpha proteins in different brain regions. *J. Neurochem*, 2001, 78: 981-990.

[43] Xu, H, Smolens, I and Gintzler, AR, Opioids can enhance and inhibit the electrically evoked release of methionine-enkephalin. *Brain Research*, 1989, 504: 36-42.

[44] Gintzler, AR, Chan, WC and Glass, J, Evoked release of methionine-enkephalin from tolerant/dependent enteric ganglia: Paradoxical dependence on morphine. *Proc. Natl. Acad. Sci. USA*, 1987, 84: 2537-2539.

[45] Wang, L and Gintzler, AR, Bimodal opioid regulation of cAMP formation: implications for positive and negative coupling of opiate receptors to adenylyl cyclase. *J. Neurochem.*, 1994, 63: 1726-1730.

[46] Wang, L and Gintzler, AR, Morphine tolerance and physical dependence: reversal of opioid inhibition to enhancement of cAMP formation. *J. Neurochem.*, 1995, 64: 1102-1106.

[47] Rivera, M and Gintzler, AR, Differential effect of chronic morphine on mRNA encoding adenylyl cyclase isoforms: relevance to physiological sequela of tolerance/dependence. *Mol. Brain Research*, 1998, 54: 165-169.

[48] Gintzler, AR and Chakrabarti, S, Opioid tolerance and the emergence of new opioid receptor-coupled signaling. *Molecular Neurobiology*, 2000, 21: 21-33.

[49] Chakrabarti, S, Rivera, M, Yan, S-Z, Tang, W-J and Gintzler, AR, Chronic morphine augments Gβγ/Gsα stimulation of adenylyl cyclase: relevance to opioid tolerance. *Mol. Pharmacol.*, 1998, 54: 655-662.

[50] Watson, AJ, Katz, A and Simon, MI, A fifth member of the mammalian G-protein β-subunit family. Expression in brain and activation of the β2 isotype of phospholipase C. *J. Biol. Chem,* 1994, 269: 22150-22156.

[51] Yoshimura, M, Ikeda, H and Tabakoff, B, mu-Opioid receptors inhibit dopamine-stimulated activity of type V adenylyl cyclase but enhance dopamine-stimulated activity of type VII adenylyl cyclase. *Mol. Pharmacol.*, 1996, 50: 43-51.

[52] Federman, AD, Conklin, BR, Schrader, KA, Reed, RR and Bourne, HR, Hormonal stimulation of adenylyl cyclase through Gi-protein βγ subunits. *Nature*, 1992, 356: 159-161.

[53] Lustig, KD, Conklin, BR, Herzmark, P, Taussig, R and Bourne, HR, Type II adenylyl cyclase integrates coincident signals from Gs, Gi, and Gq. *J.Biol.Chem.*, 1993, 268(19): 13900-13905.

[54] Avidor-Reiss, T, Nevo, I, Saya, D, Bayewitch, M and Vogel, Z, Opiate-induced adenylyl cyclase superactivation is isozyme-specific. *J. Biol. Chem.*, 1997, 272(8): 5040-5047.

[55] Chakrabarti, S, Wang, L, Tang, W-J and Gintzler, AR, Chronic morphine augments adenylyl cyclase phosphorylation: relevance to altered signaling during tolerance/dependence. *Mol. Pharmacol.*, 1998, 54: 949-953.

[56] Zimmermann, G and Taussig, R, Protein kinase C alters the responsiveness of adenylyl cyclase to G protein α and βγ subunits. *J. Biol. Chem.*, 1996, 271: 27161-27166.

[57] Tsu, RC and Wong, YH, Gi-mediated stimulation of type II adenylyl cyclase is augmented by Gq-coupled receptor activation and phorbol ester treatment. *J. Neurosci.*, 1996, 16(4): 1317-1323.

[58] Watson, PA, Krupinski, J, Kempinski, AM and Frankenfiedl, CD, Molecular cloning and characterization of the type VII isoform of mammalian adenylyl cyclase expressed widely in mouse tissues and in S49 mouse lymphoma cells. *J. Biol. Chem.*, 1994, 269: 28893-28898.

[59] Neubig, RR, Membrane organization in G-protein mechanisms. *FASEB J,* 1994, 8: 939-946.

[60] Chakrabarti, S, Oppermann, M and Gintzler, AR, Chronic morphine induces the concomitant phosphorylation and altered association of multiple signaling proteins: a novel mechanism for modulating cell signaling. *Proc. Nat'l. Acad. Sci. USA,* 2001, 98: 4209-4214.

[61] Chakrabarti, S and Gintzler, AR, Phosphorylation of Gβ is augmented by chronic morphine and enhances Gβγ stimulation of adenylyl cyclase activity. *Brain Res. Mol. Brain Res,* 2003, 119: 144-151.

[62] Chakrabarti, S, Regec, A and Gintzler, AR, Chronic morphine acts via a protein kinase Cγ-Gβ-adenylyl cyclase complex to augment phosphorylation of Gβ and Gβγ stimulatory adenylyl cyclase signaling. *Brain Res. Mol. Brain Res,* 2005, 138: 94-103.

[63] Granados-Soto, V, Kalcheva, I, Hua, X, Newton, A and Yaksh, TL, Spinal PKC activity and expression: role in tolerance produced by continuous spinal morphine infusion. *Pain*, 2000, 85: 395-404.

[64] Zeitz, KP, Malmberg, AB, Gilbert, H and Basbaum, AI, Reduced development of tolerance to the analgesic effects of morphine and clonidine in PKCγ ɣ mutant mice. *Pain*, 2001, 94: 245-253.

[65] Smith, FL, Javed, R, Elzey, MJ, Welch, SP, Selley, D, Sim-Selley, L and Dewey, WL, Prolonged reversal of morphine tolerance with no reversal of dependence by protein kinase C inhibitors. *Brain Res,* 2002, 958: 28-35.

[66] Mao, J, Price, DD, Phillips, LL, Lu, J and Mayer, DJ, Increases in protein kinase Cγ immunoreactivity in the spinal cord of rats associated with tolerance to the analgesic effects of morphine. *Brain Research*, 1995, 677: 257-267.

[67] Narita, M, Suzuki, M, Yajima, Y, Suzuki, R, Shioda, S and Suzuki, T, Neuronal protein kinase Cγ-dependent proliferation and hypertrophy of spinal cord astrocytes following repeated *in vivo* administration of morphine. *Eur. J. Neurosci*, 2004, 19: 479-484.

[68] Yasuda, H, Lindorfer, MA, Myung, CS and Garrison, JC, Phosphorylation of the G protein γ12 subunit regulates effector specificity. *J. Biol. Chem*, 1998, 273: 21958-21965.

[69] Lin, F-T, Krueger, KM, Kendall, HE, Daaka, Y, Fredericks, ZL, Pitcher,J.A. and Lefkowitz, RJ, Clathrin-mediated endocytosis of the b- β–adrenergic receptor is regulated by phsoporylation/dephosphorylation of b- βarrestin1. *J. Biol. Chem.*, 1997, 272: 31051-31057.

[70] Eisinger, DA, Ammer, H and Schulz, R, Chronic morphine treatment inhibits opioid receptor desensitization and internalization. *J. Neurosci,* 2002, 22: 10192-10200.

[71] Chakrabarti, S, Prather, PL, Yu, L, Law, PY and Loh, HH, Expression of the mu-opioid receptor in CHO cells: ability of mu-opioid ligands to promote alpha-azidoanilido[$^{32}$P]GTP labeling of multiple G protein alpha subunits. *J. Neurochem*, 1995, 64: 2534-2543.

[72] Chalecka-Franaszek, E, Weems, HB, Crowder, AT, Cox, BM and Cote, TE, Immunoprecipitation of high-affinity, guanine nucleotide-sensitive, solubilized mu-opioid receptors from rat brain: coimmunoprecipitation of the G proteins G(alpha o), G(alpha i1), and G(alpha i3). *J. Neurochem*, 2000, 74: 1068-1078.

[73] Gintzler, AR and Xu, H, Different G proteins mediate the opioid inhibition or enhancement of evoked [5-methionine]enkephalin release. *Proc. Natl. Acad..Sci USA,* 1991, 88: 4741-4745.

[74] Shen, KF and Crain, SM, Cholera toxin-A subunit blocks opioid excitatory effects on sensory neuron action potentials indicating mediation by Gs-linked opioid receptors. *Brain Res*, 1990, 525: 225-231.

[75] Szucs, M, Boda, K and Gintzler, AR, Dual effects of Tyr-D-Ala-Gly-(NMe)Phe-Gly-ol (DAMGO) and D-Phe- Cys-Tyr-D-Trp-Arg-Thr-Pen-Thr-NH2 (CTAP) on adenylyl cyclase activity; implications for μ-opioid receptor Gs coupling. *J. Pharmacol. Exp. Ther*, 2004, 310: 256-262.

[76] Burford, NT, Tolbert, LM and Sadee, W, Specific G protein activation and mu-opioid receptor internalization caused by morphine, DAMGO and endomorphin I. *Eur. J. Pharmacol*, 1998, 342: 123-126.

[77] Chakrabarti, S, Regec, A and Gintzler, AR, Biochemical demonstration of mu-opioid receptor association with Gsalpha: enhancement following morphine exposure. *Brain Res. Mol. Brain Res*, 2005, 135: 217-224.

[78] Chen, C, Xue, JC, Zhu, J, Chen, YW, Kunapuli, S, Kim de Riel, J, Yu, L and Liu-Chen, LY, Characterization of irreversible binding of beta-funaltrexamine to the cloned rat mu opioid receptor. *J. Biol. Chem*, 1995, 270: 17866-17870.

[79] Liu-Chen, LY, Chen, C and Phillips, CA, Beta-[3H]funaltrexamine-labeled mu-opioid receptors: species variations in molecular mass and glycosylation by complex-type, N-linked oligosaccharides. *Mol. Pharmacol,* 1993, 44: 749-756.

[80] Bernstein, MA and Welch, SP, mu-Opioid receptor down-regulation and cAMP-dependent protein kinase phosphorylation in a mouse model of chronic morphine tolerance. *Brain Res. Mol. Brain Res*, 1998, 55: 237-242.

[81] Tao, PL, Han, KF, Wang, SD, Lue, WM, Elde, R, Law, PY and Loh, HH, Immunohistochemical evidence of down-regulation of mu-opioid receptor after chronic PL-017 in rats. *Eur. J. Pharmacol*, 1998, 344: 137-142.

[82] Christoffers, KH, Li, H, Keenan, SM and Howells, RD, Purification and mass spectrometric analysis of the mu opioid receptor. *Brain Res. Mol. Brain Res*, 2003, 118: 119-131.

[83] Puttfarcken, PS, Werling, LL and Cox, BM, Effects of chronic morphine exposure on opioid inhibition of adenylyl cyclase in 7315c cell membranes: a useful model for the study of tolerance at mu opioid receptors. *Mol. Pharmacol,* 1988, 33: 520-527.

[84] Yabaluri, N and Medzihradsky, F, Down-regulation of mu-opioid receptor by full but not partial agonists is independent of G protein coupling. *Mol. Pharmacol,* 1997, 52: 896-902.

[85] Cruciani, RA, Dvorkin, B, Morris, SA, Crain, SA and Makman, MH, Direct coupling of opioid receptors to both stimulatory and inhibitory guanine nucleotide-binding proteins in F-11 neuroblastoma-sensory neuron hybrid cells. *Proc.Natl.Acad.Sci.U.S.A.*, 1993, 90: 3019-3023.

[86] Suh, HW, Sim, YB, Choi, YS, Song, DK and Kim, YH, Multiplicative interaction between intrathecally and intracerebroventricularly administered morphine for antinociception in the mouse: effects of spinally and supraspinally injected 3-isobutyl-1-methylxanthine, cholera toxin, and pertussis toxin. *Gen. Pharmacol,* 1995, 26: 1597-1602.

[87] Berridge, MJ and Irvine, RF, Inositol phosphates and cell signalling. *Nature*, 1989, 341: 197-205.

[88] Rhee, SG, Regulation of phosphoinositide-specific phospholipase C. *Annu. Rev. Biochem,* 2001, 70: 281-312.

[89] Smart, D, Smith, G and Lambert, DG, mu-Opioid receptor stimulation of inositol (1,4,5)trisphosphate formation via a pertussis toxin-sensitive G protein. *J. Neurochem.*, 1994, 62: 1009-1014.

[90] Nestler, EJ, Molecular mechanisms of drug addiction. *J. Neurosci.*, 1992, 12: 2439-2450.

[91] Nestler, EJ and Tallman, JF, Chronic morphine treatment increases cyclic AMP-dependent protein kinase activity in the rat locus coeruleus. *Mol.Pharmacol.*, 1988, 33: 127-132.

[92] Self, DW, McClenahan, AW, Beitner-Johnson, D, Terwilliger, RZ and Nestler, EJ, Biochemical adaptations in the mesolimbic dopamine system in response to heroin self-administration. *Synapse*, 1995, 21: 312-318.

[93] Mayer, DJ, Mao, J and Price, DD, The development of tolerance and dependence is associated with translocation of protein kinase C. *Pain*, 1995, 61: 365-374.

[94] Mayer, DJ, Mao, J and Price, DD, The association of neuropathic pain, morphine tolerance and dependence, and the translocation of protein kinase C. *NIDA Res Monogr*, 1995, 147: 269-298.

[95] Fisher, SK, Homologous and heterologous regulation of receptor-stimulated phosphoinositide hydrolysis. *Eur. J. Pharmacol,* 1995, 288: 231-250.

[96] Rebecchi, MJ and Pentyala, SN, Structure, function, and control of phosphoinositide-specific phospholipase C. *Physiol. Rev*, 2000, 80: 1291-1335.

[97] Chakrabarti, S and Gintzler, AR, Reciprocal modulation of phospholipase Cβ isoforms: adaptation to chronic morphine. *Proc. Nat'l. Acad. Sci. USA,* 2003, 100: 13686-13691.

[98] Liu, N-J, Chakrabarti, S and Gintzler, AR, Chronic morphine-induced loss of the facilitative interaction between vasoactive intestinal polypeptide and delta-opioid: involvement of protein kinase C and and phospholipase Cβs. *Brain Res*, 2004, 1010: 1-9.

[99] Smrcka, AV and Sternweis, PC, Regulation of purified subtypes of phosphatidylinositol-specific phospholipase C beta by G protein alpha and beta gamma subunits. *J. Biol. Chem*, 1993, 268: 9667-9674.

*Chapter VI*

# Opioids for Pain Management

*Howard S. Smith and Gary McCleane*
Pain Management, Albany Medical College, Albany, NY 12208

## Abstract

Of all the issues relating to persistent noncancer pain, those related to long-term opioid therapy for persistent noncancer pain remain among the most controversial. Furthermore, it may be difficult for basic scientists to appreciate some of these controversies without multiple discussions/exposures with multiple clinicians as well as clinical observations. In addition, it may be difficult to even define the issues, since what appears to be a significant clinical problem for some health care providers may not even represent a minor "speed-bump" for others. Since the medical literature on this topic is relatively inadequate at this point to provide definitive answers, clinicians may be left wrestling with various "opioid issues" based at least partly on their own training, experiences, comfort, and preferences/practice style. It is hoped that after reading the following chapter, basic scientists may begin to develop some appreciation of various issues, concerns, questions, and controversies related to long-term opioid therapy of persistent noncancer pain.

## Introduction

In 1871 William Dale, a noted physician of the time in the United Kingdom, wrote: "Opium is ... our chief medicine for relieving pain and procuring sleep, our right hand in practice, suffering humanity owes much to its virtues, and the physician could ill spare it in his battle with disease and pain. Its effects are often wonderful, translating the poor patient from a state of the most intolerable tortue to one of comparative ease and comfort" [1]. That same year, he also wrote, again referring to opium: "This remedy like every good thing is being abused" [1]. Therefore, he may have laid the framework for the so-called concept of "balance".

Since 1871 the pendulum of "opiophobia" versus "opiophilia" has swung back and forth for health care providers. Periods are marked by "opiophobia" where withholding opioids from terminally ill cancer patients because of irrational fears of addiction as well as periods marked by increased opioid abuse and diversion co-existing with an increase in the medical use of opioids for persistent noncancer pain. Recent times have seen a swing towards more extensive use of opioids. In 1997, opioid therapy for chronic pain was described as an "extension of the basic principles of good medical practice" in a consensus statement jointly published by the American Pain Society and the American Academy of Pain Medicine [2].

Studies on the use of long-acting oral opioids for chronic noncancer pain, though still relatively small, have begun to foster more accepting attitudes from mainstream American medicine regarding the use of opioids for persistent noncancer pain [3]. However, the "opioid controversy" continues to the present. Portenoy [4] has illustrated various "opiophobic" vs. "opiophilic" views in his comments predicting responses of American physicians to the recommendation for the appropriate use of opioids published by the UK's Pain Society and Royal Colleges of anaesthetists, general practitioners, and psychiatrists [5]. Kalso et al have also published recommendations for using opioids in chronic non-cancer pain [6].

Practicing in the "middle of the road" by employing the appropriate use of opioids in the context of good medical practice, as well as appropriate attention to the risk assessment and management of opioid abuse (being cognizant of potential abuse, addiction, and diversion), has become known as "balance" [7-9].

While opioids have been a mainstay of treatment for acute pain and cancer-related pain, issues surrounding opioid use for persistent noncancer pain remain somewhat controversial. Although published over a decade ago, it seems to still hold true today that physicians tend to disagree regarding the prescription of opioids for the treatment of persistent noncancer pain [PNCP] [10]. Factors that may influence the decision to prescribe opioids for PCNP may include the physician's medical specialty, geographic region of practice, and patient factors [e.g. age, diagnosis (as well as documentation of diagnosis), prognosis]. Scanlon and Chugh reported surveyed a total of 125 physicians [63 family physicians (FPs) and 62 specialists in the Calgary Health Region, CHR] in Calgary, Alberta in efforts to explore attitudes regarding the use of LTOT (long-term opioid therapy) for PNCP [11]. A minority of physicians FPs and specialists reported, "that they could handle" hydromorphone (36.7% and 13.3% respectively), fentanyl patch (30.6% and 11.1% respectively), and methadone (0% and 6.7% respectively) [11]. Scanlon and Chugh concluded that FPs in the CHR need to increase their level of comfort level toward opioids in general to adequately manage chronic non-cancer pain [11].

Although there are no easy answers to the opioid controversies, a moderate balanced approach with oversight by a qualified interdisciplinary pain team may be optimal at the current time. "There appears to be a select subpopulation of patients with chronic pain that can achieve sustained partial analgesia from opioid therapy without the occurrence of intolerable side effects or the development of aberrant drug-related behaviors" [12]. This statement appears to stand the test of time after roughly a decade. Furthermore, there are patients that appear to do well for many years on the same dose of opioid with having their primary care physician following them and writing their prescriptions. However, as the "select population" expands somewhat, the statement may need to be qualified some to include that administration of long term opioid therapy [LTOT] is optimally achieved in conjunction with a multidisciplinary multimodal approach to the evaluation and management of pain by interdisciplinary teams of pain specialists.

There appears to be general agreement that when a patient is managed by a well-coordinated multidisciplinary team (e.g. pain specialists), that compliance is better and risk of loss of control as well as complications are less than when a single doctor [especially if not a pain specialist] is managing the patient [13]. However, this may not always be possible. Additionally, close follow-up and re-assessment in multiple domains is essential and should guide continuation of, or discontinuation of opioid therapy. It is important to convey to health care providers unfamiliar with pain management and patients that opioids do not necessarily equate with pain relief. Some people seem to believe that opioids are really the only analgesics that work, that they are fine to use in most all situations as sole analgesics and should be continually increased if pain is still experienced. However, pain is extremely complex and differs for each individual. Opioids, if appropriate, may be used in conjunction with many other pharmacologic, behavioral and physical medicine approaches as well as neuromodulation techniques, along with other various analgesic strategies. Not all patients do well on opioids and subpopulations of patients may be improved when they are taken off these drugs. [14].

When given the option to discontinue opioid therapy, more than 50% of patients abandoned opioid therapy voluntarily predominantly due to intolerable side effects or suboptimal efficacy [15, 16].

## The Clinical Usage of Opioids

Cowan and colleagues performed a randomized, double-blinded, placebo-controlled, crossover pilot study to assess the effects of long-term opioid drug consumption and subsequent abstinence in chronic non-cancer pain patients receiving controlled released morphine [17]. Ten patients with PNCP taking an average daily dose of 40mg controlled-release morphine sulfate (mean 40, range 10-90; SD 21mg), for an average of two years (mean 2.175, range 2-2.25, SD 0.2 years) had their morphine substituted with placebo for 60-hour periods. Pharmacokinetic data demonstrated compliance with abstinence on all patients. Three patients (30%) reported opioid withdrawal symptoms. Cowan and colleagues had concluded their results suggested the existence of a group of PNCP patients whose long-term opioid consumption can be beneficial and remain moderate without them suffering from consequences of problematic opioid use [17].

Kalso and colleagues analyzed data from 1140 patients in fifteen randomized, placebo-controlled trials of World Health Organization (WHO) step 3 opioids for efficacy and safety in chronic non-cancer pain [15]. Four studies tested intravenous opioids in neuropathic pain in a crossover design with 115 of 120 patients completing the protocols. Eleven studies (1025 patients) compared oral opioids with placebo for four days to eight weeks and six of the 15 trials that were included had an open label follow-up of 6-24 months. The mean decrease in pain intensity in most studies was at least 30% with opioids and was comparable in neuropathic and musculoskeletal pain. Roughly 80% of patients noted at least one adverse effect. The most common adverse effects were constipation (41%), nausea (32%) and somnolence (29%). Only 44% of 388 patients on open label treatments were still on opioids after therapy for between 7 and 24 months. Adverse effects and lack of efficacy were two common reasons for discontinuation [15].

Therefore, although opioids have been touted as being "the nectar of the gods", only a minority of patients in these studies decided to go on to long-term management with opioids even though all were given that opportunity. The small number of patients and short duration of follow-up did not permit conclusions regarding issues of tolerance and addiction [15].

A significant positive correlation between pain relief during intravenous opioid testing and open label follow-up of pain relief from oral opioids were not consistently demonstrated in all four studies [18-21]. However, in three studies [18-20] intravenous opioid testing appeared reasonable at identifying those patients who did not achieve adequate analgesia from opioids: in other words, if patients responded poorly to the analgesic effects of intravenous opioids, they also tended to respond poorly to the analgesic effects of oral or transdermal opioids.

Gustorff reported on the use of intravenous remifentanil testing in a randomized placebo-controlled crossover study in 24 patients suffering from severe non-cancer pain [22]. He utilized an ascending infusion of remifentanil and placebo titrated against endpoints--- and found that the remifentanil testing allowed a distinction between eleven opioid responders and 13 non-responders. A rapid and complete recovery to the pre-testing baseline state occurred by 25 minutes in all patients. Gustorff concluded that remifentanil testing is rapid being generally completed in one hour or less and so it has potential to be used as a routine screening process in an ambulatory setting [22].

Chou and colleagues performed a systematic review of the comparative efficacy and safety of long-acting oral opioids for chronic non-cancer pain and determined that there was insufficient evidence to demonstrate that one long-acting opioid was better than another or to determine differences in efficacy between long-acting and short-acting opioids, although they reported that no randomized trials were rated as good [3]. Clinically, it appears that it is not rare that patients may respond to one opioid reasonably well and another opioid poorly. Since there is no way to predict this currently, efforts to attempt to find the opioid with maximal analgesic efficacy for an individual patient are at this point more a matter of trial and error. In terms of adverse effects there was also insuffucuent evidence to prove that different long-acting opioids are associated with different safety profiles [3], however, it appears that long-acting fentanyl is associated with less constipation than long-acting morphine.

Subsequent oral or transdermal doses that were used to achieve analgesia after intravenous testing were usually lower than equivalent intravenous doses. Therefore; in most cases intravenous opioid testing should not be used to titrate to the patients equivalent "long-term" oral or transdermal dose in persistent non-cancer pain.

In a survey of patients (N=104) prescribed opioids for mean duration of treatment 14.1 months for severe chronic non-cancer pain at a pain clinic within a National Health Service Hospital in London, United Kingdom, a total of 90 (86.5%) patients reported stopping opioid therapy at some point and, of these 59 (65%) had ceased opioid therapy permanently. This voluntary abandonment of opioids occurred despite that 72.5% of all patients initially derived some benefit from opioids, although 77% of all patients reported opioid side effects [16].

Watson and colleagues surveyed 102 patients with PNCP in a neurological practice followed by a neurologist every three months for one year or more (median 8 years, range 1-22 years) [23]. They reported that approximately one-third of patients (34 out of 102) had a change in their pain status from either severe of moderate pain, as measured by a zero to ten numerical rating scale (NRS) (mild= 1-3, moderate = 4-7, severe = 8-10); by category scale [absent, mild, moderate, severe, very severe], and by considering pain with movement. They queried patients as to whether they were satisfied with pain relief despite adverse events. Forty-five patients (44%) answered that they were satisfied, but 57 (56%) replied that they were not satisfied with their pain relief. However, of the 86 patients assessed for disability, 47 (54%) patients had significant improvement in their disability status on opioids. Also, there was some pain improvement on opioids in 78 (91%) of 102 patients and the patients chose to continue opioid therapy for some analgesia despite adverse effects [23].

Controlled-release oxycodone hydrochloride has been evaluated in post herpetic neuralgia [24] and diabetic peripheral neuropathy [25, 26]. Watson and Babul reported that a maximum dosage of 60mg/day of morphine equivalents significantly relieved pain, disability, and allodynia for patients with PHN [24]. Watson and colleagues also reported that overall pain, sleep, as well as health-related quality of life assessments were significantly improved compared with placebo at a mean daily dose of $40.0 \pm 18.5$ mg for controlled-release oxycodone [26]. Gimbel et al demonstrated that a maximum dosage of 120 mg/day of morphine equivalents significant improved pain, the performance of daily activities, and sleep [25]. Furthermore, Raja and colleagues reported that treatment with opioids and tricyclic antidepressants (TCA) resulted in greater pain relief [38% and 32%, respectively] compared with placebo (11%; p<0.001) [27]. Patients who completed the study preferred opioids over TCA treatment (54% versus 30%, P+0.02), however, more patients dropped out of the study during or after opioid treatment (e.g. 20) than during or after opioid TCA therapy (20 versus 6 patients) [27].

Rowbotham et al. demonstrated a dose-dependent analgesic effect in patients with mixed neuropathies, reporting that high-dose levorphanol yielded significantly more pain relief than lower doses of levorphanol [28].

Harke et al in a randomized controlled trial of controlled-release morphine in complex regional pain syndrome (CRPS) reported there was no difference in pain reduction compared with placebo after 8 days of use [29].

Eisenberg and colleagues examined twenty-two studies which met inclusion criteria and were classified as short-term (less than 24 hours; n=14) or intermediate-term (median=28 days; range=8-56 days; n=8) trials [30]. They reported that the short-term trials had contradictory results. However, all 8 intermediate-term trial demonstrated opioid efficacy for spontaneous neuropathic pain. A fixed-effects model meta-analysis of 6 intermediate-term studies showed mean post-treatment visual analog scale scores of pain intensity after opioids to be 14 units lower on a scale from 0 to 100 than after placebo (95% confidence interval, CI; -18 to -10; P< 0.001). As the mean initial pain intensity recorded from four of the intermediate-term trials ranged from 46-69, this 14-point difference was considered to correspond to a 20-30% greater reduction with opioids than with placebo [30].

Analysis of data from large randomized clinical trials has revealed that a roughly 30% reduction in pain intensity may be the threshold for patients to describe a reduction in chronic pain as meaningful. [31,32]. When the number needed to harm (NNH) is considered, the most common adverse event was nausea (NNH, 3.6; 95% CI, 2.9-4.8) followed by constipation (NNH, 4.6; 95% CI, 3.4-7.1), drowsiness (NNH, 5.3; 95% CI, 3.7-8.3), vomiting (NNH, 6.2; 95% CI, 4.6-11), and dizziness (NNH, 6.7; 95% CI, 4.8-10.0) [30]. Eisenberg and colleagues concluded that although short-term studies provide only equivocal evidence regarding the efficacy of opioids in reducing the intensity of neuropathic pain, intermediate-term studies demonstrate significant efficacy of opioids over placebo for neuropathic pain, which is likely to be clinically important [30]. They also concluded that further randomized controlled trials are needed in efforts to establish the long-term efficacy of opioids for neuropathic pain, the safety of long-term opioids (including addiction potential), and their effects on quality of life.

The literature appears to support the analgesic efficacy of opioids [at least in the short term] for some patients with chronic noncancer pain (especially with chronic low back pain). However, results are inconsistent regarding the effect of opioid therapy on functional status or quality of life [33] [34] [35]. Furthermore, large multi-center well-designed studies for over a decade do not exist.

There appears to be less data and more controversy surrounding the use of LTOT for various non-neuropathic PNCP, especially as pertains to chronic headaches, chronic musculoskeletal disorders and fibromyalgia syndrome.

The National Ambulatory Medical Care Survey [NAMCS] is a nationally representative yearly survey that collects information about outpatient office visits in the United States conducted by the National Center for Health Statistics (NCHS) of the Centers for Disease Control. Caudill-Slosberg and colleagues analyzed visits and prescriptions from patients of all ages for the treatment of musculoskeletal pain using NAMCS data from 1980 to 1981 (n= 89,000 visits) and 1999 to 2001 (n=45,000 visits) obtained from public files on the NCHS website (2002) [36]. They found that the use of potent opioids for the management of chronic musculoskeletal pain has dramatically increased in the United States from roughly 2% in 1980 to around 9% in 2000 [36]. During this two-decade period, NSAID prescriptions increased for both acute (19 vs. 33%, RR = 1.74; 95% CI; 1.52-1.95) and chronic (25 vs. 29%, RR = 1.16; 95% CI, 0.97 – 1.35) musculoskeletal pain visits. In 2000, one-third of the NSAID prescriptions were for COX II agents. Opioids increased for acute pain (8 vs. 11%; RR = 1.38; 95% CI, 0.92 – 1.83) and double for chronic pain (8% vs. 16%; RR – 2.0, 98% CI 1.52 – 2.48). The use of more potent opioids (hydrocodone, oxycodone, morphine) for chronic musculoskeletal pain increased from 2 to 9% of visits (RR = 4.5, 95% CI, 2.18 – 6.187). This significant increase translates into 5.9 million visits where potent opioids were prescribed in 2000, or 4.6 million visits, where potent opioids were prescribed more than 1980, assuming the total number of outpatient visits was roughly constant from 1980 to 2001 [36].

Scheman and colleagues concluded that there are patients who experience severe and disabling pain while taking opioid therapy who can experience significant improvement in pain severity and disability as well as improvement in physical and emotional functioning while participating in a pain rehabilitation program that incorporates opioid withdrawal [14].

In a study by Rome and colleagues, 274 study patients who completed a stay at the pain rehabilitation center as well as pre- and past- stay questionnaires were divided into two groups based on their pre-study "baseline" medications--- one group of 99 patients taking daily opioids and one group of 175 patients who were not taking daily opioids [14]. All patients who were taking any opioids underwent a gradual structured opioid withdrawal over two to three weeks and all 274 patients completed a three-week multidisciplinary rehabilitation program based on a cognitive behavioral model. On admission to the program, 37.9% of patients were taking daily opioids with a mean daily dose of 78.4 mg of morphine equivalent (range 3.5 – 780.0 mg). Patients taking less than the median dose (41 mg) were taking a mean daily morphine equivalent of 25.1 mg (SD:13.69 mg) and patients taking more than the median does were taking a mean daily morphine equivalent of 137.48 mg (SD:116.8) [14].

At the completion of the program, patients taking lower opioid doses, higher doses or no opioids at all prior to the program, all reported significantly reduced pain severity (P < 0.001), interference die to pain (P < 0.001), affective distress (P > 0,001), depression (P < 0.001), and catastrophizing (P > 0.001), as well as increased perceived life control (P < 0.001) and general activity (P < 0.001). Patients taking higher opioid doses reported significantly greater catastrophizing at discharge than the nonopioid group (mean difference, -2.8; SE; 1.1; P = 0.03). Patients taking higher opioid doses also reported greater pain severity at the completion of the program than the nonopioid group; however, this difference was not statistically significant (mean difference, -4.3; SE; 1.9; P+ 0.05) [14]. Although significant limitations with this study preclude clinicians to generalize the study findings, it does illustrate that at least certain patients can come off opioids and actually do better functionally as well as having less pain.

## Opioids: Clinical Background

Opioids are broad-spectrum analgesics, which are utilized for the treatment of nociceptive and neuropathic pain. Although no ideal analgesics exist and opioids are far from perfect, they may be among the best broad-spectrum analgesics currently available for many patients.

For the purposes of this chapter, persistent non-cancer pain will be arbitrarily used to refer to any pain which persists over three months in patients without a diagnosis of cancer and without a diagnosis of some advanced chronic illness which would potentially qualify them as "terminal" or "palliative care" patients with a prognosis of less than three years of life expectancy. Some have held the view that there should be no difference between the treatment approach to acute pain, cancer pain, and persistent noncancer pain. However; this does not seem to be the case for all clinicians. One key difference may be the timing of when to initiate opioid therapy, if indicated. In acute pain, cancer pain, and persistent noncancer pain, with the possible exception of end of life care, a careful history and physical examination should be performed before "just throwing analgesics at pain". Otherwise conditions such as compartment syndrome (acute pain), or deep vein thrombosis may be missed. In acute pain and cancer pain that is severe, regardless of whether the etiology of the pain is apparent or not, potent opioids for severe pain should be considered as part of the treatment plan at the initial visit. However, with persistent noncancer pain, opioids should be considered at some point into the treatment phase, but need not to be initiated at the first visit.

If a patient has three months to live or has just has major surgery performed, most clinicians would institute opioid therapy at the initial consult and would not withhold opioid therapy in an attempt to find a precise "pain diagnosis"/"pain generator"/"pain mechanism".

In persistent non-cancer pain, clinicians generally attempt to do their best to evaluate patients comprehensively including appropriate diagnostic testing and imaging in an effort to identify a precise "pain diagnosis"/ "pain generator"/ "pain mechanism". Once this work-up has been largely completed, a treatment approach may be formulated to attempt to optimally match the patient's diagnosis, situation, and concomitant co-morbidities. Opioid therapy for persistent non-cancer pain may be initiated early in this process, later in this process, or not at all. Each individual patient needs to be treated according to his or her specific situation and so management strategies should not strictly adhere to any rigorous algorithms, maximal doses, or rigid protocols.

Another issue which may be differ from acute pain to cancer pain is that of pain assessment some clinicians feel that a significant percentage of patients with PNCP on LTOT should not be managed solely on the basis of their report on the NRS-11 scale response regarding pain intensity. Although unidimensional assessments [such as the NRS-11 scale seem satisfactory for pain assessment of most patients with acute or cancer pain, multidimensional assessment tools may be especially preferred for patients with PNCP on LTOT. Additionally, other assessment instruments may potentially be helpful as well [37, 38].

The use of the term "high-dose" opioid therapy to refer to 200mg of morphine equivalents or greater per day [39] is controversial as critics maintain that there should not be any descriptors since the dose of opioids should be titrated to the effect (e.g. analgesia) and since there exists large individual variations. The appropriate dose of opioid is that dose which yields appropriate analgesia (certainly this is true in end-of-life care). Still, it would appear reasonable and potentially useful (e.g. in communication between health care providers) to employ some descriptors of opioid dose as "anchors" even though the precise doses which are labeled as low, moderate and high remains somewhat arbitrary. The authors believe that most health care providers and pain specialists would agree that 1 gram of morphine equivalents per day for persistent noncancer pain is a relatively high dose of opioids.

Even though the dose of 1 gram of morphine equivalents per day may be an appropriate dose for some patients and some patients may need significantly more, the use of the terms low-dose, moderate dose and high dose does appear to have some utility when referring to therapy and so should not be abolished. However, perhaps the dose levels should be "re-defined". Low-dose opioid therapy being less than or equal to 100 mg of morphine equivalents per day, moderate dose opioids therapy being over 100 mg but less than or equal to 300 mg of morphine equivalents per day, and high-dose opioids therapy being over 300 mg of morphine equivalents per day or greater.

Pain may be classified in many ways [40]. One approach to the classification of pain is to categorize pain according to its responsiveness to a particular treatment [40]. Utilizing this approach, pain many be divided into opioid responsive pain (ORP), moderately opioid responsive pain (MORP), and poorly responsive pain (PORP).

ORP refers to pain with a very significant response (e.g. good to excellent analgesia) to opioids (usually with low to moderate doses of opioids), MORP refers to pain with a modest response to opioids (usually with moderate to high doses of opioids), and PORP refers to pain which responds poorly to high dose opioid therapy. ORP and MORP may remain as such over many years or may wane over time (e.g. OPR becoming MORP or PORP, and MORP becoming PORP).

The old teachings of nonsteroidal anti inflammatory drugs (NSAIDs) having an analgesic ceiling effect and acting peripherally, whereas opioids have no ceiling effect and act centrally are inaccurate. Traditional views on the antinociceptive actions of opioids held that central mechanisms were primarily responsible. It has become apparent in animal models that antinociception can result from local application of opioids in the periphery in rat models of inflammation [41, 42] and rat neuropathic pain models [43]. This opioid antinociception in the periphery has been purported to be mediated via peripheral opioid receptors [44, 45] expressed on peripheral terminals of sensory neurons [46, 47]. Although, normally the opioid receptors in the periphery are sparse, they are rapidly upregulated with inflammation and attracted immune cells bringing a source of endogenous opioid receptors [47].

There is now significant evidence to show that NSAIDs have antinociceptive effects by acting in the CNS including the spinal cord [48-50] in addition to their peripheral analgesic actions. A direct effect of NSAIDs in the CNS has been established in studies demonstrating that direct CNS application of NSAID reduced pain hypersensitivity [50, 51].

Therefore, it appears that both NSAIDs and opioids work both centrally and peripherally. Additionally, opioids do not yield significant analgesic effects in all patients with various painful states. In reality, at least in certain patients, increasing the opioid dose after a certain point does not yield much more analgesic effects. In other words, in some patients by increasing the opioid dose, pain relief may "asymptotically approach" some "effective or functional" analgesic ceiling in particular patients.

## Issues for LTOT for PNCP

In spite of available opioids therapy guidelines controversies persist. LTOT (long-term opioid therapy) for persistent non-cancer pain is an area that is not easily amenable to algorithms, and "black and white" doctrines, rather this "grey zone" is better approached with individualized sound clinical judgment, balanced and appropriate approaches, and common sense.

LTOT should optimally be undertaken in conjunction with:

(a) Appropriate interdisciplinary medical care and documentation,
(b) Other appropriate pharmacologic approaches,
(c) Any appropriate physical medicine approaches,
(d) Any appropriate behavioral medicine approaches,
(e) Attention to co-morbidities,
(f) Appropriate clinician-patient relationship, and
(g) Appropriate monitoring and follow-up.

The use of LTOT for persistent non-cancer pain [PNCP] remains one of the most controversial topics in the field of pain medicine. Although it would appear that an overwhelming majority of pain specialists agree with and/or utilize LTOT for PNCP, decisions surrounding initiating LTOT, assessing LTOT, ancillary documentation (e.g. opioid contracts, urine drug testing), titration strategies as well as when to cease opioid dose escalation in a particular patient and situations warranting withdrawal of LTOT, and specific treatment goals (if any) continue to be controversial and may vary dramatically from clinician to clinician. Controversy continues to surround approaches to LTOT. There appears to exist polarization seemingly based on clinician preference, style and comfort into "opioid-stingy" clinicians (OSC) and "opioid-generous" clinicians (OGC) [52].

In efforts to illustrate the controversy regarding LTOT for PNCP the following two hypothetical "point-counterpoint" viewpoints are presented.

OGC (Opioid Generous Clinicians): These ignorant OSCs really upset me. They are opiophobic and seem to attempt to treat severe pain with acetaminophen and little or no opioids. Even if they do prescribe opioids and the patients are still in significant pain, they don't increase the opioid doses high enough. They need to go up almost exponentially for severe pain and not just from 100 mg morphine equivalents per day to 120 mg morphine equivalents per day.

OSC (Opioid Stingy Clinicians): These OGCs have no clue what they are doing. They are opiophilic and seem to have taken the WHO guidelines and concepts (e.g. believe the patient's NRS-11 report), which have utility in cancer pain and acute pain and applied this strategy to all comers with PNCP. I am not sure they even examine the patient. They don't really practice medicine. Their management seems to be based on helping the patient's pain score and consists of simplistic, mindless opioid titration. They might as well set up a drive-through opioid clinic where you tell your "pain score" into the clown's mouth and collect your script at the next window. They even tell patients that if they are still in pain they should tell me so I can increase their pain pills (e.g. opioids).

However, there does appear to be some common ground among pain specialists. The following is based on an informal verbal survey conducted with 68 certified pain specialists.

The majority of pain physicians would feel comfortable initiating and maintaining an 82 year old woman with severe pain and dysfunction from severe degenerative joint disease refractory to anti-inflammatory agents on long-term opioid therapy with a long-acting morphine sulfate preparation in a dose of 15 mg orally every 12 hours if the patient was agreeable and satisfied, had no significant adverse effects, and experienced good pain relief and improved function as evidenced by her playing golf again [which she had stopped playing secondary to pain]. Contrariwise, the majority of pain physicians may not feel comfortable initiating and maintaining a 22 year old male who is complaining only of severe lower back pain but has no other significant complaints, an entirely negative physical examination with completely non-significant diagnostic testing and diagnostic procedures/imaging studies on long-term opioid therapy with a long-acting morphine sulfate preparation in a dose of 600 mg orally every 8 hours if the patient had no changes in quality of life, function, mood, sleep, or socializing but did note that his "pain level" decreased from 9/10 to 8/10.

## LTOT Management Issues in PNCP

There are many issues surrounding LTOT for PNCP. One way of classifying various issues which may be practical [although artificial and not precise], is to categorize issues into three phases (similar analogous to the three phases of delivering an anesthetic: induction, maintenance, emergence):

(1) Initiation (Induction)
(2) Maintenance
(3) Re-assessment [increase dose, continue same dose, decrease dose, taper off (emergence)]

Decisions regarding the timing of initiation and whether to initiate LTOT for PNCP must be made on a case-by-case basis. The various factors which may enter into the clinician's decision making process may include: the patient's age, prognosis, documentation of diagnosis, previous treatments, the patient's willingness to be involved in their treatment (e.g. to help themselves), the patient's willingness to change (e.g. change of behavior/lifestyle/functioning), pain duration and intensity, history of substance use and mental health issues, patient/clinician goals, and the particular physician - patient relationship.

## Initiation of LTOT

Issues which surround the initiation and/or maintenance phase of LTOT for PNCP include: the use of opioid "contracts", the use of goal-directed therapy agreements, the use of a substance abuse history and/or "screening tool" for substance misuse, the use of urine testing, and optimally some form of psychological assessment, which could be an informal assessment by the provider as well as some sense of the "doctor-patient" relationship.

## Contracts/Agreements

Opioid contracts are also very reasonable when prescribing LTOT for patients with PNCP. However, they may not be necessary for all patients in all settings. Therefore, the use of opioid contracts should be left to clinician judgment and/or policies.

Elements of opioid contracts may include:

- only one physician prescribing opioids while being treated at a pain clinic
- use of only one pharmacy for medications
- allow random drug [blood or urine] screens and / or pill counts
- refill requests need to be made according to Pain Clinic policy and not on nights or weekends

- selling, trading or sharing opioids with anyone constitutes grounds for discontinuation of opioids and possible dismissal
- forged or abused prescriptions constitute grounds for discontinuation of opioids and dismissal
- use of any illegal controlled substances [eg marijuana, cocaine] constitutes grounds for discontinuation of opioids and possible dismissal
- safeguarding opioids from loss or theft [lost or stolen opioids will not be replaced]
- agreements to take medication exactly as prescribed
- all unused opioid medication brought to the Pain Clinic at every visit

An extension of the traditional contract is the use of a trilateral opioid contract, which is seen, agreed upon, and signed by the pain specialist, patient, and patient's primary care physician [53].

## Goal-Directed Therapy Agreements

Perhaps one of the most important principles as a clinician in initiating and maintaining LTOT for PNCP is to "know where you are and where you are going." It is crucial that the clinician has a reasonable dynamic picture of the intensity of the patient's pain, as well as its impact on social domain (family/relationships, recreational activities), emotional domain (e.g. mood) and functional domain, including physical functioning, activities of daily life, occupational issues, etc., and before the start of opioid therapy and that the patients status is continually monitored/assessed in each of these domains. It may be helpful to have some realistic and practical goals of therapy--- agreed upon by both the patient and the clinician before instituting LTOT [54]. If, in fact, the patient does not improve or deteriorates during LTOT, it may be appropriate at some point to change to a different opioid or taper the patient slowly to a lower dose of LTOT or completely off opioids and attempt different treatments.

Goal-directed therapy agreements (GDTA) also may potentially be helpful when initiating LTOT for PNCP [54]. Clinicians are sometimes faced with patients in whom opioids were started and/or exculpated in efforts to achieve analgesia--- without clearly defined endpoints. This may yield patients remaining with severe pain on relatively high-dose opioids. In efforts to clarify patient and clinician expectations and attempt to make expected treatment outcomes more finite and concrete,--- the use of some form of goal-directed therapy agreements [GDTAs] in certain circumstances may possess potential utility. As with opioid treatment agreements ["contracts"], GDTAs are not necessarily advocated for all patients or all practices but merely suggested in situations in which clinicians deem them appropriate to utilize.

GDTAs should be tailored to each individual patient, should be clear and concise, should be reasonable for the patient to attain over a finite period of time, and optimally should be agreed upon by both patient and clinician. Examples may include: Increasing daily ambulation by a defined amount, increasing social/recreational activities by a defined amount, etc. By utilizing GDTAs before instituting opioid therapy, clinicians can set defined criteria which need to be met in order to continue "Maintaining"/ titrating opioid therapy. In this manner, patients may be expected to reach certain reasonably attainable functional goals [which may need to be documented by their physical and/or behavioral therapist] in order to continue titrating or maintaining opioid therapy. The specific defined "goals" should be clearly stated in the GDTA. It appears optimal to institute the GDTA prior to instituting opioid therapy. The GDTA is essentially felt to be a "contractually" agreed upon realistic target of translational analgesia [54] which should be realized/attained in order to continue therapy as is.

It is hoped that with the use of goal-directed therapy agreements (e.g. GDTAs) in certain patients/circumstances in which the clinician feels that GDTAs are appropriate to use, that a closer match between both patient and clinician treatment expectations and outcome reality can be established [54].

## Substance Abuse History

Michna and colleagues reported that questions about substance abuse history [e.g. family history of substance abuse] and legal problems can be useful in predicting aberrant drug-related behaviors with opioid use in patients with PNCP [55].

Butler and colleagues describe a self-administered screening tool (Screener and Opioid Assessment for Patients with Pain, SOAPP) for chronic pin patients being considered for LTOT in an attempt to determine the potential risk of abuse. They have suggested that the SOAPP is a promising step toward screening risk potential for substance misuse in patients with PNCP who are being considered for LTOT [56].

## Urine Drug Testing

The use of urine drug testing (UDT) in efforts to monitor patients on LTOT treated in a pain clinic is reasonable. UDT is not mandatory for all patients on LTOT in all settings. UDT should be utilized based on the clinical judgment of the prescribing clinicians, however, some clinicians and/or clinics test all patients on LTOT sporadically based on the policies of the pain clinic. Katz and Fanciullo proposed that although further research is needed, --- it is appropriate to conduct routine urine toxicology testing in patients with chronic pain treated with opioids [57]. Caveats to the use of UDT include:

(a) ensuring the proper collection, handling, and documentation of the urine specimen
(b) being knowledgeable regarding interpretation of UDT results
(c) know exactly what your patient consumed and when it is consumed prior to the urine collection
(d) know what you are looking for and what you will do when various results come back

One of the most common urinary drug "screens" involves Fluorescence Polarization Immunoassay (FPIA), which detects the "Federal Five" of marijuana, cocaine, opiates, phencyclidine (PCP), and amphetamines/methamphetamines. This test has a relatively low sensitivity for semi-synthetic and synthetic opioids (e.g. hydrocodone, oxycodone, fentanyl). Therefore, if the test on the patient's urine is negative for the presence of the drug it does not exclude patient use. Furthermore, even if the test is positive for a specific drug a confirmatory test should follow. The confirmatory urine drug test is based on principles of gas chromatography and mass spectrometry (GC/MS), or high performance liquid chromatography (HPLC). GC/MS is considered to be the "gold standard".

## Psychological Assessment

Although there may not be any specific need for psychological/psychiatric evaluations by mental health professionals or for any psychological testing prior to LTOT, it seems prudent that clinicians should "know" a patient and have an established provider-patient relationship before initiating LTOT. Wasan and colleagues reported that high levels of psychopathology [comprised mainly of depression] anxiety, and high neuroticism] are associated with diminished opioid analgesia in patients with discogenic low back pain [58].

## Maintenance Re-Assessment of LTOT

Issues, which surround the maintenance of LTOT for PNCP, include: continued documentation, side effects, tolerance, discontinuation of LTOT, and aberrant drug taking behaviors.

Although the maintenance phase of many patients may be very smooth, there are other patients who will experience "turbulence" during the LTOT maintenance phase for PNCP. There are many factors which may contribute to turbulence in LTOT for PNCP including: increased pain, increased side effects, new pain, new adverse effects, behavioral [alterations, changes, in patient's goals/expectations, and aberrant drug behaviors. The first four [increased pain, increased side effects, new pain, new side effects] should prompt a comprehensive history and physical examination in efforts to search for new etiologies of pain/side effects. Other considerations include: progression of disease [which may lead to the phenomenon of pseudo addiction], opioid-induced hyperalgesia/pain, analgesic tolerance, non-compliance/ "dyscompliance" (e.g. taking the medicine prescribed but not in the exact manner prescribed), and increased function/physical activity.

## Documentation Issues and Documentation Tools

Regulatory agencies, state medical boards, and various peer-review groups among others not only expect appropriate medical care but also require proper documentation. In cases of LTOT for PNCP, aside from the usual "SOAP", style medical progress notes--- various other issues may deserve documentation.

Passik and colleagues have proposed the use of "The Four A's", a documentation scheme which may be helpful to clinicians in the office who are prescribing LTOT for PNCP [59]. The four A's are: Analgesia (pain relief), Activities of daily living (psychosocial functioning), Adverse effects (side effects), and Aberrant drug taking (addition-related outcome) [59]. Passik and Weinreb concluded that the four A's check list was a valuable instrument for tracking outcomes in patients receiving LTOT for PNCP [60]. Passik et al evaluated 388 patients with an instrument called the Pain Assessment and Documentation Tool (PADT)- which was modified from 59 items to 41 items in 4 domains [pain relief, patient functioning, adverse events, and drug-related behavior] [61]. Passik and colleagues concluded that the PADT appeared to be a useful tool for clinicians to guide the evaluation of various outcomes during LTOT [61].

Patients with persistent pain on oral opioid therapy sometimes ask to "come off" the opioids because of adverse effects, even if they perceived that opioids were providing reasonable analgesic effects. The distress which may be caused by opioid adverse effects may also be seen with acute postoperative pain patients who may occasionally ask to stop their opioids despite them being perceived as effective analgesics, because of the significant distress and suffering that they perceive they are experiencing from an opioid adverse effect.

It therefore appears crucial to assess opioid adverse effects and optimally this should be done in a manner as to be able to follow trends as well as compare the patients perceived intensity of the adverse effects versus the intensity of pain and/or other symptoms or adverse effects.

One reasonable short and simple patient-administered quantitative tool which can be rapidly be utilized clinically with the patient completing it in the waiting room is termed the Numerical Opioid Side Effect [NOSE] assessment tool [62]. The NOSE instrument is self-administered, can be completed by the patient in minutes, and can be entered into electronic databases or inserted into a hard-copy chart on each patient visit. The NOSE assessment tool is easy to administer as well as easy to interpret and may provide clinicians with important clinical information that could potentially impact various therapeutic decisions. Although most clinicians probably routinely assess adverse effects of treatments, it is sometimes difficult to find legible, clear, and concise documentation of such information in outpatient records. Furthermore, the documentation that does exist may not always attempt to "quantify" the intensity of treatment-related adverse effects or lend itself to looking at trends.

It has been proposed that the use of a collection of various tools may provide adjunct information and help clinicians to create a more complete picture regarding longitudinal trends of overall progress/functioning for their patients with PNCP on LTOT [63].

## **Translational Analgesia**

A recent concept that may possess potential utility for clinicians is translational analgesia [38, 52]. Translational analgesia refers to improvements in physical, social or emotional function which are realized by the patient as a result of improved analgesia--- or essentially what did the pain relief experienced by the patient "translate" into in terms of perceived improved quality of life. In most cases, a sustained and significant improvement in pain perception that is deemed worthwhile to the patient should "translate" into improvement in quality of life or improved social, emotional or physical function. Improvements in social, emotional, or physical domains are often spontaneously reported by patients, but in most cases should be able to be ascertained or elicited via "focused" interview techniques with the patient and/or significant others/family and/or "focused" physical exam. Improvements may be subtle and could include: going out more with friends, making more contact with family/friends, taking more frequent walks, doing more activities of daily living (laundry) or improved mood/relations with family members. This concept is certainly not exclusive to opioid therapy and is thought to apply to other treatments.

The TAS (Translational Analgesic Score) is a patient-generated tool that attempts to quantify the degree of "translational analgesia" [38]. It is simple, rapid, and user-friendly and therefore can be utilized in a busy pain clinic. The patient can be handed the TAS sheet with questions to fill out at each visit while in the waiting room and the responses are e averaged for an overall score that is recorded in the chart.

It is not necessarily inappropriate or inhumane to taper relatively "high-dose" opioid therapy in a patient with PNCP who notes that his numerical rating scale-11 (NRS-11) "pain score" has dropped from 9/10 to 8/10 after escalating to over a gram of long-acting morphine preparation per day but in whom the patient as well as the patient's family/significant other cannot describe [and the clinician cannot elicit] any significant "translational analgesia". A patient with PNCP who remains a "hermit/couch potato" despite equivocal or minimally improved analgesia should not be considered as a therapeutic success.

Rome and colleagues have demonstrated that at least a subpopulation of patients seems to do better after tapering off opioids [14]. Furthermore, more evidence regarding the hyperalgesic actions of opioids in certain circumstances is mounting [64, 65].

The periodic assessment of the patient with persistent noncancer pain should be performed in multiple domains (e.g. social domain, analgesia domain, functional domain, emotional domain). The author believes that the relatively common practice of evaluating patients with persistent noncancer pain by obtaining a NRS-11 pain score at each assessment and basing opioid analgesic treatment on this score suboptimal. Although there exist multiple tools which assess multiple domains used in research, there is no widely accepted and used simple, convenient, and universally acceptable instrument, which is utilized in busy clinical pain practices. The SAFE (see below) score [37] is a multi-domain assessment tool that may have potential utility for rapid dynamic assessment in the busy clinic setting. The SAFE Score is a clinician-generated tool and may be best utilized in conjunction with the TAS as an adjunct [38].

The SAFE score is obtained after four individual ratings that are documented by the clinician after evaluating the patient. The ratings in each of the four domains are then added to yield the "SAFE score". Each individual rating ranges from 1 to 5 with a possible total score of 4 to 20. A SAFE score is documented at each visit. The domains assessed include the following:

S = Social [social functioning]
A = Analgesia [pain relief]
F = Function [physical functioning]

E = Emotional [emotional functioning].

The patient's status in each of the four domains is rated as follows:
1 - Excellent    2 - Good    3 – Fair    4 - Borderline    5 – Poor

The SAFE Tool (see figure 1) can be flowed by longitudinally looking at trends globally or in specific domains.

|  | Rating | Criterion |  |  |  |  |
|---|---|---|---|---|---|---|
| *Social* Marital, family, friends, leisure, recreational |  | 1 supportive harmonious socializing engaged | 2 | 3 | 4 | 5 conflictual discord isolated bored |
| *Analgesia* Intensity, frequency, duration |  | 1 comfortable effective controlled | 2 | 3 | 4 | 5 intolerable ineffective uncontrolled |
| *Function* Work, ADL's, home management school training physical activity |  | 1 independent active productive energetic | 2 | 3 | 4 | 5 dependent unmotivated passive deconditioned |
| *Emotional* Cognitive, stress, attitude, mood, behavior, neuro-vegetative signs |  | 1 clear relaxed optimistic upbeat composed | 2 | 3 | 4 | 5 confuse tense pessimistic depressed distressed |
| Total Score |  |  |  |  |  |  |

Figure 1. Sample S.A.F.E. Form

## Opioid Analgesic Agents

There is significant variability in the responses of different patients to different opioids. Patient factors which may have an impact on opioid activity include: body fat content, body mass, organ function, age, volume of distribution, and presence and activity of various metabolic enzymes. Additional factors may include: gender, genetics, opioid receptor sub-type mix [quantity, distribution, and intrinsic affinity], previous medication/ drug history/ recreational alcohol, and status/environment history of nociceptive pathways/receptors.

The Cancer Unit of the World Health Organization [WHO] convened an expert committee in 1986 and proposed a useful approach to cancer pain known as the WHO 3-step analgesic ladder, which relied heavily on the use of potent opioids for severe cancer pain. (See figure 2).

Dworkin and colleagues have reviewed randomized clinical trials of various analgesic potent agents and opioids as a "first-line" agent in their evidence –based approach to the treatment of neuropathic pain [66].

Opioids can be categorized into different families:

- Phenanthrenes
- Benzomorphans
- Phenylpiperidines
- Diphenylheptanes

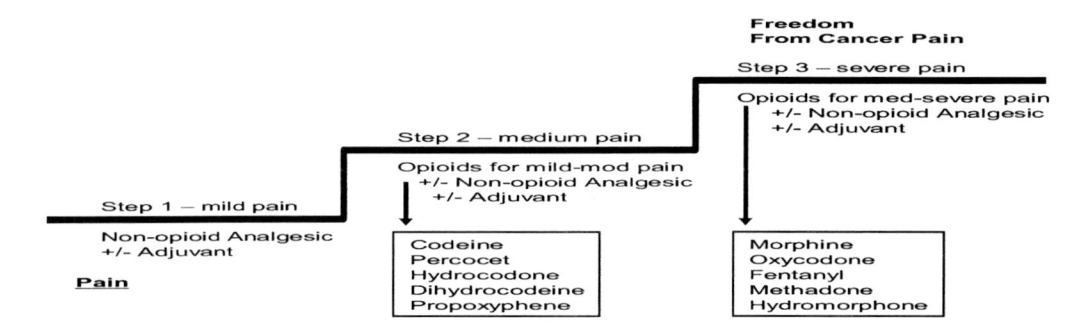

Figure 2. WHO 3-step Analgesic Ladder

The phenanthrenes have a 5-ringed structure and include: morphine, codeine, hydromorphone, buprenorphine, nalbuphone and butorphanol. The 6-OH group on morphine may lead to side effects such as nausea. Phenanthrenes, which lack the 6-OH group (e.g. oxycodones, hydromorphone, hydrocodone), may be better tolerated in patients with nausea from morphine. If a patient cannot tolerate a dehydroxylated phenanthrene, it will not be worthwhile giving the patient a trial of a hydroxylated phenanthrene.

The benzomorphans have a 3-ringed structure and the prototype is pentazocine. The phenylpiperidines have a 2-ringed structure and include: meperidine, fentanyl, sufentanil, alfentanil and remifentanil. The diphenylheptanes are unlike the other groups in that they can be considered somewhat linear in structure.

In general, agents such as the agonist-antagonist group (agents such as nalbuphone and pentazocine which are antagonists at the Mu opioid receptor and agonists at the Kappa opioid receptor), meperidine, and propoxyphene have little to no role in the long-term management of persistent noncancer pain.

Morphine sulfate (considered by some the "prototype opioid") is the best known and most commonly used opioid for pain relief. Morphine belongs to the phenanthrene opioid class and absorption post oral administration is approximately 20-30% [67]. After intramuscular administration of morphine sulfate, the analgesic onset is about 10-20 minutes, the time to peak analgesia is roughly 30-60 minutes, the analgesic duration is about 3-5 hours, and the elimination half-life is 203 hours [67]. It is a relatively hydrophilic opioid with slow elimination from the brain compartment relative to plasma. The oral-to-parental ratio for long term dosing is 3:1. When initiating therapy it may be as high as 6:1. The major metabolic pathways of morphine are in the liver via glucuronidation. Although there may be a small unmetabolized fraction present, some of the metabolites of morphine include morphine-3-glucuronide (M3G) [60%], morphine-6-glucuronide (M6G) [10%], morphine-3-sulfate [5%], normorphine [4%], and morphine 3, 6 diglucuronide (<1%) [67].

M6G possesses analgesic qualities and when administered intrathecally as an infusion to humans, is more potent than morphine [68]. There is dramatic delay in the rate of the rise of M6G plasma concentrations probably resulting from slow and incomplete transfer of M6G through the blood-brain barrier. This could conceivably help explain the increased analgesic efficacy which can be occasionally encountered over the initial titration period of morphine.

M3G is devoid of analgesic activity [69], however, intracerebroventricular or intraperitoneal M3G has been reported to induce allodynia and hyperalgesia, with higher doses potentially leading to behavior excitation, myoclonus, and seizures [70, 71]. These efforts may occur via "non-opioid" mechanisms--- perhaps involving the NMDA receptor. Additionally, M3G may actually antagonize the analgesic effects of morphine perhaps partly via non-opioid mechanisms, e.g. facilitating dynorphin actions and/or direct or indirect effects on the NMDA receptor complex [67]. It is conceivable that patients' analgesic response to morphine may be related to their M3G-to-M6G ratio [67]. However, Goucke and colleagues reported that the M3G-to-M6G ratios in 11 patients with "morphine-resistant pain receiving long-term morphine were similar to published values in patients with well-controlled pain [72]. Clearly, there are no easy answers in attempts to explain opioid analgesic efficacy but it is hoped that in the future the more that clinicians appreciate the various pharmacokinetic/pharmacodynamic differences among opioids and patients, the better equipped they may be to approaches issues of suboptimal opioid analgesia.

If a patient had abnormal differential induction and/or function of the various uridine glucuronosyl transferase (UGT) enzymes, conceivably this could lead to altered M3G-to-M6G ratios and resultant inadequate analgesia. Furthermore, if a patient on high doses of morphine exhibits hyperalgesia, agitation and/or myoclonus, this could conceivably be due to M3G and switching the use of non-UGT-metabolized opioids (e.g. methadone) should be considered. Morphine glucuronides are eliminated from the body via urinary excretion. In patients with renal failure, the retention of plasma M6G induces a progressive accumulation of this active metabolite in cerebrospinal fluid; this accumulation may contribute to the increased susceptibility and increased side effects (e.g. respiratory depression, sedation, vomiting) to morphine in patients with renal failure [67].

Hydromorphone is a phenanthrene-derivative structural analog of morphine, which is essentially "dehydroxylated morphine". It may be produced in the body by N-demethylation of hydrocodone. The oral bioavailability is roughly 30-40% [67]. After intramuscular administration of hydromorphone, the analgesic onset is about 10-20 minutes, the time to peak analgesic is roughly 30-60 minutes, the analgesic duration is about 3-5 hours; and the elimination half-life is roughly 2-3 hours [67]. Hydromorphone has a strong affinity for the mu opioid receptor and is as relatively hydrophilic as morphine sulfate. The oral-to-parental ratio is about 5:1 and when administered parenterally, roughly 1.5 mg of hydromorphone is equivalent to 10mg of morphine.

The major metabolic pathways of hydromorphone are similar to morphine and predominantly in the liver via glucuronidation (e.g. hydromorphone-3-glucuronide, H3G), hydromorphone-6 glucuronides (H6G). H3G is similar to M3G, being devoid of analgesic activity and potentially leading to a range of dose-dependent neuro excitatory side effects [e.g. allodynia, myoclonus, seizures]. Hydromorphone appears to be especially well suited to use cautiously renal failure.

Methadone is a racemic mixture of two enantiomers ("L" or "D"/"S" or "R", 50:50), which is being increasingly used for long-term analgesia and also in opioid rotation schedules. Methadone is a synthetic, open chain mu opioid receptor agonist which is equipotent to morphine after parenteral administration. The pharmacokinetics and pharmacodynamics of methadone are extremely variable. Therefore; titration should be performed slowly, cautiously, and tailored to the individual patient and their responses. Oral bioavailability of methadone is highly variable and may range from 40% to 99% [67]. Intestinal metabolism by cytochrome P-450 3A4 (CYP3A4) located in the intestinal wall may contribute to marked variability in presystemic methadone inactivation [73]. L-methadone provides analgesia through actions at the mu opioid receptor and d-methadone exhibits n-methyl-d-aspartate [NMDA] receptor antagonist activities in vitro and in vivo, --- therefore, it may conceivably diminish the development of opioid tolerance and opioid induced hyperalgesia [74]. It appears that morphine and methadone when used in combination may exhibit analgesic synergy [75].

Methadone pharmacokinetics follows a biexponential model (2-3 hours of initial phase and an extremely variable 9-87 hours of terminal phase), which appears to account for the discrepancy between moderate length (6 to 8 hours) of analgesic action and the tendency for drug accumulation with repeated dosing [67].

Methadone is metabolized via CYP3A4 in the liver, yielding essentially no active metabolites. It is sequentially N-demethylated to the inactive metabolites 2-ethylidene-1, 5-dimethyl-3, 3-diphenylpyrrolidine (EDDP) and 2-ethyl-5-methyl-3, 3-diphenylpyraline (EMDP) and is excreted largely in the feces [67]. When urine pH is greater than 6.0, the remaining renal clearance of methadone is decreased significantly [this decrease in renal clearance may also occurs in the elderly and oncology patients] [67].

Fentanyl is a synthetic phenyl piperidine mu opioid receptor agonist. It is roughly 80 times more potent than morphine, is highly lipophilic, and binds avidly to plasma proteins. After intra muscular administration of fentanyl citrate, the analgesic onset time is roughly 7-15 minutes; the time to peak analgesia may be extremely variable but could be approximated by 15-45 minutes, the analgesic duration is about 1-2 hours, and the elimination half-life is about 2-4 hours [67].

The predominate pathway of fentanyl metabolism is by piperidine N-dealkylation to norfentanyl via hepatic microsomal CYP3A4 [67]. Amide hydrolysis to desproprionyl fentanyl and alkyl hydroxylation to hydroxyfentanyl are relatively minor pathways [67]. Hydroxynorfentanyl is a minor, secondary metabolite arising from N-dealkylation of hydroxyfentanyl [67].

Oral transmucosal fentanyl citrate (OTFC), a candied matrix formulation administered orally as a palatable lozenge on a stick, is applied against the buccal mucosa and as it dissolves in saliva a proportion of the drug diffuses across the oral mucosa with the rest being swallowed and partially absorbed in the stomach and intestine. The bioavailability is about 50%.

OTFC appears to be particularly well suited for breakthrough pain [which is present in roughly two-thirds of cancer patients with pain] due to its rapid onset. Meaningful analgesia may occur between 5 to 10 minutes after initiating OTFC use. Peak plasma concentrations are achieved at 20 minutes and the duration of analgesia is roughly 2 hours [76].

Oxycodone is a phenanthrene, which likes hydromorphone lacks the 6-hydroxyl group of morphine, and is generally well tolerated. After oral administration of oxycodone the analgesic onset is about 30-60 minutes, the time to peak analgesia [median t max] is roughly 60 minutes, and the analgesic duration may be about 3-6 hours and can be about 3-6 hours and can be variable, and the elimination half-life may vary but is usually about 2-3 hours [77, 78]. The bioavailability of oral relative to intramuscular oxycodone was 60% [77].

The metabolism of oxyxodone is extensive (about 95%) and complex with many "minor" routes. Oxycodone and its phase I metabolites produced by O-demethylation, N-demethylation, 6-Ketoreduction, and N-oxidation yield oxymorphone, noroxycodone, noroxymorphone, 6- oxycodol, nor-6-ocycodol, oxycodone-N-oxide, and 6-oxycodol-N-oxide. Phase II conjugates with glucuronic acid of several of these compounds appear in the urine as well as the N-oxidized derivative of 6-oxycodol and an O-glucuronide of this compound [79]. Ten percent (about 8-14%) of the administered dose is excreted essentially unchanged [conjugated or unconjugated] in the urine [77]. Oxymorphone, a 3-0-demethylation metabolite of oxycodone, is a potent opioid that has a 3 to 5 times higher mu opioid receptor affinity than morphine [80]. Oxymorphone is not currently available in the United States. Oxymorphone has been studied for postsurgical pain in an oral immediate-release formulation and appears to be effective [81]. Oxymorphone has also been studied as an oral extended-release formulation and it appears that oxymorphone may be effective for moderate to severe pain secondary to osteoarthritis [82]. It also seems that oxymorphone extended-release may be equianalgesic to oxycodone controlled-release at half the milligram daily dosage [with comparable safety] [83, 84] and may be more potent than morphine at equianalgesic doses [85]. Noroxymorphone demonstrated a 3- and 10-fold higher affinity for the mu opioid receptor than oxycodone and noroxycodone, respectively [86]. Genetic polymorphism in the expression of CYP3A5 is a significant issue that contributes to the intersubject variability of CYP3A activity in vivo [87]. Thus, CYP3A expression and activity may be major determinants of oxycodone clearance in vivo, and inhibitors of or inducers of CYP3A expression and/or activity may significantly affect the activities/actions of oxycodone.

The O-demethylation pathway represents a relatively minor metabolic pathway for oxycodone with CYP2D6 being the major O-demethylase most likely accounting for 79% to 90% of O-demethylase activity in human hepatic microsomes [86]. Significant individual variation in oxycodone metabolism may account for wide variability in clinical responses [88].

## Drug Interactions with Opioids

The majority of significant pharmacokinetic drug interactions appear to involve drug metabolism or protein binding. Codeine is metabolized to morphine [which is the "active" analgesic agent] via the cytochrome P450 enzyme CYP2D6. Codeine has essentially no analgesic activity in people lacking CYP2D6 (up to roughly 27% of Caucasians) or in people taking CYP2D6 inhibitors (e.g. quinidine) [89]. Acceleration of methadone metabolism due to induction of CYP3A4 by antiretroviral drugs or vifampin has lead to methadone withdrawal symptoms [89]. Additionally, alkylating agents which may impair $\alpha_1$ – acid glycoprotein synthesis may significantly affect the protein binding and therefore the activity of methadone [89].

Chemotherapeutic agents could result in altered transmembrane transport of morphine, methadone, or fentanyl secondary to inhibition of P-glycoprotein [89]. However, the clinical significance of this is uncertain.

## Opioid Tolerance, Dependence, and Addiction

Physical dependence on opioids, which may occur after just two weeks of opioid therapy, is typically manifested in an abstinence syndrome or withdrawal symptoms, typically occurring with abrupt cessation of opioid or with the administration of an opioid antagonist (e.g. naloxone). Symptoms and/or signs may include: anxiety, irritability, chills, hot flashes, arthalgias, lacrimation, rhinorrhea, diaphoresis, nausea, vomiting, abdominal cramps, goose flesh, hypertension, tachycardia, tachypnea, and diarrhea. The onset of withdrawal symptoms may occur with 6 to 12 hours and peak at 24 to 72 hours after opioid discontinuation for short-acting opioids (e.g. morphine sulfate immediate release), but onset may be delayed for 24 hours or longer and may be milder in severity for patients taking long acting agents (e.g. methadone). Agents that have been used to ameliorate the severity of the withdrawal syndrome include: clonidine and buprenorphine.

Addiction is extremely uncommon and in general should not deter clinicians from initiating opioids if appropriate. Although it is vanishingly small (e.g. less than 1%) when opioid administered to patients with acute pain for a short period in the hospital, the incidence of addiction when opioids are administered long-term to patients with persistent noncancer pain in the setting of an outpatient chronic pain clinic is higher. It is unknown how much higher but probably at least approaches or somewhat surpasses that of other substances of abuse. Careful monitoring is suggested and the use of urine drug testing, opioid "contracts"/agreements, as well as techniques such as unscheduled pill counting and writing prescriptions of small quantities (i.e. 2 to 3 days) with having patients pick up new prescriptions every 2 to 3 days may be employed by clinicians under certain circumstances.

Although the precise incidence and prevalence of controlled substance abuse and addiction is unknown in a chronic pain clinic setting, it appears to be significant and estimates of 5% to 10% may actually be on the conservative side [90, 91]. Katz and colleagues analyzed the results of behavioral monitoring and urine toxicology in patients receiving long-term opioid therapy, and reported that 43% presented with either a positive urine toxicology or one or more aberrant drug-taking behaviors [92]. Furthermore, controversy surrounds the issue of whether the use of short-acting or long-acting opioids has any impact on the risk of abuse/addiction. It is the author's belief that the idea that long-acting opioid preparations are causally associated with less abuse/addiction is not supported by definite evidence and has been "overplayed". Following 200 patients (100 who received hydrocodone for analgesia and 100 who received methadone) over a three month period, utilizing urine rapid drug screens revealed no significant difference in prescription opioid abuse or illicit drug abuse between patients who received hydrocodone or methadone, suggesting that the use of long-acting opioid preparations by patients in chronic pain does not reduce the risk of drug abuse [93].

## Opioid Abuse

The epidemiology of prescription use and abuse is not precisely known but the trends have been analyzed. In 2001, the College on Problems of Drug Dependence (CPDD) commissioned a Taskforce on Prescription Opioid Abuse in efforts to develop a position statement to address issues surrounding the non-medical use and abuse of prescription opioids. [9].

The National Household Survey on Drug Abuse (NHSDA) collects incidence and prevalence data of abused drugs by administering questionnaires each year to a randomized sample of the population that live in households. Although the prevalence of lifetime, past year, and past month non-medical use of prescription opioids in people aged 12 years and older was stable from 1999 to 2000, significantly increased lifetime and past year usage were noted from 2000 to 2001 [94, 95].

The Monitoring the Future (MTF) project which has assessed non-medical use of prescription opioids in 12$^{th}$ graders since 1991, noted that past 30-day usage of prescription opioids has increased from 1.1 % in 1991 to 3% in 2001, a 173% increase [9, 96].

The Drug Abuse Warning Network (DAWN), an ongoing national data system initiated in 1988, collects information on drug-related visits to emergency departments (Eds) from a national probability of samples [9, 97]. DAWN attempts to ascertain the health consequences of drug use reflected in ED visits with the number of mentions of drugs during a drug-related visit being a key endpoint [9]. The number of mentions of opioid analgesics from 44,518 in 1994 to 99,317 in 2001, an increase of 123% (P < 0.05) [9, 97].

The Treatment Episode Data Set (TEDS) collects treatment admissions for drug abuse and demographic data on the abusers [98]. Since 1994, a steady increase can be seen in the number of treatment admissions in which prescription opioids (not including methadone) are listed as the primary drug of abuse. The 14,044 admissions in 1994 were increased 45% to 20,394 in 1999 [98]. Joranson focusing on the four opioids [morphine, fentanyl, oxycodone, and hydromorphone], concluded that increases in the medical use of prescription opioids did not lead to an increase in abuse [99]. However, Zacny and colleagues, analyzing the DAWN as data did not concur [97].

One issue which has been thought to be an important consideration in the relative ease of abuse potential between various opioid analgesics is the ease with which the active opioid ingredient can be extracted from the prescription opioid product. Katz and colleagues developed an extractability rating system for prescription opioid analgesic products in preliminary efforts to assess the abuse liability of various prescription opioid products [100].

The term pseudoaddiction has been coined [101] to describe specific behaviors in individuals who experience inadequate pain management. This condition may manifest itself when inappropriate doses or dosing intervals are established, which may occur more often in opioid-tolerant patients, or in cancer patients with unrecognized rapid progression of disease.

The phenomenon of tolerance and opioid-induced hyperalgesia remains controversial in terms of their clinical significance. Although it is easy to produce and appreciate tolerance in animal studies some investigators doubt that is highly clinically studies in humans since clinical studies designed to diminish the incidence of tolerance--- were unable to demonstrate its occurrence.

Portenoy [4] has commented on the consensus statement of the UK Pain Society, the Royal College of Anaesthestics, General Practitioners, and Psychiatrists [5] stating that their "recommendations properly emphasize that tolerance seems to be a minor problem in practice". Although the authors agree with this statement for cancer pain and pain approaching end-of-life care, the authors believe that there exists a subpopulation of patients with persistent noncancer pain in whom tolerance represents a significant clinical challenge.

The authors believe that opioid-induced hyperalgesia and tolerance can present a major clinical dilemma, the incidence of tolerance is unknown, tolerance may exist as a wide clinical spectrum being barely perceptible to dramatic (both in its severity as well as in its time course), and although it seems to be an issue to reckon with in many patients over time, it may only occur and/or be clinical significant in a minority of the population. Strategies emerging to address the issue of tolerance which are appearing in the clinical arena include: opioid rotation (however, if the patient's pain is well-controlled without side effects, this may not be optimal), co-administration of an NMDA antagonist (e.g. methadone, dextromethorphan), co-administration of an ultra-low dose of a mu opioid receptor antagonist, and perhaps in the future among other agents co-administration of cholecystokinin antagonists.

## Intrathecal Long-Term Opioid Therapy

Opioids have been administered by most routes including: oral, rectal, transdermal, intratracheal, oral transmucosal, sublingual, intra nasal, subcutaneous, intra muscular, subcutaneous, intravenous, epidural, and intrathecal. Although morphine is the only opioid approved for intrathecal use in a continuous pump many other opioids have been used intrathecally in various clinical circumstances (e.g. fentanyl, hydromorphone).

Intraspinal drug infusion is an available option that may be used for the treatment of intractable persistent pain that is unresponsive to less invasive approaches. In efforts to review current literature, revise the algorithm for drug selection developed in 2000, and develop current guidelines among other goals, the Polyanalgesia Consensus Conference 2003 was organized. Opioids have been and continue to be a mainstay agent for intraspinal therapy. In fact, the guideline developed at the Polyanalgesia Consensus Conference 2003 suggests that the first line intraspinal agent should be an opioid alone such as morphine sulfate or hydromorphone switching from one agent to another if the maximum dose is reached or side effects occur [102]. If a maximum dose of 15 mg/day of morphine and/or maximum concentration 30 mg/ml for morphine, or for hydromorphone 10 mg/d and/or maximum concentration of 30 mg/ml, or perhaps in selected cases of "predominant" neuropathic pain, the guidelines would suggest that the clinician could proceed to "step 2" (the addition of bupivacaine or clonidine to the opioid) of the six step algorithm [102].

Smith and colleagues evaluated 202 patients life-limiting cancer and pain scores consistently over 5 despite 200 mg of morphine or more daily in a multicenter, multinational randomized controlled study of comprehensive medical management versus drug delivery systems and concluded that implantable intrathecal drug delivery systems (IDDS) reduced pain, significantly relieved common drug toxicities, and was possibly associated with improved survival in patients with refractory cancer pain [103].

One criticism [104] of the study by Smith and colleagues [103] was that the authors arbitrarily defined refractory cancer pain for purposes of patient eligibility, as patients with a pain score of ≥ 5/10 despite 200 mg per day of oral morphine or the equivalent, which did not seem to be an especially high dose of opioids (at least by oncology standards).

Smith et al further evaluated IDDS in a six-month clinical trial of IDDS plus comprehensive medical management versus comprehensive medical management alone [105]. Smith et al concluded that IDDS improved clinical success, reduced pain scores, alleviated analgesic toxicities, as well as potentially contributing to improved survival for the duration of the six-month trial [105].

Smith and Coyne went onto describe 30 patients who crossed over from unsuccessful comprehensive medical management to implantable drug delivery systems and concluded that it is possible for even the most refractory of cancer pain patients to derive clinically important pain relief as well as relief of drug toxicities by crossing over from comprehensive medical management intrathecal implantable drug delivery system [106].

## Opioid Side Effects

Increasing evidence suggest a useful analgesic effect when a variety of strong opioids are used in the treatment of neuropathic and nonneuropathic pain. That said, they are neither universally effective nor universally well tolerated by patients. Although, some investigators have referred to common opioid side effects as generally benign, they appear to be significantly unpleasant and quite severe to at least some patients and they may contribute to discontinuation of opioid therapy in a significant number of patients. Therefore, it may be useful to have patients fill out an assessment tool (e.g. the NOSE Assessment) [62] in the waiting rooms in efforts to longitudinally follow opioid effects so as to be in a better position to attempt pro-active strategies to combat opioid side effects. Common opioid side effects may include: nausea and vomiting, pruritus, sedation, and constipation. Potential future agents such as methylnaltrexone or avilmopan may offer promise in the management of opioid-associated constipation without the risk of opioid withdrawl or reversal of opioid analgesic effects.

There exist no large well-designed double blind randomized controlled multicenter prospective studies which carefully examine the effects of opioids on libido, the immune system or other potential side effects over many years. Although there are no known obvious detrimental effects of long-term opioid therapy on major organ functions (e.g. kidneys, liver, etc.), a complete picture of the effects of LTOT has not been fully established.

Opioids and/or opioid-like substance have been used for many centuries, however various effects of specific agents re only recently becoming appreciated [e.g. buprenorphine hepatotoxicity] [107, 108], codeine phosphate-induced hypersensitivity syndrome [109].

Although, overall gross clinical safety of opioids is appreciated, there may be subtle changes that are not fully appreciated. In this decade of pain research, the association of high dose methadone and the potential for $QT_c$ prolongation with possible Torsade-de-Pointes has been noted [110]. Although there have been no overt organ toxicities appreciated with opioids, it is conceivable if animal data can be applied to humans [111-113] that over many years in certain predisposed patients morphine and its metabolites or other opioids may, via the risk of increased lipid peroxidation, potentially facilitate certain subtle unrecognized subclinical changes in normal organ structure and/or function.

The biologic consequences of other effects of opioids are also incompletely elucidated. Immunologic effects of opioids appear to differ: with different opioid agents [114]; with short-term versus long-term administration [114]; as well as with the state of the organism (presence of inflammation versus absence of inflammation, presence of pain versus absence of pain).

While a number of strong opioid preparations have been introduced over the last few years, these tend to be new formulations rather than new compounds. For example, oxycodone, fentanyl and buprenorphine have a long pedigree as analgesics. The new aspect of them is their presentation as a controlled release preparation in the case of oxycodone and as transdermal preparations in the case of fentanyl and buprenorphine. It is arguable whether any individual opioid offers significant analgesic benefit over the other members of this class. They do, however, differ to a certain extent in the incidence and frequency of side effects associated with their use. For example, Staats and colleagues [115] retrospectively studied 1,836 patients receiving treatment with transdermal fentanyl, sustained release oxycodone and sustained release morphine. Those receiving transdermal fentanyl had a lower risk of developing constipation than those taking either of the other two strong opioids (3% as opposed to a 6% risk with oxycodone and 5% with morphine) [115]. The incidence these authors quote for the occurrence of constipation is significantly lower than other others report with transdermal fentanyl. For example, Milligan and colleagues [116] found that with transdermal fentanyl use over a 12-month period in an open label trial in which 301 patients continued use for the 12 months, constipation was noted as a side effect in 19% [116]. Menten and colleagues [117] suggest that in terms of patients treated with transdermal fentanyl for cancer-related pain, the incidence of constipation is related not to the dose of transdermal fentanyl used, but rather on the amount of morphine used as a rescue analgesic [117]. Van Seventer and colleagues [118] give support to the impression of a lower risk of constipation with transdermal fentanyl. They enrolled 131 patients and commenced them on transdermal fentanyl or controlled release morphine. Doses were titrated until effect was apparent. The quality of analgesia achieved in both groups was equal. Constipation was less common in those treated with fentanyl: at the end of one week 27% in the fentanyl group reported constipation as opposed to 57% in the controlled release morphine group. In general terms other side effects were more common, or severe, in the morphine group. Of the patients enrolled in the study, 36% in the controlled release morphine group withdrew because of side effects as opposed to only 4% in the transdermal fentanyl group. Of those who continued with the trial, 14% in the fentanyl group reported troublesome side effects as opposed to 36% in the morphine group [118].

Quigley [119] has reviewed the available studies examining the use of hydromorphone in the treatment of cancer and noncancer pain. He concludes that of the limited number of studies available, hydromorphone differs little in its effect or side effect profile to the other strong opioid analgesics [119].

When incomplete relief or unacceptable side effects are apparent with opioid therapy, substitution to another opioid is suggested as an option. While this approach has gained popularity, Quigley [120] in his systematic review of available studies published up until January 2003 concludes that the evidence for this strategy is "... largely anecdotal or based on observational and uncontrolled studies" [120].

A variety of issues influence the tolerability of opioids. Well known side effects such as nausea, vomiting, constipation and cognitive impairment can all reduce their tolerability in the short term to the extent that sustained use is impractable. Efficacy and incidence of side effects seems to be, at least in part, dose related [28]. Furthermore, the incidence of side effects decreases with sustained use (i.e. tolerance usually develops to most opioid side effects with the notable exception of constipation) [121]. With extended release preparations these side effects may be more gradual in onset, as may be their initial analgesic effect. That said, Watson and colleagues [26] studied patients with painful diabetic neuropathy. Patients were treated for 4 weeks with controlled release oxycodone or placebo. The only side effects in which side effects occurred on a statistically more significant basis in the oxycodone treated group were dry mouth and constipation [26].

A recurrent anxiety associated with chronic strong opioid administration is its effect on cognition and motor tasks as exemplified by driving safety. Schinder and colleagues [122] examined this issue in opioid addicts (not with chronic pain) using an Austrian standard test battery for measurement of performance related to driving ability, the Act and React Test (ART) system. Subjects were taking either methadone or buprenorphine and were compared to healthy controls. They found that those taking these strong opioids did not differ significantly in comparison with the healthy controls in the majority of the ART standard tests [122].

Jamison and colleagues [123] examined the psychomotor effects of long-term opioid [oxycodone and fentanyl] use in 144 patients with low back pain. They measured the results of two neuropsychological tests (Digit Symbol and Trail Making Test-B) on all subjects prior to institution of the strong opioid and again 90 and 180 days after opioid commencement. They found that sustained use was not associated with impairment of the neuropsychological variables measured. Indeed, memory, incidental learning and psychomotor performance were improved in many of the subjects. They also noted that a minority of patients had a decrease in performance. This tended to occur in older patients and in those with lower pre-treatment pain scores. There were no differences in neuropsychological performance between patients taking oxycodone or transdermal fentanyl [123].

Tassain and colleagues [124] studied 28 patients with chronic noncancer pain in whom sustained release morphine was prescribed. Eighteen stayed on this therapy and the other 10 discontinued treatment because of unacceptable side effects but acted as a control group. They found that when baseline, pre-treatment neuropsychological variables were compared in these patients with results obtained after 3, 6 and 12 months treatment that there were no significant differences. Indeed in two measures of information processing (the Stroop interference score and the digit symbol test) the results were actually better after 6 and 12 months treatment. The most frequent side effects with treatment were gastrointestinal in nature with almost 50% of patients still reporting constipation after 12 months of morphine therapy [124].

Similarly, Sabatowski and colleagues [125] assessed attention, reaction, visual orientation, motor coordination and vigilance in 30 subjects using a stable dose of transdermal fentanyl for non-cancer pain and compared these to 90 healthy volunteers. Non of the results from the measures differed significantly between the fentanyl treated and volunteer subjects and they concluded that in patients treated with stable doses of transdermal fentanyl, the threshold for fitness to drive did not differ significantly between the groups [125]. In contrast, when morphine and oxycontin are administered on a one off basis to volunteers and compared to placebo, both morphine and oxycontin produce effects on psychomotor performance and these effects are dose related [126].

Long-term administration may be complicated by other factors that can influence their long term tolerability. For example, acute administration of opioids increases prolactin, growth hormone, thyroid stimulating hormone and ACTH while inhibiting leutenising hormone (LH) release [127-129]. When administered on a long-term basis different endocrine results are observed. Abs and colleagues [130] have extensively investigated 73 patients receiving intrathecal opioids for chronic nonmalignant pain. Their average duration of opioid treatment was 26 months. Decreased libido and impotence was present in 23 of the 24 men studied. Nine of the men had a significantly reduced testosterone level and most had a decreased LH level. All of the premenopausal females had either amenorrhea or an irregular cycle with ovulation in only one patient. All postmenopausal women had a decreased LH and FSH level when compared to controls. The twenty-four hour urinary cortisol excretion was significantly lower than controls in 14 of the 73 patients. Fifteen percent of all patients developed growth hormone deficiency. Therefore, in patients receiving intrathecal opioids on a long term basis the majority of men and all women developed hypogonadotrophic hypogonadism, 15% developed central hypocorticism and about 15% developed growth hormone deficiency [130].

A single case report highlights a different possible side effect of fentanyl use. Kokko and colleagues [131] report apparent inappropriate antidiuretic hormone (ADH) release in a patient with a known lung tumour treated with fentanyl. Withdrawal of fentanyl terminated the ADH release, while reinstitution of fentanyl at a latter date triggered of a further inappropriate ADH release [131].

As with TCAs, paradoxical pain can complicate opioid use [64, 65, 132-146]. If such pain occurs and remains unidentified, it may lead to an increase in opioid dose with a potential increase in opioid related side effects and consequent reduction in tolerability. Opioid induced paradoxical pain may be caused by opioid induced release of spinal dynorphin and cholecystokinin.

## Summary

Overall, the use of LTOT for PNCP may provide significant analgesia patients with minimal side effects for many years, however, it must be kept in mind that:

(a) LTOT may not be optimal for all patients
(b) LTOT does not provide good or excellent analgesia in all patients
(c) LTOT is not devoid of side effects
(d) LTOT should be monitored in efforts to assess efficacy, side effects and aberrant drug behavior
(e) LTOT can be successfully withdrawn in selected patients who may do better without opioids
(f) Prescribing LTOT for PNCP remains very much an art which may be used successfully alone or in conjunction with other therapeutic options but typically not as a first-line agent for patients who have not tried previous treatments

## Opioid Glossary

| | |
|---|---|
| GDTA | Goal Directed Therapy Agreement |
| LTOT | Long Term Opioid Therapy |
| ORP | Opioid Responsive Pain |
| M3G | Morphine 3 Glucuronide |
| M6G | Morphine 6 glucuronide |
| MORP | Moderately Opioid Responsive Pain |
| NOSE | Numerical Opioid Side Effect assessment tool |
| OTFC | Oral Transmucosal Fentanyl Citrate |
| OGC | Opioid Generous Clinicians |
| OSC | Opioid Stingy Clinicians |
| PNCP | Persistent Non Cancer Pain |
| PORP | Poorly Opioid Responsive Pain |
| SAFE | Social, Analgesia, Function, Emotional score |
| SOAPP | Screener and Opioid Assessment for Patients with Pain |
| TAS | Translational Analgesic Score |
| UDT | Urine Drug Testing |

## References

[1] Dale W. On pain, and some of the remedies for its relief. *Lancet* 1871; [13 May]: 641-642; [20 May]: 679-690; [3 June]: 739-741; [17 June]: 816-817.

[2] American Academy of Pain Medicine, American Pain Society, The use of opioids for the treatment of chronic pain [http://www.painmd.org/productpub/statements/pdfs/opioids.pdf] [Assessed August 4, 2004]
[3] Chou R, Clark E, Helfan M, et al. Comparative efficacy and safety of long-acting oral opioids for chronic non-cancer pain: a systematic review. *J. Pain Symptom. Manage.* 2003; 26: 1026-1048.
[4] Portenoy RK. Appropriate use of opioids for persistent non-cancer pain. *Lancet.* 2004; 364: 739-40.
[5] A consensus statement prepared on behalf of the Pain Society, the Royal College of Aneasthetists, the Royal College of General Practitioners, and the Royal College of Psychiatrists, *Recommendations for the appropriate use of opioids for persistent non-cancer pain,* the Pain Society, London [March 2004][http://www.painsociety.org/pdf/opioids_doc_2004.pdf] [assessed August 9, 2004]
[6] Kalso E, Allan L, Dellemijn PL, et al. Recommendations for using opioids in chronic non-cancer pain. *Eur. J. Pain.* 2003; 7: 381-6.
[7] A joint statement from 21 health organizations and the Drug Enforcement Administration, *Promoting pain relief and preventing abuse of pain medications: a critical balancing act.* [http://www.medsch.wisc.edu/painpolicy/Consensus 2.pdf] [accessed August 4, 2004]
[8] World Health Organization. Achieving balance in nation opioids control policy: guidelines for assessment, *WHO*, Geneva [2000]
[9] Zacny J, Bigelow G, Compton P, et al. College on problems of drug dependence task force on prescription opioid non-medical use and abuse: position statement. *Drug Alcohol Depend.* 2003; 69: 215-232.
[10] Turk, DC, Brody MC, Okifuji EA: Physicians' attitudes and practices regarding the long-term prescribing of opioids for non-cancer pain. *Pain.* 1994; 59: 201-8.
[11] Scanlon MN, Chugh U. Exploring physicians' comfort level with opioids for chronic noncancer pain. *Pain Res. Manag.* 2004; 9: 195-201.
[12] Portenoy RK. Opioid therapy for chronic nonmalignant pain: a review of the critical issues. *J. Pain Symptom Manage.* 1996; 11: 203-17.
[13] Breivik H. Opioids in chronic non-cancer pain, indications and controversies. *Eur. J. Pain.* 2005; 9: 127-130.
[14] Rome JD, Townsend CO, Bruce BK, et al. Chronic noncancer pain rehabilitation with opioid withdrawal: comparison of treatment outcomes based on opioid use status at admission. *Mayo Clinic Proc.* 2004; 79: 759-68.
[15] Kalso E, Edwards JE, Moore RA, McQuay HJ. Opioids in chronic non-cancer pain: a systematic review of efficacy and safety. *Pain* 2004; 112: 372-80.
[16] Cowan DT, Wilson-Barnett J, Griffiths P, et al. A survey of chronic noncancer pain patients prescribed opioid analgesics. *Pain Med.* 2003; 4: 340-51.
[17] Cowan DT, Wilson-Barnett J, Griffiths P, et al. A randomized, double-blind, placebo-controlled, cross-over pilot study to assess the effects of long-term opioid drug consumption and subsequent abstinence in chronic noncancer pain patients receiving controlled-release morphine. *Pain Med.* 2005; 6: 113-21.

[18] Dellemijn PLI, Vanneste JAL. Randomized double-blind active-placebo-controlled crossover trial of intravenous fentanyl in neuropathic pain. *Lancet.* 1997; 349: 753-758.
[19] Dellemijn PLI, van Duijn H, Vanneste JAL. Prolonged treatment with transdermal fentanyl in neuropathic pain. *J. Pain Symptom Manage.* 1998; 16: 220-229.
[20] Attal NA, Guirimand F, Brasseur L, et al. Effects of IV morphine in central pain. A randomized placebo-controlled study. *Neurology.* 2002; 58: 554-563.
[21] Huse E, Larbig W, Flor H, et al. The effect of opioids on phantom limb pain and cortical reorganization. *Pain.* 2001; 90: 47-55.
[22] Gustorff B. Intravenous opioid testing in patients with chronic non-cancer pain. *Eur. J. Pain.* 2005; 9: 123-5.
[23] Watson CP, Watt-Watson JH, Chipman ML. Chronic noncancer pain and the long term utility of opioids. *Pain Res. Manag.* 2004; 9: 19-24.
[24] Watson CP, Babul N. Efficacy of oxycodone in neuropathic pain: A randomized trial in post herpetic neuralgia. *Neurology.* 1998; 50: 1837-41.
[25] Gimbel JS, Richards P. Portenoy RK. Controlled-release oxycodone for diabetic neuropathy: A randomized controlled trial. *Neurology.* 2003; 60: 927-34.
[26] Watson CP, Moulin D, Watt-Watson J, Gordon A, Eisenhoffer J. Controlled-release oxycodone relieves neuropathic pain: a randomized controlled trial in painful diabetic neuropathy. *Pain.* 2003; 105: 71 – 8.
[27] Raja SN, Haythornwaite JA, Pappagallo M, et al. Opioids versus antidepressants in post herpetic neuralgia: A randomized placebo-controlled trial. *Neurology.* 2002; 59: 1015-21.
[28] Rowbotham MC, Twilling L, Davies PS, Reisner L, Taylor K, Mohr D. Oral opioid therapy for chronic peripheral and central neuropathic pain. *N. Engl. J. Med.* 2003; 348: 1223 – 32.
[29] Harke H, Gretenkort P, Ladleif HU, et al. The response of neuropathic pain and pain in complex regional pain syndrome to carbamazapine and sustained-release morphine in patients pretreated with spinal cord stimulation: A double-blinded randomized study. *Anesth. Analg.* 2001; 92: 488-95.
[30] Eisenbrg E, McNicol ED, Carr DB. Efficacy and safety of opioid agonists in the treatment of neuropathic pain of nonmalignant origin: systematic review and meta-analysis trials. *JAMA.* 2005; 293: 3043-52.
[31] Farrar JT, Portenoy RK, Berlin JA, et al. Defining the clinically important difference in pain outcome measures. *Pain.* 2000; 88: 287-294.
[32] Farrar JT, Young JP Jr, LaMoreaux L, et al. Clinical importance of changes in chronic pain intensity measured on an 11-point numerical pain rating scale. *Pain.* 2001; 94: 149-158.
[33] Rashig S, Koller M, Haykowsky M, et al. The effect of opioid analgesia on exercise test performance in chronic low back pain. *Pain.* 2003: 106: 199-25.
[34] Moulin DE, Iezzi A, Amireh R, et al. Randomized trial of oral morphine for chronic non-cancer pain. *Lancet.* 1996; 347: 143-7.
[35] Bartleson JD. Evidence for and against the use of opioid analgesics for chronic nonmalignant low back pain: A review. *Pain Med.* 2002; 3: 260-71.

[36] Caudill-Slosberg MA, Schwartz LM, Woloshin S. Office visits and analgesic prescriptions for musculoskeletal pain in U.S.: 1980 vs. 2000. *Pain.* 2004; 109: 514-9.
[37] Smith HS, Audette J, Witkower A. Playing It "SAFE". *J. Cancer Pain Symptom Palliation.* 2005; 1: 3 –10.
[38] Smith HS. Translational Analgesia and Translational Analgesia Score. *Journal of Cancer Pain and Symptom Palliation.* 2005: 1:
[39] Ballantyne JC, Mao J. Opioid therapy for chronic pain. *N. Eng. J. Med.* 2003; 349: 1943-53.
[40] Smith HS. Taxonomy of Pain Syndromes. In: *The Neurological basis of pain.* Ed Pappagallo M. 2005, pp 289-300, McGraw-Hill Companies, Inc., New York, New York.
[41] Stein C, Millan MJ, Yassouridas A, et al. Antinocieceptive effects of mu- and kappa-agonists in inflammation are enhanced by a peripheral opioid receptor-specific mechanism. *Eur. J. Pharmacol.* 1988; 155: 255-264.
[42] Perrot S, Guilbaud G, Kayser V. Effects of intraplantar morphine on paw edema and pain–related acute inflammation. *Pain.* 1999; 83: 249-57.
[43] Obara I, Przewlocki R, Przewlocka B. Local peripheral effects of mu-opioid agnostics in neuropathic pain in rats. *Neurosci. Lett.* 2004; 360: 85-9.
[44] Stein C, Machelska H, Binder W, et al. Peripheral opioid analgesia. *Curr. Opin. Pharmacol.* 2001; 1: 62-5.
[45] Stein C, Schafer M, Machelska H. Attacking pain at its source: new perspectives on opioids. *Nat. Med.* 2003; 9: 1003-8.
[46] Zhou L, Zhang Q, Stein C, et al. Contribution of opioid receptors on primary afferent versus sympathetic neurons to peripheral opioid analgesia. *J. Pharmacol. Exp. Ther.* 1998; 286: 1000-6.
[47] Stein C. Opioid receptors on peripheral sensory neurons. *Adv. Exp. Med. Biol.* 2003; 521: 69-76.
[48] Dirig DM, Konin GP, Isakson PC, et al. Effect of spinal cyclooxygenase inhibitors in rat using the formalin test and in vitro prostaglandin E2 release. *Eur. J. Pharmacol.* 1997; 331: 155-160.
[49] Dirig DM, Isakson PC, Yaksh TL. Effect of COX-1 and COX-2 inhibition on induction and maintenance of carrageenan-evoked thermal hyperalgesia in rats. *J. Pharmacol. Exp. Ther.* 1998; 285: 1031-1038.
[50] Malmberg AB, Yaksh TL. Cyclooxygenase inhibition and the spinal release of prostaglandin E2 and amino acids evoked by paw formalin injection: A microdialysis study in unanesthetized rats. *J. Neurosci.* 1995; 15: 2768-2776.
[51] Samad TA, Moore KA, Sapirstein A, et al. Interleukin-1 beta-mediated induction on COX-2 in the CNS contributes to inflammatory pain hypersensitivity. *Nature.* 2001; 410: 471-475.
[52] Smith HS. Introduction. In: *Drugs For Pain.* Ed: Smith HS. 2003; pp 1-8; Hanley and Belfus, Philadelphia, Pennsylvania.
[53] Fishman SM, Mahajan G, Jung SW, et al. The trilateral opioid contract. Bridging the pain clinic and the primary care physician through the opioid contract. *J. Pain Symptom Manage.* 2002; 24: 335-44.

[54] Smith HS. Goal-Directed Therapy Agreements. *Journal of Cancer Pain and Symptom Palliation*. 2005; 1.

[55] Michna E, Ross EL, Hynes WL, et al. Predicting aberrant drug behavior in patients treated for chronic pain: importance of abuse history. *J. Pain Symptom Manage*. 2004; 28: 250-8.

[56] Butler SF, Budman SH, Fernandez K, et al. Validation of a screener and opioid assessment measure for patients with chronic pain. *Pain*. 2004; 112: 65-75.

[57] Katz N, Fanciullo G. Role of urine toxicology testing in the management of chronic opioid therapy. *Clin. J. Pain*. 2002; 18: 576-82.

[58] Wasan AD, Davar G, Jamison R. The association between negative affect and opioid analgesia in patients with discogenic low back pain. *Pain*. 2005; 177: 450-61.

[59] Passik SD, Whitcomb LA, Dodd S, et al. Pain outcomes in long-term treatment with opioids: *Preliminary results with a newly developed physician checklist*. Presented at the Fourth Conference on Pain Management and Chemical Dependency, Washington, DC, December 7-9, 2000.

[60] Passik SD, Weinreb HJ. Managing chronic non-malignant pain: Overcoming obstacles to the use of opioids. *Adv. Ther*. 2000; 17: 70-83.

[61] Passik SD, Kirsh KL, Whitcomb L, et al. A new tool to assess and document pain outcomes in chronic pain patients receiving opioid therapy. *Clin. Ther*. 2004; 26: 552-61.

[62] Smith HS. The Numerical Opioid Side Effect [NOSE] Assessment Tool. *Journal of Cancer Pain and Symptom Palliation*. 2005; 1.

[63] Smith HS. Perspectives in persistent non-cancer pain. *Journal of Cancer Pain and Symptom palliation*. 2005; 1.

[64] Yaksh TL, Harty GJ, Onofrio BM. High dose of spinal morphine produce a non-opiate receptor mediated hyperaesthesia: clinical and theoretical implications. *Anesthesiology*. 1986; 64: 590 – 7.

[65] Ossipov MH, Lai J, Vanderah TW, Porreca F. Induction of pain facilitation by sustained opioid exposure: relationship to opioid antinociceptive tolerance. *Life Sciences*. 2003; 73: 783 – 800.

[66] Dworkin RH, Backonja M, Rowbotham MC, et al. Advances in neuropathic pain: diagnosis, mechanisms, and treatment recommendations. *Arch. Neurol*. 2003; 60: 1524-34.

[67] Janicki PK, Parris WC. Clinical Pharmacology of opioids. In: *Drugs For Pain*. Ed: Smith HS. 2003; pp 97-118; Hanley and Belfus, Philadelphia, Pennsylvania.

[68] Grace D, Fee JP. A comparison of intrathecal morphine-6-glucuronide and intrathecal morphine sulfate as analgesics for total hip replacement. *Anesth. Analg*. 1996; 83: 1055-9.

[69] Hewett K, Dickenson AH, McQuay HJ. Lack of effect of morphine-3-glucuronide on the spinal antinociceptive actions of morphine in the rat: an electrophysiological study. *Pain*. 1993; 53: 59-63.

[70] Gong QL, Hedner J, Bjorkman R, et al. Morphine-3-glucuronide may functionally antagonize morphine-6-glucuronide induced antinociception and ventilatory depression in the rat. *Pain*. 1992; 48: 249-55.

[71] Igawa Y, Westerling D, Mattiasson A, et al. Effects of morphine metabolites on micturation in normal, unanesthetized rats. *Br. J. Pharmacol.* 1993; 110: 257-62.
[72] Goucke CR, Hackett LP, Ilett KF. Concentrations of morphine, morphine-6-glucuronide and morphine-3-glucuronide in serum and cerebrospinal fluid following morphine administration to patients with morphine-resistant pain. *Pain.* 1994; 56: 145-9.
[73] Oda Y, Kharasch ED. Metabolism of methadone and levo-alpha-aetylmethadol [LAAM] by human intestinal cyctochrome 3A4 [CYP3A4]: a potential complication of intestinal metabolism to presystemic clearance and bioactivation. *J. Pharmacol. Exp. Ther.* 2001; 298: 1021-32.
[74] Inturrisi CE. Pharmacology of methadone and its isomers. *Minerva Anestesiol.* 2005; 71: 435-7.
[75] Bolan EA, Tallarida RJ, Pasternak GW. Synergy between mu opioid ligands: evidence for functional interactions among mu opioid receptor subtypes. *J. Pharmacol. Exp. Ther.* 2002; 303: 557-62.
[76] Lichtor JL, Sevarino FB, Joshi GP, et al. The relative potency of oral transmucosal fentanyl citrate compared with intravenous morphine in the treatment of moderate to sever post-operative pain. *Anesth. Analg.* 1999; 89: 732-38.
[77] Poyhia R, Seppala T, Olkkola KT, et al. The pharmacokinetics and metabolism of oxycodone after intramuscular and oral administration to healthy subjects. *Br. J. Clin. Pharmacol.* 1992; 33: 617-21.
[78] Poyhia R, Vainio A, Kalso E. A review of oxycodone's clinical pharmacokinetics and pharmacodynamics. *J. Pain Symptom Manage.* 1993; 8: 63-7.
[79] Baldacci A, Caslavska J, Wey AB, et al. Identification of new oxycodone metabolites in human urine by capillary electrophoresis--- mu stage ion-trap mass spectrometry. *J. Chromatogr. A.* 2004; 1051: 273-82.
[80] Childers SR, Creese I, Snowman AM, et al. Opiate receptor binding affected differentially by opiates and opioid pep tides. *Eur. J. Pharmacol.* 1979; 55: 11-8.
[81] Gimbel J, Ahdieh H. The efficacy and safety of oral immediate release oxymorphone for postsurgical pain. *Anesth. Analg.* 2004; 99: 1472-7.
[82] Matsumoto AK, Babul N, Ahdieh H. Oxymorphone extended-release tablets relieve moderate to severe pain and improve physical function in osteoarthritis: results of a randomized double-blind, placebo--- and active--- controlled Phase III trial. *Pain Med.* 2005; 6: 357-66.
[83] Gabrail NY, Dvergsten C, Ahdieh H. Establishing the dosage equivalency of oxymorphone extended release and oxycodone controlled release in patients with moderate to severe cancer pain. *Curr. Med. Res. Opin.* 2004; 20: 911-8.
[84] Hale ME, Dvergsten C, Gimbel. Efficacy and safety of oxymorphone extended release in chronic low back pain: results of a randomized, double-blind, placebo--- and active-controlled phase III study. *J. Pain.* 2005; 6: 21-8.
[85] Sloan P, Slatkin N, Ahdieh H. Effectiveness and safety of oral extended-release oxymorphone for the treatment of cancer pain: a pilot study. *Support Care Cancer.* 2005; 13: 57-65.

[86] Lalovic B, Phillips B, Risler LL, et al. Quantitative contribution of CYP2D6 and CYP3A to oxycodone metabolism in human liver and intestinal microsomes. *Drug Metab. Dispos.* 2004; 32: 447-54.

[87] Lamda JK, Lin YS, Schuetz EG, et al. Genetic contribution to variable human CTP3A-mediated metabolism. *Adv. Drug Deliv. Rev.* 2002; 54: 1271-94.

[88] Heiskanen TE, Ruismaki PM, Seppala TA, et al. Morphine or oxycodone in cancer pain? *Acta Oncol.* 2000; 39: 941-7.

[89] Smith HS. Potential Analgesic Interactions. In: *Drugs for Pain.* Ed Smith HS. 2003; pp 453-463. Hanley and Belfur, Philadelphia, Pennsylvania.

[90] Manchikanti L, Pampati V, Damron KS, et al. Prevalence of prescription drug abuse and dependency in patients with chronic pain in western Kentucky. *J. Ky. Med. Assoc.* 2003; 101: 511-7.

[91] Manchikanti, L. Fellows B, Damron KS, et al. Prevalence of illicit drug use among individuals with chronic pain in the Commonwealth of Kentucky: am evaluation of patterns and trends. *J. Ky. Med. Assoc.* 2005; 103: 55-62.

[92] Katz N, Sherburne S, Beach M, et al. Behavioral monitoring and urine toxicology testing in patients receiving long-term opioid therapy. *Anes. Analg.* 2003; 97: 1097-102.

[93] Manchikanti L, Manchukonda R, Pampati V, et al. Evaluation of abuse of prescription and illicit drugs in chronic pain patients receiving short-acting [hydrocodone] or long-acting [methadone] opioids. *Pain Physician.* 2005; 8: 257-261.

[94] Substance Abuse and Mental Health Services Administration [SAMHSA], Office of applied studies; *Summary of findings from the 2000 National Household Survey on Drug Abuse NHSDA Series H-13*, DHHS Publication No. [SMA] 01-3549, 2001. Rockville, MD.

[95] Substance Abuse and Mental Health Services Administration [SAMHSA], Office of applied studies; results from the 2001 *National Household Survey on Drug Abuse*: Volume II. Technical Appendices and selected data tables. [Office of Applied Studies, NHSDA Series H-18, DHHS. Publication No. SMA 02-3759], 2002. Rockville, MD.

[96] Johnston LD, O'Malley PM, Bachman JG. *Monitoring the future national results on adolescent drug use: Overview of key findings*, 2001. [NIH Publication No. 02-5105]. 2002. National Institute on Drug Abuse, Bethesda, MD.

[97] Substance Abuse and Mental Health Services Administration [SAMHSA], Office of applied studies; *Emergency Department Trends from the Drug Abuse Warning Network*, Final estimates 1994-2001. *SWAN Series D-21*, DHHS Publication No. [SMA] 02-3635, 2002, Rockville, MD

[98] Substance Abuse and Mental Health Services Administration [SAMHSA], Office of applied studies; Treatment Episode Data Set [TEDS]: 1994-1999. *National Admissions to Substance Abuse Treatment Services, DASIS series: S-14*, DHHS. Publication No. [SMA] 01-3550, 2001. Rockville, MD.

[99] Joranson DE, Gilson AM, Dahl JL, et al. Pain management, controlled substances, and state medical board policy: a decade of change. *J. Pain Symptom Manage.* 2002; 23: 138-147.

[100] Katz N. Development of an Extractability Rating System for Prescription Opioid Analgesic Products. *Abstract presented at American Pain Society meeting*; Boston, MA, March 30-April 2, 2005.

[101] Weissman DE, Haddox JD. Opioid pseudoaddiction--- an iatrogenic syndrome. *Pain*. 1989; 36: 362-6

[102] Hassenbusch SJ, Portenoy RK, Cousins M, et al. Polyanalgesic Consensus Conference 2003: an update on the management of pain by intraspinal drug delivery-report of an expert panel. *J Pain Symptom Manage*. 2004; 27: 540-63.

[103] Smith TJ, Staats PS, Deer T, et al. Randomized clinical trial of an implantable drug delivery system compared with comprehensive medical management for refractory cancer pain, drug-related toxicity, and survival. *J. Clin. Oncol*. 2002; 20: 4040-9.

[104] Davis, MP, Walsh D, Lagman R, et al. Randomized clinical trial of an implantable drug delivery system. *J. Clin. Oncol*. 2003; 21: 2800-1.

[105] Smith TJ, Coyne PJ, Staats PS, et al. An implantable drug delivery systems [IDDS] for refractory cancer pain provides sustained pain control, less drug-related toxicity, and possibly better survival medical management [CMM]. *Ann. Oncol*. 2005; 16: 825-33.

[106] Smith TJ, Coyne PJ. Implantable drug delivery systems [IDDS] after failure of comprehensive medical management [CMM] can palliate symptoms in the most refractory cancer pain patients. *J. Palliat. Med*. 2005; 8: 736-42.

[107] Berson A, Fau D, Fornacciari R, et al. Mechanisms for experimental buprenorphine hepatotoxicity: major role of mitochondrial dysfunction versus metabolic activation. *J. Hepatol*. 2001; 34: 261-9.

[108] Herve S, Riachi G, Noblet C, et al. Active hepatitis due to buprenorphine administration. *Eur. J. Gastroenterol. Hepatol*. 2004; 16: 1033-7.

[109] Enomoto M, Ochi M, Teramae K, et al. Codeine phosphate-induced hypersensitivity syndrome. *Ann. Pharmacother*. 2004; 38: 799-802.

[110] Krantz MJ, Lewkowiez L, Hays H, et al. Torsade de pointes associated with very high-dose methadone. *Ann. Intern. Med*. 2002; 137: 501-4.

[111] Todaka T, Ishida T, Kita H, et al. Bioactivation of morphine in human liver: isolation and identification of morphinone, a toxic metabolite. *Biol. Pharm. Bull*. 2005; 28: 1275-80.

[112] Atici S, Cinel I, Cinel L, et al. Liver and kidney toxicity in chronic use of opioids: an experimental long term treatment model. *J. Biosci*. 2005; 30: 245-52.

[113] Zhang YT, Zheng QS, Pan J, et al. Oxidative damage of biomolecules in mouse liver induced by morphine and protected by antioxidants. *Basic Clin. Pharmacol. Toxicol*. 2004; 95: 53-8.

[114] Martucci C, Panerai AE, Sacerdote P. Chronic fentanyl or buprenorphine infusion in the mouse: similar analgesic profile but different effects on immune responses. *Pain*. 2004; 110: 385-92.

[115] Staats PS, Markowitz J, Schein J. Incidence of constipation associated with long-acting opioid therapy: a comparative study. *South Med. J*. 2004; 97: 129 – 34.

[116] Milligan K, Lanteri-Minet M, Borchert K et al. Evaluation of long-term efficacy and safety of transdermal fentanyl in the treatment of chronic noncancer pain. *J. Pain*. 2001; 2: 197 – 204.

[117] Menten J, Desmedt M, Lossignol D, Mullie A. Longitudinal follow up of TTS-fentanyl use in patients with cancer-related pain: results of a compassionate use study with special focus on elderly patients. *Curr. Med. Res. Opin.* 2002; 18: 488 – 98.

[118] Van Seventer R, Smit JM, Schipper RM, Wicks MA, Zuurmond WW. Comparison of TTS-fentanyl with sustained-release oral morphine in the treatment of patients not using opioids for mild-to-moderate pain. *Curr. Med. Res. Opin.* 2003; 19: 457 – 69.

[119] Quigley C. Hydromorphone for acute and chronic pain. *Cochrane Database Syst. Rev.* 2002; 1: CD003447.

[120] Quigley C. Opioid switching to improve pain relief and drug tolerability. *Cochrane Database Syst. Rev.* 2004; 3: CD004847.

[121] Mystakidou K, Parpa E, Tsilika E et al. Long-term management of noncancer pain with transdermal therapeutic system-fentanyl. *J. Pain.* 2003; 4: 298 – 306.

[122] Schindler SD, Ortner R, Peternell A, Eder H, Opgenoorth E, Fischer. Maintenance therapy with synthetic opioids and driving aptitude. *Eur. Addict. Res.* 2004; 10: 80 – 7.

[123] Jamison RN, Schein JR, Vallow S, Ascher S, Vorsanger GJ, Katz NP. Neuropsychological effects of long-term opioid use in chronic pain patients. *J. Pain. Symptom Manage.* 2003; 26: 913 – 21.

[124] Tassain V, Attal N, Fletcher D et al. Long term effects of oral sustained release morphine on neuropsychological performance in patients with chronic non-cancer pain. *Pain.* 2003; 389 – 400.

[125] Sabatowski R, Schwalen S, Rettig K, Herberg KW, Kasper SM, Radbruch L. Driving ability under long-term treatment with transdermal fentanyl. *J. Pain Sympt. Mange.* 2003; 25: 38 – 47.

[126] Zacny JP, Gutierrez S. Characterizing the subjective, psychomotor, and physiological effects of oral oxycodone in non-drug abusing volunteers. *Psychopharmacology.* 2003; 170: 242 – 54.

[127] Grossman A. Brain opiates and neuroendocrine function. *Clin Endocrinol. Metab.* 1983; 12: 725 – 46.

[128] Su CF, Liu MY, Li MT. Intraventricular morphine produces pain relief, hypothermia, hyperglycemia and increased prolactin and growth hormone levels in patients with cancer pain. *J. Neurol.* 1987; 235: 105 – 8.

[129] Paice JA, Penn RD, Ryan WG. Altered sexual function and decreased testosterone in patients receiving intraspinal opioids. *J. Pain Symptom Manage.* 1994; 9: 126 – 31.

[130] Abs R, Verhelst J, Maeyaert J, Van Buyten J-P, Opsomer F, Adriaensen H, Verlooy J, Van Havenbergh, Smet M, Van Acker K. Endocrine consequences of long term intrathecal administration of opioids. *J. Clin. Endocrinol. Metab.* 2000; 85: 2215 – 22.

[131] Kokko H, Hall PD, Afrin LB. Fentanyl associated syndrome of inappropriate antidiuretic hormone secretion. *Pharmacotherapy.* 2002; 22: 1188 – 92.

[132] Compton P, Athanasos P, Elashoff D. Withdrawal hyperalgesia after acute opioid physical dependency in non addicted humans: a preliminary study. *J. Pain.* 2003; 4: 511–9.

[133] De Conno F, Caraceni A, Martini C, Spoldi E, Salvetti M, Ventafridda V. Hyperalgesia and myoclonus with intrathecal infusion of high-dose morphine. *Pain.* 1991; 47: 337–9.

[134] Heger S, Maier C, Otter K, Helwig U, Suttorp M. Morphine induced allodynia in a child with brain tumour. *BMJ.* 319: 627 – 9.

[135] Parisod E, Siddall PJ, Viney M, McClelland JM, Cousins MJ. Allodynia after acute intrathecal morphine administration in a patient with neuropathic pain after spinal cord injury. *Anesth. Analg.* 2003; 97: 183 – 6.

[136] Sjogren P, Jensen N-K, Jensen TS. Disappearance of morphine induced hyperalgesia after discontinuing or substituting morphine with other opioid analgesics. *Pain.* 1994; 59: 313 – 6.

[137] Sjogren P, Jonsson T, Jensen N-K, Drenck N-E, Jensen TS. Hyperalgesia and myoclonus in terminal cancer patients treated with continuous intravenous morphine. *Pain.* 1993; 55: 93 – 7.

[138] Woolf CJ. Intrathecal high dose morphine produces hyperalgesia in the rat. *Brain Res.* 1981; 209: 491 – 5.

[139] Guignard B, Bossard AE, Coste C et al. Acute opioid tolerance: intraoperative remifentanil increases postoperative pain and morphine requirement. *Anesthesiology.* 2000; 93: 409 – 17.

[140] Hood DD, Curry R, Eisenach JC. Intravenous remifentanil produces withdrawal hyperalgesia in volunteers with capsaicin-induced hyperalgesia. *Anesth. Analg.* 2003; 97: 810 – 5.

[141] Devulder J. Hyperalgesia induced by high-dose intrathecal sufentanil in neuropathic pain. *J. Neurosurg. Anesthesiol.* 1997; 9: 146 – 8.

[142] Wang Z, Gardell LR, Ossipov MH et al. Pronociceptive actions of dynorphin maintain chronic neuropathic pain. *J. Neurosci.* 2001; 21: 1779 – 86.

[143] Vanderah TW, Gardell LR, Burgess SE, Ibrahim M, Dogrul A, Zhong C-M, Zhang E-T, Malan TP, Ossipov MH, Lai J, Porreca F. Dynorphin promotes abnormal pain and spinal opioid antinociceptive tolerance. *J. Neurosci.* 2000; 20: 7074 – 9.

[144] Vanderah TW, Ossipov MH, Lai J, Malan TP, Porreca F. Mechanisms of opioid induced pain and antinociceptive tolerance: descending facilitation and spinal dynorphin. *Pain.* 2001; 92: 5 – 9.

[145] Vanderah TW, Suenaga NM, Ossipov MH, Malan TP, Lai J, Porreca F. Tonic descending facilitation from the rostral ventromedial medulla mediates opioid induced abnormal pain and antinociceptive tolerance. *J. Neurosci.* 2001; 21: 279 - 86.

[146] Yaksh TL, Harty GJ. Pharmacology of the allodynia in rats evoked by high dose intrathecal morphine. *J. Pharmacol. Exp. Ther.* 1988; 244: 501 – 7.

*Chapter VII*

# Inflammatory Mediators in the Mechanisms of Nociception - Preclinical Studies

*Tarek A. Samad*

Neural Plasticity Research Group, Department of Anesthesia and Critical Care,
Massachusetts General Hospital, Harvard Medical School
149 13th Street, Room 4309, Boston, MA 02129

## Abstract

Multiple mechanisms control the occurrence of neural plasticity, the cellular basis of painful sensation manifested in the ability of neurons to change their function, chemical profile, or structure. The sensory inflow that is generated in primary sensory neurons by intense or noxious peripheral stimuli is transferred, via their central axons, to second order neurons in the spinal cord. The synaptic contacts between afferent central terminals and dorsal horn neurons are highly organized, both topographically, to reflect their location, and by sensory fiber type. Inflammation results in the production of a soup of cytokines, growth factors and inflammatory mediators that regulate and often alter the somatosensory system by amplifying responses and increasing sensitivity to stimuli. These inflammatory mediators act at several levels both peripherally and centrally to regulate functional and chemical properties of peripheral and central neurons. Enormous progress has been made in elucidating the molecular and cellular mechanisms for plasticity in sensory and spinal cord neurons. This has expanded our understanding of both pain mechanisms and of the mechanism of action of currently used analgesics, and more importantly will lead to the identification of new targets for novel forms of therapy.

# Introduction

Pain symptoms comprise two categories: physiological and pathological pain. Physiological pain represents an essential early alert to the presence in the environment of damaging stimuli. Pathological pain can be further divided into two groups: inflammatory pain, initiated by tissue damage/inflammation, and neuropathic pain, initiated by nervous system lesions. Both groups of pathological pain are characterized by hypersensitivity at the site of damage and in adjacent normal tissue. Pain may appear spontaneously or after a stimulus that normally does not produce pain (allodynia). Moreover, noxious stimulus may evoke greater and more prolonged pain (hyperalgesia) [1].

Inflammatory pain manifests as spontaneous pain and pain hypersensitivity. Spontaneous pain reflects direct activation of specific receptors on nociceptor terminals by inflammatory mediators. Pain hypersensitivity is the consequence of early post-translational changes, both in the peripheral terminals of the nociceptor and in spinal cord dorsal horn neurons, as well as later transcription-dependent changes in effector genes, again in primary sensory and dorsal horn neurons. Inflammatory regulates neuroplasticity via a combination of activity-dependent changes in the neurons and inflammatory mediators initiating particular signal transduction pathways. These pathways phosphorylate membrane proteins changing their function, and activate transcription factors, altering gene expression. Two distinct aspects of sensory neuron function are changed as a result of these processes, basal sensitivity, or the capacity of peripheral stimuli to evoke nociception, and stimulus-evoked hypersensitivity, the capacity of certain inputs to generate prolonged alterations in the sensitivity of the system. Transcriptional and post-translational changes potentiate the system and alter pain sensitivity.

After inflammation or nerve injury, dramatic alterations in the somatosensory system occur, amplifying responses and increasing sensitivity to peripheral stimuli resulting in the activation of pain by normally innocuous or low intensity stimuli. Clinical pain is then an expression of plasticity in the somatosensory system, operating at multiple sites via diverse mechanisms.

The contribution of sensory neurons to inflammatory pain is complex. Inflammation results in the production of a soup of cytokines, growth factors and inflammatory mediators such as interleukin-1β, nerve growth factor (NGF), bradykinin and prostanoids. Many of those elements directly activate the nociceptors by interacting with membrane receptors expressed on the peripheral afferent. These receptors activate intracellular signal pathways that converge on calcium-dependent protein kinase C (PKC) and cAMP-dependent protein kinase A (PKA). Two major targets for these kinases are the TRPV1 heat sensor and the sodium channel Nav1.8 [2]. Postranslational modification of these channels modulates their activity and therefore modulates, for example, peripheral heat hypersensitivity and excitability and responsiveness of the nociceptor. NGF, in addition to its direct sensitizing action in the peripheral terminal of the nociceptor, is retrogradely transported to the cell body in the dorsal root ganglion (DRG) where it modulates p38 and ERK MAP kinase and CREB pathways, and therefore modulates expression of genes such as substance P, CGRP, BDNF, ASIC and TRPV1 channels [4].

Enhanced signaling leads to sensitization of the nociceptor by reducing its transduction threshold. Although nociceptors are highly specialized and differentiated, their phenotype can change such that the functional and signaling capacity of the neuron alters. Tissue injury leads also to changes at the level of the spinal cord dorsal horn, including induction of new genes, sprouting of primary sensory neurons, upregulation of a variety of neurotransmitters and neuromodulators, their receptors, as well as second messenger systems. These changes cause a prolonged increase in the excitability of dorsal horn neurons leading to central sensitization.

Inflammation involves intense nociceptor activity, leading to an enhanced spinal release of various neurotransmitters, neuromodulators and trophic factors such as glutamate, substance P and BDNF. This results in the activation of ligand gated ion channels and receptors including NMDA, metabotropic glutamate, neurokinin (NK1), and tyrosine kinase B (TrkB) receptors in the dorsal horn, which in turns will activate various intracellular signal transduction pathways including PKA, PKC and ERK MAP kinase. Induction of these pathways can lead to increase in expression of the immediate early genes such as c-Fos and COX-2 (cyclooxygenase-2) and late response genes such as prodynorphin, NK1 and TrkB in dorsal horn neurons. Response elements present in the promoter region of these genes mediate their transcriptional induction in response to major intracellular signaling pathways. These activity dependent transcriptional changes in spinal cord are also accompanied by transcriptional changes in primary sensory neurons.

Moreover, and in addition to triggering activity-dependent transcriptional changes in dorsal horn neurons, several lines of evidence suggest that inflammation also generates a systemic humoral signal that acts via endothelial cells of the cerebrovascular system to induce an inflammatory response in the CNS, the proinflammatory cytokine interleukin 1 β (IL-1β) was shown to play a pivotal role in the central inflammatory cascade [5,6] There are then two forms of input from peripheral inflamed tissue to the CNS. The first is mediated by electrical activity in sensitized nerve fibers innervating the inflamed area, which signal the location of the inflamed tissue, and the onset, duration and nature of any stimulus applied to this tissue. The second is a humoral signal originating from the inflamed tissue, which acts to produce a widespread induction of inflammatory response in the CNS. Both inputs are sensitive to NSAIDs and COX-2 inhibitors as well as to opioid derived anesthetics. Other classes of drugs such as TNFα and IL-1 receptor antagonists were also shown to modulate these inputs [7, 8].

## Prostanoids in Pathological Pain

Tissue injury and inflammation are associated with increased prostanoid synthesis and pain hypersensitivity. Soon after their initial isolation, prostanoids were shown to influence inflammation and immune responses and their administration was found to reproduce the major signs of inflammation, including augmented pain sensitivity [9]. Peripheral inflammation increases prostanoid levels at the site of inflammation, and this local release contributes directly to inflammation and pain. More recently, peripheral inflammation was also shown to increase central prostanoid levels [10, 11], thus mediating more wide spread changes in pain perception, such as the sickness syndrome invloving fever, anorexia, altered mood and sleep patterns [12].

Basal levels of prostanoids are important for homeostatic functions in many tissues, particularly in the kidney, gastric mucosa and platelets [13]. In other tissues, constitutive production of prostanoid is low, but can be increased within minutes by inflammatory stimuli [13] acting on constitutively expressed prostanoid synthetic enzymes. Pro-inflammatory signals trigger multiple transcriptional and post-translational changes that alter the synthetic enzyme levels and activity, and this leads to early, massive and sustained increases in prostanoid levels [5].

Advances in our understanding of the molecular biology of the phospholipase A2, cyclooxygenase and prostaglandin synthase enzymes, as well as the development of new pharmacological tools that inhibit these enzymes, the signals that regulate them, and the prostanoid receptors through which prostanoids act, promise to rapidly expand our understanding and the treatment of clinical inflammatory pain states.

## Prostanoids Synthesis

Prostanoids derive from arachidonic acid that is liberated from phospholipids in the cell membrane by the action of phopholipase A2 enzymes (PLA2s). COX is the enzyme that catalyzes the first two reactions of the prostaglandin (PG) pathway leading to the formation of PGH2, an intermediate metabolite. Tissue-specific isomerases (prostaglandin synthases) metabolize PGH2 into the prostaglandin isoforms PGE2, PGD2 and PGF2, prostacyclin (PGI2) or thromboxane (TxA2) [14, 15], which then exert their biological actions via seven transmembrane domain, G-protein coupled receptors, classified as DP, EP, FP, IP and TP receptors according to their respective prostanoid ligand [16-19]. Differential tissue expression and induction patterns of PLA2, COX, isomerases and prostanoid receptors, play the major role in determining and modulating the cellular effects of the prostanoids.

## Cyclooxygenase

The existence of an inducible COX isoform whose expression was regulated by endogenous cytokines and glucocorticoids was long suggested, but it was not until the early 1990s when a new COX isoenzyme (COX-2) was successfully cloned [20-22]. This finding marked the beginning of a new era in the treatment of pain and inflammation. The recognition that two isoforms of cyclooxygenase exist has led to intense efforts to characterize the relative contribution of each isoform to prostanoid production in specific systems in order to develop specific antagonists that provide anti-inflammatory action with minimal side effects compared to currently used NSAIDs.

COX-1 is expressed constitutively and generally produces prostanoids in response to fine-tune physiological processes requiring instantaneous, continuous regulation (e.g. Hemostasis) [14, 21]; in contrast, COX-2 is inducible and typically produces prostanoids that mediate responses to physiological stress such as injury, infection and inflammation [14, 21]. These two cyclooxygenase isoforms reveal a differential gene expression profile, distinct kinetic properties and subcellular compartmentation and interactions with phospholipases and synthases [13, 23].

The general consensus is that COX-1 is present in many cell types and is constitutively expressed, whereas COX-2 is induced as an immediate early gene and is strongly regulated at both transcriptional and translational levels [21]. It is important to note that COX-1 expression could be induced in stress conditions such as nerve injury while the constitutive expression of COX-2 in many tissues including the central nervous system and the kidney is well established.

Regulation of COX-2 messenger RNA has been shown to represent a key mechanism for control of COX-2 levels. Since its discovery, COX-2 expression has shown to be induced by numerous factors including neurotransmitters, growth factors, proinflammatory cytokines, lipopolysaccharide, calcium, phorbol esters and small peptide hormones [21].

The anti-inflammatory and analgesic benefits of NSAIDs have been proposed to derive from inhibition of COX-2 isoform induced at the site of injury/inflammation. Prostanoids contribute to the development of peripheral sensitization by acting on sensory nerve terminals by contributing to protein kinase-mediated phosphorylation of sodium channels in nociceptor terminals, increasing excitability, reducing the pain threshold and potentiating action of pain producing molecules such as bradykinin. The new knowledge about the functional properties of COX-1 and COX-2 has had a major impact in the last decade on the development of compounds that specifically target and inhibit COX-2 activity while sparing COX-1 at therapeutic doses. COX-2 specific inhibition would alleviate pain and inflammation without disrupting the homeostatic functions mediated by COX-1-derived prostanoids, suggesting that many of the deleterious side effects of conventional NSAIDs, which cannot distinguish between COX-1 and COX-2 isoforms could be avoided.

## Peripheral and Central Induction of COX-2

Inflammatory diseases such as rheumatoid arthritis are characterized by an exudative and proliferative inflammatory response that is accompanied by spontaneous pain and excessive pain sensitivity, movement of a joint within a normal range becomes painful and there are systemic changes in mood and behavior that constitute the sickness syndrome.

Marked increases in PLA2 and COX-2 expression occur at the site of local inflammation, and the original hypothesis for the mechanism of action of NSAIDs formulated by John Vane in his Nobel prize winning work, was that they inhibited prostanoid production in the periphery preventing a sensitizing action of PGE$_2$ on the peripheral terminals of sensory fibers. More recently, peripheral inflammation has been shown also to induce a widespread increase in COX-2 and prostaglandin E synthase (PGES) expression in CNS. The proinflammatory cytokine IL-1β is upregulated at the site of inflammation and plays the major role in inducing COX-2 in local inflammatory cells by activating the transcription factor NFκB. IL-1β is also responsible for the induction of COX-2 in the CNS in response to peripheral inflammation, but this interestingly is not the consequence either of neural activity arising from the sensory fibers innervating the inflamed tissue, or of systemic IL-1β in the plasma. Instead, peripheral inflammation produces some other signal molecule that enters the circulation, crosses the blood brain barrier and acts to elevate IL-1β, leading to COX-2 expression in neurons and non-neuronal cells in many different areas of the spinal cord [6]. An elevation of COX-2 also occurs at many levels in the brain, mainly in the endothelial cells of the brain vasculature [24].

Inflammatory mediators including prostanoids contribute to the development of pain by acting both in the periphery and in the central nervous system. Peripherally, they increase the sensitivity of nociceptors and facilitate the establishment of peripheral sensitization, thereby reducing the pain threshold and potentiating the action of painful mechanical and thermal stimuli or irritant molecules such as bradykinin [5]. Centrally, inflammatory mediators increase excitability in pain transmission neuronal pathways in the spinal cord by altering the release of neurotransmitters and neuromodulators from central terminals of pain fibers and from dorsal horn neurons and the activity of their respective receptors and transporters in the spinal cord [4]. The time course of increase in prostanoid levels corresponds well with the development of allodynia and hyperalgesia in animal models of peripheral inflammation, moreover pharmacologic analysis and nociceptive behavior studies using NSAIDs and COX-2 inhibitors has shown the involvement of both peripheral and central prostanoids in inflammatory pain hypersensitivity [25, 26]. Using different animal models of peripheral inflammation using different inflammatory agents such as formalin, CFA, carrageenan, and zymosan, peripheral and central prostanoids have been shown to contribute to both mechanical and thermal pain hypersensitivity [25]. The induction of COX-2 expression is more widespread than the spinal projection of the inflamed tissue, in neuronal and non-neuronal cells of the central nervous system, has been shown to occur primarily as a response to interleukins [6]. Inhibition of prostanoid production by prevention of COX-2 gene induction via inhibition of production/action or signaling of peripheral and central cytokines represents a future prospect for therapeutic intervention in inflammatory pain. The activated cytokine cascade such as IL-1β and IL-6 could be inhibited using enzyme inhibitors, neutralizing agents, or receptor antagonists [6]. This approach, unlike the use of COX-2 and COX-1/COX-2 inhibitors, should leave constitutive activity of COX-2 and COX-1 intact, and by preventing the production of other effector molecules that participate in the prostanoid synthesis casacade such as PGES, will lead to better inhibition of prostanoid levels.

# References

[1] Woolf CJ, Mannion RJ: Neuropathic pain: aetiology, symptoms, mechanisms, and management. *Lancet.* 1999, 353:1959-64.

[2] Lee SY, Lee JH, Kang KK, Hwang SY, Choi KD, Oh U. Sensitization of vanilloid receptor involves an increase in the phosphorylated form of the channel. *Arch. Pharm. Res.* 2005 Apr;28(4):405-12.

[3] Vijayaragavan K, Boutjdir M, Chahine M. Modulation of Nav1.7 and Nav1.8 peripheral nerve sodium channels by protein kinase A and protein kinase C. *J. Neurophysiol.* 2004 Apr;91(4):1556-69.

[4] M. Costigan, J. Scholz, T. A. Samad, and C. J. Woolf. Pain. In: Siegel G.J., Albers R.W., Brady S.T., Price D.L., editors. *Basic Neurochemistry*, Seventh Edition.

Amsterdam, Boston, Heidelberg, London, New York, Oxford, Paris, San Diego, San Francisco, Singapore, Sydney, Tokyo. Elsevier, Academic Press, 2006. p. 927-937.

[5] Samad, T.A., Sapirstein, A, and Woolf, C.J. (2002) Prostanoids and pain: unraveling mechanisms and revealing therapeutic targets. *Trends Mol. Med.* 2002 Aug;8(8):390.

[6] Samad, T.A., *et al.* (2001) Interleukin-1beta-mediated induction of Cox-2 in the CNS contributes to inflammathory pain hypersensitivity. *Nature* 410, 471-475.

[7] Yocum D. Effective use of TNF antagonists. *Arthritis Res. Ther.* 2004;6 Suppl 2:S24-30.

[8] Furst DE. Anakinra: review of recombinant human interleukin-I receptor antagonist in the treatment of rheumatoid arthritis. *Clin. Ther.* 2004 Dec;26(12):1960-75.

[9] Tilley, S.L., Coffman, T.M., and Koller, B.H. (2001) Mixed messages: modulation of inflammation and immune responses by prostaglandins and thromboxanes. *J. Clin. Invest.* 108(1), 15-23.

[10] Dirig, D.M., and Yaksh, T.L. (1999) Spinal synthesis and release of prostanoids after peripheral injury and inflammation. *Adv. Exp. Med. Biol.* 469, 401-8.

[11] Vanegas, H., and Schaible, H. (2001) Prostaglandins and cycloxygenases in the spinal cord. *Prog.Neurobiol.* 64, 327-363.

[12] Dantzer, R. *et al.* (1998) Molecular basis of sickness behavior. *Ann. NY Acad. Sci.* 856, 132-138.

[13] Funk, C.D. (2001) Prostaglandins and leukotrienes: advances in eicosanoid biology. *Science* 294(5548), 1871-5.

[14] Smith, W.L., Dewitt D.L., and Garavito, R.M. (2000) Cyclooxygenases: structural, cellular, and molecular biology. *Annu.Rev.Biochem.* 69, 145-182.

[15] Garavito, R.M., and Dewitt, D.L. (1999) The cyclooxygenase isoforms: structural insights into the conversion of arachidonic acid to prostaglandins. *Biochim.Biophys.Acta* 1441, 278-287.

[16] Minami, T. *et al.* (2001) Characterization of EP receptor subtypes responsible for prostaglandin E2-induced pain responses by use of EP1 and EP3 receptor knockout mice. *Br.J.Pharmacol.* 133, 438-444.

[17] Narumiya, S., Sugimoto, Y., and Ushikubi, F. (1999) Prostanoid receptors: structures, properties, and functions. *Physiol. Rev.* 79, 1193-1226.

[18] Sugimoto, Y., Narumiya, S., and Ichikawa, A. (2000) Distribution and function of prostanoid receptors: studies from knockout mice. *Prog.Lipid. Res.* 39, 289-314.

[19] Breyer, R.M. *et al.* (2001) Prostanoid receptors: subtypes and signaling. *Annu.Rev.Pharmacol.Toxicol.* 41, 661-690.

[20] Herschman HR, Fletcher BS, Kujubu DA: TIS10, a mitogen-inducible glucocorticoid-inhibited gene that encodes a second prostaglandin synthase/cyclooxygenase enzyme. *J.Lipid. Mediat.* 1993, 6:89-99.

[21] O'Banion MK, Sadowski HB, Winn V, Young DA: A serum- and glucocorticoid-regulated 4-kilobase mRNA encodes a cyclooxygenase-related protein. *J.Biol.Chem.* 1991, 266:23261-23267.

[22] Xie WL, Chipman JG, Robertson DL, Erikson RL, Simmons DL: Expression of a mitogen-responsive gene encoding prostaglandin synthase is regulated by mRNA splicing. *Proc.Natl.Acad.Sci.U.S.A*,1991,88:2692-2696.

[23] Fitzpatrick FA, Soberman R: Regulated formation of eicosanoids. *J.Clin.Invest* 2001, 107:1347-1351.
[24] Laflamme, N., Lacroix, S., and Rivest, S. (2001) Effects of selective COX-1 and -2 inhibition on formalin-evoked nociceptive behaviour and prostaglandin E(2) release in the spinal cord. *J. Neurochem.* 79(4):777-86.
[25] T.A. Samad, S. Abdi. Cyclooxygenase-2 and antagonists in pain management. *Current Opinion in Anaesthesiology,* 2001, 14, 527-532.
[26] Warner TD, Mitchell JA. Cyclooxygenases: new forms, new inhibitors, and lessons from the clinic. *FASEB J.* 2004 May;18(7):790-804.

*Chapter VIII*

# Antiinflammatory Medications in Pain Management

*Ezekiel Fink and Gary J. Brenner*
Department of Anesthesia and Critical Care,
Massachusetts General Hospital, 55 Fruit Street, Boston, MA 02114

## Abstract

The non steroidal anti-inflammatory drugs (NSAIDs) comprise a large group of commonly used analgesics that are employed in the treatment of a variety of pain complaints. The analgesic properties and side effects of the NSAIDs are largely due to the inhibition of peripheral and central prostaglandin synthesis via the blockade of the enzyme cyclooxygenase (COX). Recent research suggests that the efficacy of the NSAIDs in treating osteoarthritis, low back pain, and migraines may be due to the role the COX cascade plays in the pathophysiology of these conditions.

## Introduction

The medicinal properties of acetylsalicylate were observed in *1763* by the clergyman Edmund Stone. He found that dried willow bark helped treat "agues" or fevers of those living in the damp areas of his hometown of Chipping Norton, England. In 1971, over two centuries later, John Vane identified the mechanism of action of aspirin for the first time, well after it had become one of the most widely used medications in the world [1]. In 1991 the COX-2 gene was cloned. The selective COX-2 inhibitors were developed shortly thereafter and were heralded as the next wonder drug. The evolution of the non-steroidal anti-inflammatory drugs (NSAIDs) juxtaposes great scientific achievement with lessons in humility on limits of human understanding of the molecular universe. In this chapter we will review the clinical applications of NSAIDs as they relate to pain management.

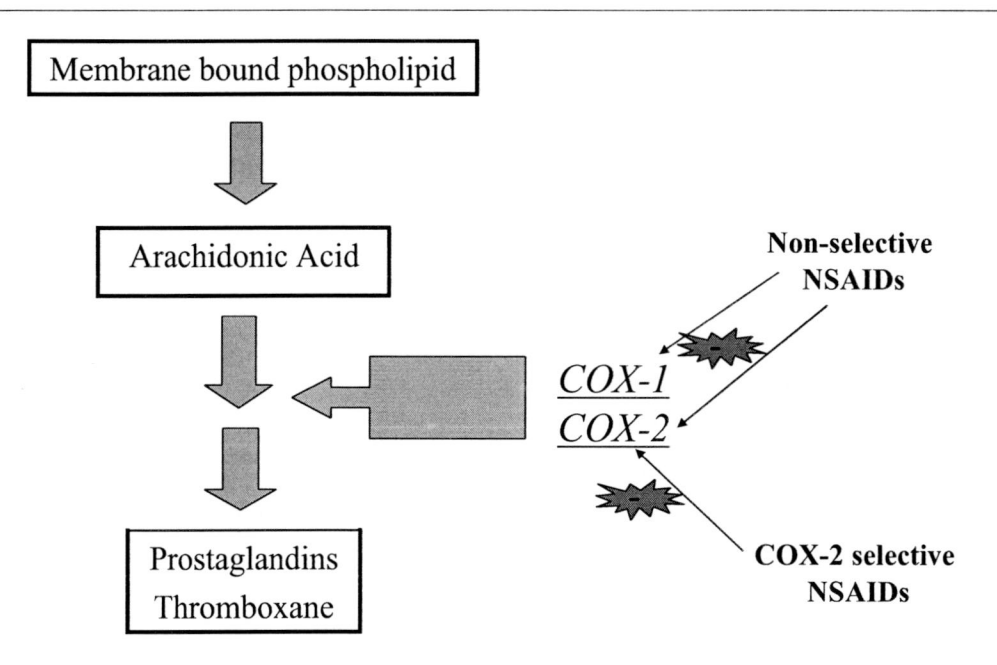

Figure 1. NSAIDs inhibit the cyclooxygenase cascade

| NON-SELECTIVE COX INHIBITORS | *Anthranilic acids (fenamates)* |
| --- | --- |
| |     Mefenamic acid |
| *Salicylic acid derivatives* |     Meclofenamic acid |
|     Aspirin | *Alkanones* |
|     Sodium salicylate |     Nabumetone |
|     Choline magnesium | |
| *Trisalicylate* | |
|     Salsalate | |
|     Diflunisal | SELECTIVE COX-2 INHIBITORS |
|     Sulfasalazine | |
|     Osalazine | *Coxibs* |
| *Para-aminophenol derivatives* |     Rofecoxib |
|     Acetaminophen |     Celecoxib |
| *Indole and indene acetic acid* |     Valdecoxib |
|     Indomethacin | *Enolic acid* |
|     Sulindac |     Piroxicam |
| *Heteroaryl acetic acid* |     Meloxicam |
|     Tolmetin | *Indole acetic acid* |
|     Diclofenac |     Etodolac |
|     Ketorolac | *Sulfonanilides* |
| *Arylpropionic acids* |     Nimesulide |
|     Ibuprofen | |
|     Naproxen | |
|     Flurbiprofen | |
|     Ketoprofen | |
|     Fenoprofen | |
|     Oxaprozin | |

Figure 2. Classes of COX inhibitor drugs

## Mechanisms of Action

The analgesic property of aspirin and other NSAIDs is largely due to the inhibition of peripheral and central prostaglandin synthesis via the blockade of the enzyme cyclooxygenase (COX) (Figure 1). NSAIDs are also thought to prevent cytokine-induced hyperalgesia via inhibition of the release of tumor necrosis factor-alpha (TNF-α). There are two classes of NSAIDs (Figure 2). The older, non-selective NSAIDs, also known as traditional NSAIDs, inhibit both COX-1 and COX-2. The newer selective NSAIDS specifically target COX-2 and were developed to treat pain and inflammation while reducing the risk of the serious gastrointestinal side effects seen with the nonselective nonsteroidal anti-inflammatory drugs.

On a molecular level, both types of NSAIDs inhibit COX-1 and COX-2 to variable degrees (Figure 3).

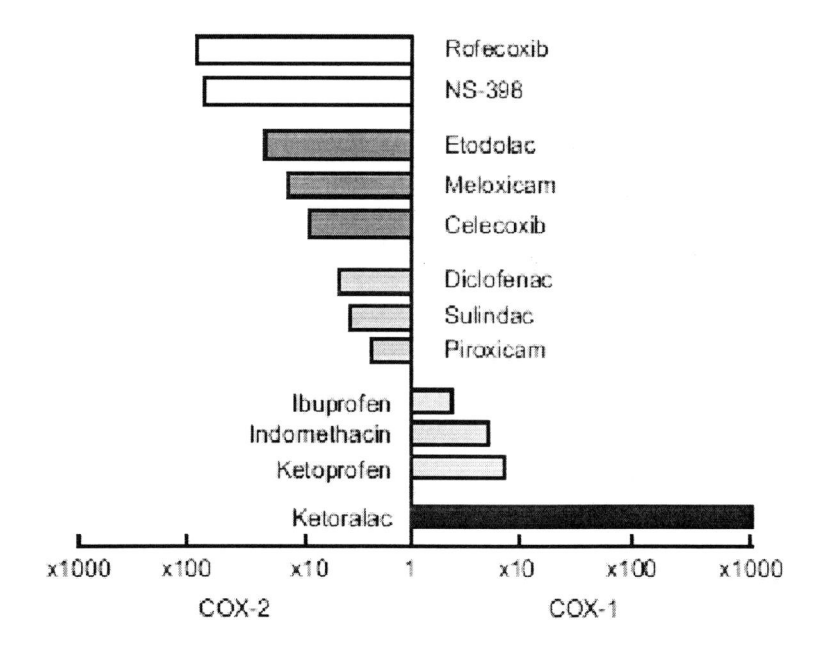

Figure 3. Selectivity of the various NSAIDs COX isoform inhibition (Reprinted with permission from Hawkey CJ. Best Pract Res Clin Gastroenterol. 200;15(5):801-20. which was derived from Warner TD, Giuliano F, Vojnovic I, Bukasa A, Mitchell JA, Vane JR. Nonsteroid drug selectivities for cyclo-oxygenase-1 rather than cyclo-oxygenase-2 are associated with human gastrointestinal toxicity: a full in vitro analysis. Proc Natl Acad Sci U S A. 1999;96(13):7563-8.)

Cyclooxygenases are a group of bi-functional enzymes that mediate the cascade of prostanoids, a class of proteins that are formed by most cells and act as autocrine and paracrine mediators of inflammation and sensitivity to pain, among other functions. A variety of stimuli – trauma, cytokines, etc. – can cause a cell's outer membrane to synthesize arachidonic acid, which is converted by COX enzymes into precursors of several prostanoids. The products of the COX cascade were first thought to be a product of the prostate gland (thus named *pros*tanoids) and they are synthesized in all vertebrate tissues. Prostanoid isomers act on G-protein coupled cell-surface receptors and have short half-lives [2].

Cyclooxygenase has two isoforms, COX-1 and COX-2. COX-1 is constitutively expressed at far higher levels in most cells than COX-2, which is induced in a variety of tissues following injury. Nonetheless, COX-1 does play a role in modulating peripheral inflammatory responses. The expression of COX-2 increases dramatically in the central nervous system (CNS) following injury and is also a major mediator of the inflammatory response. Modulation of both COX-1 and COX-2 genes are thought to play a role in a wide range of normal and pathophysiological conditions [3].

COX-2 is the isoform more highly expressed in the cervical and lumbar spinal cord, primarily in neurons of laminae II-III, motor neurons of lamina IX and in glial cells, though both COX isoforms are constitutively present in the CNS [4]. CNS COX-2 is upregulated in the CNS with both central and peripheral injury. CNS prostaglandins play an important role in nociceptive processing and hyperalgesia [5] and there is evidence that agents that inhibit prostaglandin synthesis prevent or reverse pain states [6].

## Adverse Events

Non-selective NSAIDs are associated with a variety of adverse effects. Compared with the selective inhibitors, there are increased risks of GI complications, such as bleeding and perforation, especially if patients are over age 65, have a history of peptic ulcer disease or upper gastrointestinal bleeding, and are using corticosteroids or anticoagulants. There may be an increase in GI complications with smoking and alcohol consumption. Non-selective NSAIDs also increase the risk of nephrotoxicity, including hypertension and renal insufficency, in patients with intrinsic kidney disease or hypertension, or with the use of a diuretic or ACE inhibitor [7].

The selective COX-2 inhibitors appear to have several advantages over the non-selective NSAIDs. COX-2 inhibitors are thought to cause less gastrointestinal irritation because, unlike the non-selective NSAIDs, they do not cause inhibition of either the COX-1 derived gastroprotective prostaglandins or platelet COX-1 derived thromboxane A2. Subsequent investigation has shown that COX-2 plays a role in resolving mucosal inflammation and ulcer healing in the gastrointestinal tract [8] and clinical trials largely support an improved GI profile with the selective COX-2 inhibitors. A meta-analysis of all 8 double blind, randomized phase 2b/3 rofecoxib osteoarthritis trials conducted from December 1996 through March 1998 demonstrated a lower incidence of GI bleeding with COX-2 inhibitors versus traditional NSAIDS. This analysis indicated that treatment with rofecoxib was associated with a significantly lower incidence of upper GI bleeding incidents than treatment with traditional NSAIDs [9]. These results were supported by another large study [10] but not all studies have found a significant difference between COX-2 and non-selective NSAIDs in GI toxicity [11]. A recent meta-analysis of 31 randomized controlled trials to investigate the adverse events seen with the COX-2 inhibitor celecoxib confirmed that there were less GI ulcers, bleeding events, and less GI upset than with traditional NSAIDs [12]. The COX-2 inhibitors do cause renal toxicity [7] and have been shown to raise blood pressure [8].

The COX-2 inhibitors are now thought to increase the risk of thrombotic events, including myocardial infarction and stroke. In the Vioxx Gastrointestinal Outcome Research

(VIGOR) study, which compared rofecoxib and naproxen, a five-fold increase in the number of myocardial infarctions was found in the rofecoxib group [10]. There were several follow-up studies, including the Celecoxib Long-term Arthritis Safety Study (CLASS), that did not support the VIGOR study results, perhaps due to methodological inconsistencies [11, 13]. The Adenomatous Polyp Prevention on Vioxx (APPROVe) study found that out of 2586 randomized into a rofecoxib treatment group and placebo, a total of 46 patients in the rofecoxib group had a confirmed thrombotic event (myocardial infarctions and ischemic cerebrovascular events) as compared with 26 patients in the placebo group after 18 months [14]. The APPROVe study led to the withdrawal of rofecoxib from the market. Randomized controlled trials demonstrated similar risks for thrombotic events with the other coxibs, despite their structurally distinct nature. In retrospect, the difficulties with these medications may have been due to the duration of the clinical studies and the small sizes of the study prior to approval. COX-2 dependent formation of prostaglandin I2 is felt to be the mechanism responsible for the prothrombotic state. There are no placebo controlled randomized controlled trials to determine the cardiovascular safety of traditional NSAIDs. There is some evidence to suggest that certain traditional NSAIDs, including ibuprofen and naproxen, may undermine the cardioprotective effect of aspirin [8].

# NSAID Use in Three Common Pain States

## Osteoarthritis

Joint pain caused by osteoarthritis is one of the most common complaints in the adult population. Osteoarthritis is an age related disease characterized by degeneration of multiple synovial joints, usually in the hands, spine, hips, and knees. Gross examination of the joints reveals focal areas of damage to cartilage that disproportionately affects the load bearing areas. Other gross pathological findings include new bone formation at the joint margins, changes in the subchondral bone, variable degrees of mild synovitis, and thickening of the joint capsule [15].

Within a synovial joint, most structures (bone, periosteum, synovium, ligaments, and the joint capsule) are richly innervated. Cartilage is not innervated and therefore cannot be the primary source of perception of arthritic joint pain [16]. Furthermore, recent studies have suggested that radiographic evidence of joint damage is associated with increased probability of joint pain, but the extent of damage does not necessarily correlate with the severity of pain [17]. Damage to other structures that comprise the joint may play a larger role in producing pain. A correlation has been found between pain and both synovitis and subchondral bone changes seen on radiography, suggesting that these two tissues could be sources of pain in osteoarthritis [18]

Recent research suggests that joint destruction in OA has a significant inflammatory component and alterations in the COX cascade play an important role in the disease etiology. Prostaglandin-E2 (PGE2) regulates interleukin-1 beta (IL-1B) stimulated human synovial fibroblasts to produce interleukin-6, interleukin-8, interleukin-11, macrophage colony stimulating factor, and vascular endothelial growth factor, all chemical mediators of the inflammatory response and joint destruction [19]. One of the mechanisms of degradation of cartilage proteoglycan is through induction of IL-1 by COX –2 derived synovial PGE2 [20]. COX-2 derived prostanoids have been found to mediate apoptosis in human synovial fibroblasts [21]. Leukotrienes (COX products) are thought to mediate the increase of expression of collagenases and the decrease of chondrocyte repair of cartilage by increasing the expression of the cytokines tumor necrosis factor (TNF) and IL-1. Leukotrienes have been directly implicated in causing bone resorption in the joint space as well [22].

Current understanding of the pathophysiology of OA would suggest that NSAIDs target essential components of the destructive pathway, however, many of the molecular effects of the medication are poorly understood. Ibuprofen and other NSAIDs routinely used for the treatment of OA have been shown to double the amount of synovial collagenases released by cells while aspirin does not. It appears that the presence of prostaglandin E, which is produced by the COX cascade, may prohibit the cytokine-induced upregulation of certain collagenase [23]. Furthermore, both selective and non-selective COX inhibitors cause the upregulation of leukotrienes due to shunting of the lipoxygenase pathway; the effects of this on cartilage remains to be determined.

COX levels are the major current indicator used to assess NSAID activity. The NSAIDs, however, regulate the function of many other genes [24]. Some animal studies have suggested that use of NSAIDs may accelerate disease progression in OA. In vivo studies in dogs have demonstrated that some of the NSAIDs suppress proteoglycan biosynthesis in normal and degenerating articular cartilage [25]. Recent evidence suggests that NSAIDs are not disease modifying in OA because they fail to inhibit the COX enzyme hydroperoxidase dependent free radical formation. It is hypothesized that this may lead to tissue destruction [8]. The clinical implications of the full biological effects of NSAIDs are unclear.

One major clinical trial implicates non-selective COX inhibitors as a cause of progression of OA. A randomized controlled trial compared indomethacin with placebo and tiaprofenic acid with placebo in treating OA of the knee by following the rate of radiographic progression of OA of the knees. 376 of the 812 enrolled patients (46%) completed at least one year of study and were included in the results. More than twice as many patients showed radiographic deterioration in the indomethacin group as in the placebo group, thus the study was ended early. No statistically significant difference was found in disease progression between tiaprofenic acid and placebo [26].

NSAIDs have been prescribed for OA for over 30 years and there are many years of literature support for efficacy of all NSAIDs for short-term management of OA pain. There is good evidence for the efficacy of non-selective NSAIDs compared to both placebo and acetaminophen in patients with OA. However, there is no consistent evidence suggesting that one non-selective NSAID is the most efficacious in treating OA. Review of topical NSAIDs has also demonstrated efficacy in patients with OA but no trials have compared the oral and topical route [7]. The COX-2 inhibitors have shown similar efficacy to non-selective NSAIDs in treating OA [27].

The support in the literature for long-term NSAIDs use in OA is not ubiquitous. A meta-analysis of 23 randomized controlled trials that examined the efficacy of all NSAIDs (non-selective and COX-2 inhibitors) in treating knee OA found that NSAIDs work slightly better than placebo for short term pain relief (15.6% better than placebo on visual analogue scale for 2-13 weeks) but long-term use could not be supported because of the significant adverse events [28]. The amount of improvement found in this study may not justify the use of NSAIDs in a chronic pain population, as chronic pain patients have reported that a pain reduction of 30% is considered meaningful [29]. There are a number of other of individual trials and meta-analysis that find NSAIDs to be less efficacious than acetaminophen or comparable to placebo in short term treatment of OA [30].

It is important to note that many of the clinical trials that have assessed the efficacy of NSAIDs in OA have high dropout rates due to either lack of efficacy or adverse events. Thus, these data must be interpreted with caution.

## Low Back Pain

Low back pain is one of the most common complaints seen in medical practice and effects up to 80% of adults at some time in their lives. The majority of therapies for low back pain remain unsubstantiated by clinical trials. This may be because low back pain encompasses a heterogeneous group of syndromes with different underlying etiologies.

Low back pain is a complex clinical problem that may be categorized by the duration of symptoms. Acute back pain has been defined as lasting no more than several weeks and usually recovers spontaneously. Persistent/chronic back pain lasts longer than 3-6 months. Many of the individuals with persistent/chronic back pain have high levels of pain, exaggerated pain behaviors, other psychological disturbances, and accompanying disability. While psychological symptoms certainly contribute to the back pain complaint, it is rarely the case that back pain is due exclusively to psychological causes. It is not uncommon for back pain to be present with no readily identifiable cause, and a large segment of the population has spine pathology but is essentially asymptomatic [31].

There are multiple structural causes of low back pain including lumbar disc disease, root compression and inflammation, facet joint arthropathy, and sacroiliac joint dysfunction. The COX cascade has been shown to be involved in the inflammatory processes associated with many of these lumbar spinal pathologies. The culture media from the herniated lumbar discs from humans showed increased levels of prostaglandin E2, in addition to other eicosanoids, when compared with the control discs [32]. Further, cells from humans herniated lumbar discs express mRNA for COX-2, IL-1 beta and TNF alpha following in vitro cytokines stimulation, and PGE2 production is suppressed by a selective inhibitor of COX-2 in these cells [33]. Herniated disc material and facet joint bone and cartilage from patients requiring fusion surgery have been found to contain high prostaglandin levels [34]. Cytokines also play an important role in the initiation and maintenance of back pain. Recent studies have identified interleukins and tumor necrosis factor in herniated discs and degenerating facet joints [35, 36]. In addition, there are numerous other spinal and spine-associated (ligaments, nerves, vessels, and muscle) structures whose contribution to low back pain is poorly understood.

NSAIDs are widely used to treat low back pain - both for their analgesic and anti-inflammatory properties. In a randomized, controlled trial the efficacy of nimesulide, a COX-2 inhibitor, was compared with ibuprofen in 104 patients with acute low back pain. There was a comparable improvement in all measured parameters of the pain and back function parameters measured from the third day of treatment onward in both groups [37]. A meta-analysis of 51 RCT's and double blind control trials found that all NSAIDs are effective for short term symptomatic relief in acute low back pain and no specific NSAID, non-selective or COX-2 inhibitor, is clearly more effective than any other [38]. There is similar literature support for the use of NSAIDs in treatment of chronic low back pain [39], however evidence of efficacy and safety with long-term use of NSAIDs is still lacking.

## Migraine Headache

Migraine is a common episodic headache disorder that affects approximately 8% of men and 25% of woman. In 1988, the International Headache Society defined diagnostic criteria for migraine and differentiated between migraine with aura and migraine without aura. Moderate to severe pulsatile pain that affects one side of the head and lasts for 4 – 72 hours characterizes migraine headaches. Nausea, vomiting, photophobia, and phonophobia often accompany the headaches. In at least 30% of patients, the headaches are preceded by an aura, which is a transient neurological symptom that most frequently affects the vision [40].

The development of a migraine headache is thought to be as a result of activation of the nociceptive sensory afferent fibers from the ophthalmic division of the trigeminal nerve that are restricted to the meningeal blood vessels. Activation of these nociceptive fibers leads to the activation of the second order neurons in the trigeminocervical complex, which ultimately leads to peripheral and then central sensitization. This sensitization is thought to be required for generating and maintaining migraine pain [40, 41]. The prevailing former explanation for the pathophysiology of migraines was thought to be vasospasm leading to mechanical excitation of cranial vessel sensory fibers ("vascular theory"). Recent evidence has shown that there is no change in blood flow velocity in cranial vessels during migraine attacks and a consistent relationship between vessel caliber, cerebral blood flow, and headache has not been established [42].

Migraine is now considered a neurovascular pain syndrome in which there is abnormal neuronal excitability in the brain parenchyma and peripheral sensitization of the trigeminal vascular system. This encompasses the idea the cortical spreading depression (CDS) as the cause of visual aura [43]. Emerging evidence in this new model for migraine supports neurogenic inflammation within cephalic tissue as an important mechanism in the development of head pain in migraine. This inflammation causes activation of meningeal afferents, release of neuropeptides, vasodilation, and extravasation of plasma proteins. The resultant ions and inflammatory agents act upon the sensory fibers innervating the meninges, activating and sensitizing peripheral nociceptors which leads to head pain [44]. The source of the inflammatory agents is unclear, but may come from parenchymal or meningeal tissue, or blood. Exogenous precipitants in the air, food, and medications may activate similar pathways in a susceptible individual [42].

There is some evidence that implicates products of the COX cascade in the pathogenesis of migraine headaches. Electrical or inflammation mediated stimulation of rat trigeminal ganglia in vitro causes release of prostaglandin E2 from the dura mater. Levels of prostaglandin E2 are elevated in the plasma, saliva, and venous blood in patients during migraine attacks. Administration of pro-inflammatory prostaglandins causes migrainous symptoms in migraineurs. Also, the established efficacy of the NSAIDs for migraine headaches is relevant in establishing the pathophysiology of migraine headaches. A possible mechanism of the COX-2 selective agents involves suppression of the central sensitization associated with migraine [50]. The cytokines also may play a role in mediating migraine pain. Cytokines and their receptors are nearly ubiquitously found in the CNS and have been shown to play a role in the development (and reduction) of hyperalgesia and the hypersensitivity of primary afferents that leads to inflammation [42].

A substantial body of data supports the acute treatment of migraine headaches with NSAIDs. In 1999, a placebo controlled randomized controlled study that compared acetylsalicylate and sumatriptan for treatment of acute migraine attacks found that both treatments were highly effective compared to placebo ($p < 0.0001$) in decreasing headache from severe or moderate to mild or none. Sumatriptan showed a significantly ($p = 0.001$) better initial response (91.2%) compared to the NSAID response (73.9%), but the NSAID was significantly better tolerated (7.6%) than sumatriptan (37.8%). There was no significant difference between treatment groups in recurrence of headache in responders within 24 h (18.2% L-ASA, 23.1% sumatriptan, 20% placebo) and improvement of accompanying symptoms (nausea, vomiting; photophobia, phonophobia, and visual disturbances) [45]. Furthermore, ibuprofen, ketoprofen and aspirin have all been found to be two to threefold more effective than placebo in randomized controlled trials examining efficacy in treating migraine headaches [46-48]. COX-2 inhibitors have been found to be equally efficacious to non-selective NSAIDs in treating acute migraine attacks [49]. These results are encouraging as population based studies estimate that up to 57% of migraineurs take exclusively over the counter NSAIDs for migraine treatment [51].

## Conclusion

NSAIDs comprise a large group of commonly used analgesics that are employed in the treatment of a variety of pain complaints. The recent generally unexpected demonstration of increased risk for thrombotic events with COX-2 inhibitors underscores that we do not yet have a complete understanding of the full biologic effects or clinical implications of the NSAIDs. A better understanding of the molecular mechanisms underlying both physiological and pathophysiological pain would also aid in understanding the efficacy and limitations of cyclooxygenase inhibition.

## References

[1] Cronstein BN. Cyclooxygenase-2-selective inhibitors: translating pharmacology into clinical utility. *Cleve. Clin. J. Med.* 2002;69 Suppl 1:SI13-9.
[2] Chandrasekharan NV, Simmons DL. The cyclooxygenases. *Genome Biol.* 2004;5(9):241.

[3] Burian M, Geisslinger G. COX-dependent mechanisms involved in the antinociceptive action of NSAIDs at central and peripheral sites. *Pharmacol. Ther.* 2005 Aug;107(2):139-54.

[4] Beiche F, Klein T, Nusing R, Neuhuber W, Goppelt-Struebe M. Expression of cyclooxygenase isoforms in the rat spinal cord and their regulation during adjuvant-induced arthritis. *Inflamm. Res.* 1998 Dec;47(12):482-7.

[5] Scheuren N, Neupert W, Ionac M, Neuhuber W, Brune K, Geisslinger G.Peripheral noxious stimulation releases spinal PGE2 during the first phase in the formalin assay of the rat. *Life Sci.* 1997;60(21):PL 295-300.

[6] Dirig DM, Isakson PC, Yaksh TL. Effect of COX-1 and COX-2 inhibition on induction and maintenance of carrageenan-evoked thermal hyperalgesia in rats. *J. Pharmacol. Exp. Ther.* 1998 Jun;285(3):1031-8.

[7] Hochberg MC, Dougados M. Pharmacological therapy of osteoarthritis. *Best Pract. Res. Clin. Rheumatol.* 2001 Oct;15(4):583-93.

[8] Grosser T, Fries S, FitzGerald GA. Biological basis for the cardiovascular consequences of COX-2 inhibition: therapeutic challenges and opportunities. *J. Clin. Invest.* 2006 Jan;116(1):4-15.

[9] Langman MJ, Jensen DM, Watson DJ, Harper SE, Zhao PL, Quan H, Bolognese JA, Simon TJ.Adverse upper gastrointestinal effects of rofecoxib compared with NSAIDs. *JAMA.* 1999 Nov 24;282(20):1929-33.

[10] Bombardier C, Laine L, Reicin A, Shapiro D, Burgos-Vargas R, Davis B, Day R, Ferraz MB, Hawkey CJ, Hochberg MC, Kvien TK, Schnitzer TJ; VIGOR Study Group.Comparison of upper gastrointestinal toxicity of rofecoxib and naproxen in patients with rheumatoid arthritis. VIGOR Study Group. *N. Engl. J. Med.* 2000 Nov 23;343(21):1520-8, 2 p following 1528.

[11] Silverstein FE, Faich G, Goldstein JL, Simon LS, Pincus T, Whelton A, Makuch R, Eisen G, Agrawal NM, Stenson WF, Burr AM, Zhao WW, Kent JD, Lefkowith JB, Verburg KM, Geis GS. Gastrointestinal toxicity with celecoxib vs nonsteroidal anti-inflammatory drugs for osteoarthritis and rheumatoid arthritis: the CLASS study: A randomized controlled trial. Celecoxib Long-term Arthritis Safety Study. *JAMA.* 2000 Sep 13;284(10):1247-55.

[12] Moore RA, Derry S, Makinson GT, McQuay HJ. Tolerability and adverse events in clinical trials of celecoxib in osteoarthritis and rheumatoid arthritis: systematic review and meta-analysis of information from company clinical trial reports. *Arthritis Res. Ther.* 2005;7(3):R644-65.

[13] Ray WA, Stein CM, Daugherty JR, Hall K, Arbogast PG, Griffin MR. COX-2 selective non-steroidal anti-inflammatory drugs and risk of serious coronary heart disease. *Lancet.* 2002 Oct 5;360(9339):1071-3.

[14] Bresalier RS, Sandler RS, Quan H, Bolognese JA, Oxenius B, Horgan K, Lines C, Riddell R, Morton D, Lanas A, Konstam MA, Baron JA; Adenomatous Polyp Prevention on Vioxx (APPROVe) Trial Investigators. Cardiovascular events associated with rofecoxib in a colorectal adenoma chemoprevention trial. *N. Engl. J. Med.* 2005 Mar 17;352(11):1092-102.

[15] Dieppe PA, Lohmander LS. Pathogenesis and management of pain in osteoarthritis. *Lancet.* 2005 Mar 12-18;365(9463):965-73.

[16] Kidd BL, Photiou A, Inglis JJ. The role of inflammatory mediators on nociception and pain in arthritis. *Novartis Found Symp* 2004; 260: 122–33; discussion 133–38, 277–79.

[17] Davis MA, Ettinger WH, Neuhaus JM, Barclay JD, Segal MR.Correlates of knee pain among US adults with and without radiographic knee osteoarthritis. *J. Rheumatol.* 1992 Dec;19(12):1943-9.

[18] McCrae F, Shouls J, Dieppe P, Watt I.Scintigraphic assessment of osteoarthritis of the knee joint. *Ann. Rheum. Dis.* 1992 Aug;51(8):938-42.

[19] Inoue H, Takamori M, Shimoyama Y, Ishibashi H, Yamamoto S, Koshihara Y.Regulation by PGE2 of the production of interleukin-6, macrophage colony stimulating factor, and vascular endothelial growth factor in human synovial fibroblasts. *Br. J. Pharmacol.* 2002 May;136(2):287-95.

[20] Hardy MM, Seibert K, Manning PT, Currie MG, Woerner BM, Edwards D, Koki A, Tripp CS. Cyclooxygenase 2-dependent prostaglandin E2 modulates cartilage proteoglycan degradation in human osteoarthritis explants. *Arthritis Rheum.* 2002 Jul;46(7):1789-803.

[21] Jovanovic DV, Mineau F, Notoya K, Reboul P, Martel-Pelletier J, Pelletier JP.Nitric oxide induced cell death in human osteoarthritic synoviocytes is mediated by tyrosine kinase activation and hydrogen peroxide and/or superoxide formation. *J. Rheumatol.* 2002 Oct;29(10):2165-75.

[22] He W, Pelletier JP, Martel-Pelletier J, Laufer S, Di Battista JA. Synthesis of interleukin 1beta, tumor necrosis factor-alpha, and interstitial collagenase (MMP-1) is eicosanoid dependent in human osteoarthritis synovial membrane explants: interactions with antiinflammatory cytokines. *J. Rheumatol.* 2002 Mar;29(3):546-53.

[23] Pillinger MH, Rosenthal PB, Tolani SN, Apsel B, Dinsell V, Greenberg J, Chan ES, Gomez PF, Abramson SB. Cyclooxygenase-2-derived E prostaglandins down-regulate matrix metalloproteinase-1 expression in fibroblast-like synoviocytes via inhibition of extracellular signal-regulated kinase activation. *J. Immunol.* 2003 Dec 1;171(11):6080-9.

[24] Abramson SB. Inflammation in osteoarthritis. *J. Rheumatol Suppl.* 2004 Apr;70:70-6.

[25] Brandt KD, Palmoski MJ.Effects of salicylates and other nonsteroidal anti-inflammatory drugs on articular cartilage. *Am. J. Med.* 1984 Jul 13;77(1A):65-9.

[26] Huskisson EC, Berry H, Gishen P, Jubb RW, Whitehead J.Effects of antiinflammatory drugs on the progression of osteoarthritis of the knee. LINK Study Group. Longitudinal Investigation of Nonsteroidal Antiinflammatory Drugs in Knee Osteoarthritis. *J. Rheumatol.* 1995 Oct;22(10):1941-6.

[27] Bensen WG, Fiechtner JJ, McMillen JI, Zhao WW, Yu SS, Woods EM, Hubbard RC, Isakson PC, Verburg KM, Geis GS. Treatment of osteoarthritis with celecoxib, a cyclooxygenase-2 inhibitor: a randomized controlled trial. *Mayo. Clin. Proc.* 1999 Nov;74(11):1095-105.

[28] Bjordal JM, Ljunggren AE, Klovning A, Slordal L.Non-steroidal anti-inflammatory drugs, including cyclo-oxygenase-2 inhibitors, in osteoarthritic knee pain: meta-analysis of randomised placebo controlled trials. *BMJ.* 2004 Dec 4;329(7478):1317.

[29] Rowbotham MC. What is a "clinically meaningful" reduction in pain? *Pain.* 2001 Nov;94(2):131-2.

[30] Wegman A, van der Windt D, van Tulder M, Stalman W, de Vries T. Nonsteroidal antiinflammatory drugs or acetaminophen for osteoarthritis of the hip or knee? A systematic review of evidence and guidelines. *J. Rheumatol.* 2004 Feb;31(2):344-54.

[31] Kidd BL, Richardson PM. How does neuropathophysiology affect the signs and symptoms of spinal disease? *Best. Pract. Res. Clin. Rheumatol.* 2002 Jan;16(1):31-42.

[32] Kang JD, Georgescu HI, McIntyre-Larkin L, Stefanovic-Racic M, Donaldson WF 3rd, Evans CH Herniated lumbar intervertebral discs spontaneously produce matrix metalloproteinases, nitric oxide, interleukin-6, and prostaglandin E2. *Spine.* 1996 Feb 1;21(3):271-7.

[33] Miyamoto H, Saura R, Harada T, Doita M, Mizuno K. The role of cyclooxygenase-2 and inflammatory cytokines in pain induction of herniated lumbar intervertebral disc. *Kobe. J. Med. Sci.* 2000 Apr;46(1-2):13-28.

[34] Willburger RE, Wittenberg RH. Prostaglandin release from lumbar disc and facet joint tissue. *Spine.* 1994 Sep 15;19(18):2068-70.

[35] Takahashi H, Suguro T, Okazima Y, Motegi M, Okada Y, Kakiuchi T. Inflammatory cytokines in the herniated disc of the lumbar spine. *Spine.* 1996 Jan 15;21(2):218-24.

[36] Igarashi A, Kikuchi S, Konno S, Olmarker K. Inflammatory cytokines released from the facet joint tissue in degenerative lumbar spinal disorders. *Spine.* 2004 Oct 1;29(19):2091-5.

[37] Pohjolainen T, Jekunen A, Autio L, Vuorela H. Treatment of acute low back pain with the COX-2-selective anti-inflammatory drug nimesulide: results of a randomized, double-blind comparative trial versus ibuprofen. *Spine.* 2000 Jun 15;25(12):1579-85.

[38] van Tulder MW, Scholten RJ, Koes BW, Deyo RA. Non-steroidal anti-inflammatory drugs for low back pain. *Cochrane Database Syst. Rev.* 2000;(2):CD000396.

[39] Zerbini C, Ozturk ZE, Grifka J, Maini M, Nilganuwong S, Morales R, Hupli M, Shivaprakash M, Giezek H; The Etoricoxib CLBP Study Group. Efficacy of etoricoxib 60 mg/day and diclofenac 150 mg/day in reduction of pain and disability in patients with chronic low back pain: results of a 4-week, multinational, randomized, double-blind study. *Curr. Med. Res. Opin.* 2005 Dec;21(12):2037-49.

[40] Pietrobon D. Migraine: new molecular mechanisms. *Neuroscientist.* 2005 Aug;11(4):373-86.

[41] Malick A, Burstein R. Peripheral and central sensitization during migraine. *Funct. Neurol.* 2000;15 Suppl 3:28-35.

[42] Waeber C, Moskowitz MA. Migraine as an inflammatory disorder. *Neurology.* 2005 May 24;64(10 Suppl 2):S9-15.

[43] Silberstein SD. Migraine pathophysiology and its clinical implications. *Cephalalgia.* 2004;24 Suppl 2:2-7.

[44] Moskowitz MA. Neurogenic versus vascular mechanisms of sumatriptan and ergot alkaloids in migraine. *Trends Pharmacol. Sci.* 1992 Aug;13(8):307-11.

[45] Diener HC. Efficacy and safety of intravenous acetylsalicylic acid lysinate compared to subcutaneous sumatriptan and parenteral placebo in the acute treatment of migraine. A

double-blind, double-dummy, randomized, multicenter, parallel group study. The ASASUMAMIG Study Group. *Cephalalgia.* 1999 Jul;19(6):581-8

[46] Codispoti JR, Prior MJ, Fu M, Harte CM, Nelson EB. Efficacy of nonprescription doses of ibuprofen for treating migraine headache. a randomized controlled trial. *Headache.* 2001 Jul-Aug;41(7):665-79.

[47] Dib M, Massiou H, Weber M, Henry P, Garcia-Acosta S, Bousser MG; Bi-Profenid Migraine Study Group. Efficacy of oral ketoprofen in acute migraine: a double-blind randomized clinical trial. *Neurology.* 2002 Jun 11;58(11):1660-5.

[48] MacGregor EA, Dowson A, Davies PT. Mouth-dispersible aspirin in the treatment of migraine: a placebo-controlled study. *Headache.* 2002 Apr;42(4):249-55.

[49] Misra UK, Jose M, Kalita J. Rofecoxib versus ibuprofen for acute treatment of migraine: a randomised placebo controlled trial. *Postgrad. Med. J.* 2004 Dec;80(950):720-3.

[50] Jakubowski M, Levy D, Goor-Aryeh I, Collins B, Bajwa Z, Burstein R. Terminating migraine with allodynia and ongoing central sensitization using parenteral administration of COX1/COX2 inhibitors. *Headache.* 2005 Jul-Aug;45(7):850-61.

[51] Lipton RB, Stewart WF, Diamond S, Diamond ML, Reed M. Prevalence and burden of migraine in the United States: data from the American Migraine Study II. *Headache.* 2001 Jul-Aug;41(7):646-57.

*Chapter IX*

# Chronic Pain and the Sympathetic Nervous System: Mechanisms and Potential Implications for Pain Therapies

*Amit Sharma[1] and Srinivasa N. Raja[2]*
[1]Assistant Professor, Department of Anesthesiology,
College of Physicians and Surgeons of Columbia University, New York, NY
[2]Professor, Director, Division of Pain Medicine, The Johns Hopkins University
Department of Anesthesiology/CCM, Baltimore, MD

## Abstract

Role of autonomic nervous system in generation or maintainance of chronic pain had been debated for many decades. One pertinent example of this association is Raynaud's phenomenon in which cold induced exaggerated reflex sympathetic vasoconstriction can induces ischemic pain. By virtue of some inexplicable mechanisms, sympathetic nervous system had also been impugned in protracting non-ischemic variety of chronic pain in certain diseases like phantom limb pain, post-herpetic neuralgia, metabolic neuropathies, fibromyalgia and complex regional pain syndrome. Although a clear understanding of this variety of pain has still not been achieved, some changes at receptor level have been elucidated. The purpose of this chapter is to review the current conception regarding the pathophysiology and treatment of this variety of pain.

---

[1] Assistant Professor, Department of Anesthesiology, College of Physicians and Surgeons of Columbia University 622 West 168th Street, PH 5, Room 500, New York, NY 10032. Email: as2298@columbia.edu

# Introduction

The nervous system is broadly divided into the somatic nervous system and the autonomic nervous system (ANS). The somatic nervous system processes perceptive inputs and provides voluntary control of musculature. The ANS regulates individual organ functions and homeostasis; and for the most part is not subject to voluntary control. ANS dysfunction may cause ischemic pain in certain conditions, which is truly an indirect effect secondary to reduction in blood flow to the involved extremity. Although ANS has no direct role in the transmission of sensory input, certain disease states have been shown to have its involvement in the generation or maintenance of pain. The mechanisms and therapeutic interventions to treat this variety of ANS dysfunction will be discussed in this chapter.

# Autonomic Nervous System

## Anatomy and Physiology

Although ANS is mostly considered an efferent system, its activity is influenced by afferent input to the central nervous system, analogous to the reflex arc in the somatic nervous system. The afferent visceral inputs transmit impulses at various segments of central nervous system, which in turn modulate the 'autonomic outflow'. This 'autonomic outflow' is divided into 'sympathetic' and 'parasympathetic' components anatomically. Sympathetic preganglionic fibers originate in the spinal cord, travel via the first thoracic to third or fourth lumbar ventral spinal nerves and synapse with ganglions in 'sympathetic chain' or in 'collateral ganglion' close to the viscera. The parasympathetic nervous system, on the other hand, takes origin in the midbrain or medulla (cranial outflow) or sacral segments of spinal cord (sacral outflow). The postganglionic fibers of both these divisions then supply numerous visceral organs like eye, facial glands, heart, airways and lungs, gastrointestinal tract, adrenals, kidneys, bladder and genitalia.

Chemically, the autonomic nervous system is divided into noradrenergic and cholinergic divisions. Most postganglionic sympathetic fibers, with few exceptions, are noradrenergic. Noradrenergic discharge often occurs in "fight or flight" situations leading to widespread responses like mydriasis, tachycardia, and constriction of peripheral vessels, bronchodilation, decreased gastrointestinal motility and piloerection. On the other hand, cholinergic discharge leads to more limited response and stimulate anabolic responses in the body [1].

## Role of Sympathetic Nervous System in Pain: Studies in Humans

Initial suggestions of involvement of sympathetic nervous system (SNS) in pain disorder were made in patients suffering from complex regional pain syndrome (CRPS). The clinical picture of this disease with vascular (vasodilation or vasoconstriction, skin temperature asymmetries or skin color changes) and sudomotor abnormalities (swelling, hyper or hypohidrosis) probably generated this initial hypothesis [2].

Pain dependent on the discharge of sympathetic nerves is referred to as sympathetically maintained pain (SMP). Since pain involved in CRPS patients was observed to improve with blockade of the SNS, increased autonomic discharge was proposed as a potential mechanism for SMP. Numerous scientific data like presence of warm painful extremity in early part of the disease and sub-normal catecholamine levels in the venous return of the affected extremity alienated this hypothesis. Subsequently, these findings were explained by three distinct phases in CRPS. They included an initial phase involving warm, erythematous skin (Stage I or Acute Stage) presumably due to SNS under-activity; an intermittent phase of both warm and cold sensation (Stage II or Dystrophic Stage) followed by chronic cold sensation (Stage III or Atrophic Stage) due to SNS hyper-activity. Many studies have shown reduction in vasomotor tone in very early stages of the disease [3, 4] but not in later stages. There is also a reduction in plasma norepinephrine and neuropeptide Y concentration on the affected extremity in early phase of the disease strengthening this theory [5].

Although the idea of these distinct stages explained many scientific theories, it was constantly debated due to variable clinical presentations of CRPS patients [6]. It was later recognized that the apparent increase in vasomotor tone in later stages of CRPS (as evident by vasoconstriction or cold skin) is due to increased sensitivity (hyper or super-sensitivity) of skin microvessels to catecholamines [4] or secondary changes in neurovascular transmission while actual sympathetic tone is still depressed. Possible mechanisms for this hightened sensitivity might be decreased neuronal uptake of norepinephrine in the sympathetic neuroeffector junction [7] or increased number of peripheral α-receptors [8, 9].

The interaction of the sympathetic nervous system and catecholamines on primary afferents has been examined using experimental models in human. For example, cutaneous application of the algogenic agent capsaicin causes neurogenic inflammation by activating and sensitizing nociceptors. The heat hyperalgesia that develops after topical application of capsaicin in human volunteers was enhanced following iontophoresis of noradrenaline suggesting an adrenergic effect on sensitized cutaneous nociceptors [10]. Phentolamine, a mixed $α_1$- and $α_2$- antagonist inhibited the norepinephrine-induced pain and mechanical hyperalgesia in capsaicin-sensitized skin [11, 12]. Control studies with non-adrenergic vasoconstrictors, angiotensin II and vasopressin as well as occlusion of blood flow indicated that a part of the norepinephrine-induced enhancement of hyperalgesia in capsaicin treated skin may be secondary to changes in cutaneous blood flow [13, 14]. However, when sympathetic cutaneous vasoconstrictor activity was modulated in physiological ranges by thermoregulatory stress, capsaicin-induced hyperalgesia was not significantly altered [15]. Similarly, Pedersen et al. [16], while using a cutaneous heat injury model, observed that sympathetic blocks with bupivacaine did not alter spontaneous pain and heat hyperalgesia. In patients with rheumatoid arthritis, however, regional intravenous guanethidine produced a decrease in pain and an increase in pinch strength [17]. Thus, studies provide conflicting evidence for a possible interaction of the sympathetic and the sensory nervous systems in inflammation.

A number of clinical studies demonstrate that sympathetic activity and catecholamines influence the activity of primary afferents in patients with neuropathic pain and CRPS. Studies in humans support the concept that nociceptors develop catecholamine sensitivity after complete or partial nerve lesions. Injection of epinephrine or norepinephrine around a stump neuroma is reported to be more painful than injections of saline [18, 19]. In addition, intravenous phentolamine, but not propranolol, relieves SMP [20, 21]. The pain relief resulting from both procedures in patients subjected to both a local anesthetic sympathetic ganglion block and a phentolamine infusion shows good correlation [21, 22]. The detection of autoantibodies against the autonomic nervous system in certain CRPS patients provides further evidence for a role of the sympathetic nervous system in pain [23].

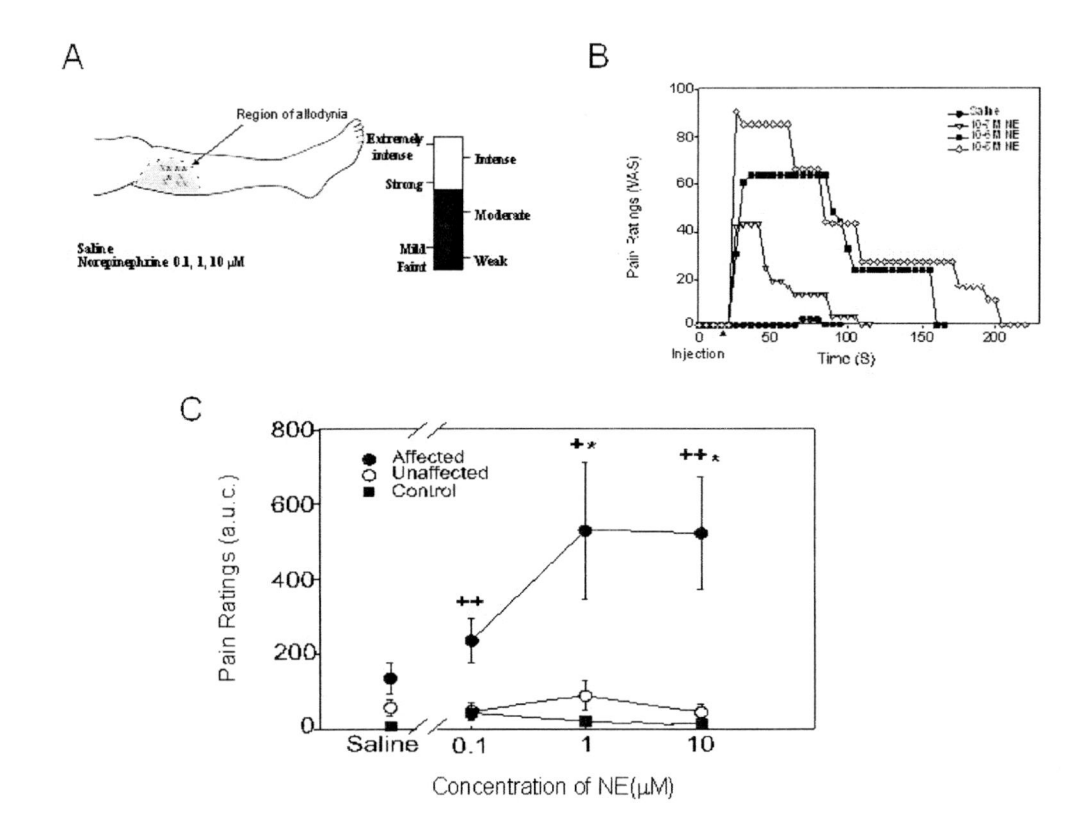

Figure 1. The pain induced by intradermal injections of norepinephrine in normal subjects and patients with sympathetically maintained pain. A) Experimental paradigm: The region of allodynia was mapped using a camel's hairbrush. Sites for intradermal injections were marked on the skin (x) within the allodynic region, and the mirror-image contralateral extremity, such that they were separated by at least 3 cm. The patient underwent a sympathetic ganglion block with a 0.25% bupivacaine solution. Intradermal injections of saline and incremental concentrations of norepinephrine (NE) were made at different sites first on the unaffected extremity. The patient rated the pain induced by the injection continuously using a computerized visual analog scale with descriptive markers as shown in the figure. B) Pain ratings to saline and NE in the affected limb of a patient with SMP. This patient experienced no pain to the saline injection but had a dose-related increase in intensity and duration of pain to NE. C) Mean pain ratings to the different concentrations of NE in control subjects and the affected and unaffected limbs of patients with SMP. Note that the pain ratings to the NE injections are significantly increased in the affected limb compared to the saline injections. (* = $p < 0.05$) and compared to the unaffected limb and control subjects (+ = $p < 0.05$; ++ = $p < 0.01$, ANOVA) [8]

Additional studies in CRPS and postherpetic neuralgia patients support the postulate that noradrenergic sensitivity of human nociceptors develops after injury to the nervous system. In CRPS and post-traumatic neuralgias, intracutaneous application of norepinephrine into a symptomatic area rekindles spontaneous pain and dynamic mechanical hyperalgesia that had been relieved by sympathetic blockade [24, 25]. A potential criticism of the above studies were that the doses of exogenous norepinephrine (NE) used were much higher than are likely to exist *in vivo*. Therefore, the algesic effects of peripheral administration of NE in physiologically relevant doses were compared in patients with SMP and normal subjects [8]. Intradermal NE, in physiologically relevant doses, was demonstrated to evoke greater pain in the affected regions of patients with SMP, than in the contralateral unaffected limb, and in control subjects (Figure 1). Moreover, the majority of the patients who had an increase in pain to injection of NE in the affected extremity also reported a decrease in pain to systemic administration of phentolamine. These observations support a role for cutaneous adrenergic receptors in the mechanisms of sympathetically maintained pain. Consistent with this hypothesis, in patients with CRPS spontaneous pain and mechanical hyperalgesia was augmented when sympathetic cutaneous vasoconstrictor neurons were activated physiologically by thermoregulatory stress (Figure 2) [26, 27, 28].

Additional lines of evidence from pharmacological studies also support a peripheral $\alpha$-adrenergic mechanism in SMP. Topical application of the $\alpha_2$-adrenergic agonist, clonidine relieves hyperalgesia at the site of application in SMP, but not SIP patients [9]. This effect was considered to be secondary to a reduction in the release of NE via activation of the $\alpha_2$-adrenergic receptor on the sympathetic terminal. Injection of NE and the $\alpha_1$-adrenergic agonist, phenylephrine, into clonidine-treated area produced marked pain and hyperalgesia. Quantitative autoradiographic studies indicate that the number of $\alpha_1$-adrenoceptors in hyperalgesic skin of patients with SMP is significantly greater than in the skin of normal subjects [13]. Finally, an increase in venous $\alpha$-adrenoceptor responsiveness has been observed in patients with CRPS [29].

## Animal Models of Sympathetically Maintained Pain

A number of animal models of neuropathic pain have been developed to study the mechanism of chronic neuropathic pain. Initial studies used transection of a peripheral nerve resulting in the formation of a neuroma, while subsequent models involved partial injury to a peripheral nerve, e.g., sciatic nerve, or transection or tight ligation of spinal nerve(s). These experimental models may mimic the clinical syndrome of CRPS 2 (Causalgia). Although earlier studies indicated that the sympathetic nervous system might play an important role in the maintenance of pain in these animal models of neuropathic pain, later studies have indicated that the role of the sympathetic nervous system is not consistent in these models [30, 31, 32]. More recently animal models have been developed that do not involve a direct injury to nerves and may be more representative of CRPS 1. The chronic post-ischemia pain (CPIP) syndrome model used prolonged hind limb ischemia followed by reperfusion [33]. Another model resembling CRPS 1 involved a distal tibial fracture and cast immobilization for 4 weeks [34]. Whether the pain behavior in these models is mediated by the sympathetic nervous system is uncertain.

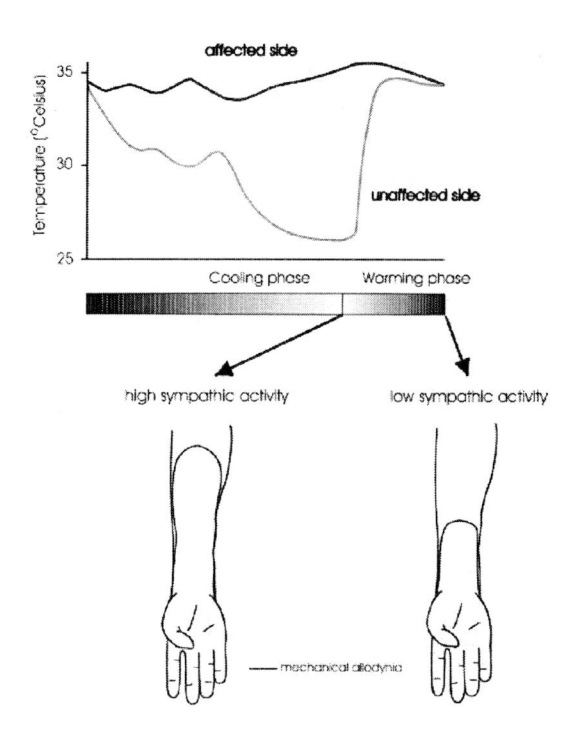

Figure 2. *Influence of cutaneous sympathetic vasoconstrictor activity on pain in patients with CRPS.* Physiological reflex stimuli were used to induce an activation of sympathetic efferents and release of noradrenaline: To alter sympathetic skin nerve activity, whole body cooling and warming was performed with the help of a thermal suit. The subject was lying in a suit supplied by tubes, in which water at 12°C and 50°C temperature respectively was circulated (inflow temperature) to cool or warm the whole body. Cooling induces a massive tonic activation of these neurons. In contrast warming leads to a considerable decrease of activity. Sympathetic activity can thus be switched on and off in a controlled manner and simultaneous measurement of pain sensations made. High sympathetic activity during cooling induces a decrease of skin temperature due to vasoconstriction (unaffected side). During the experiment the forearm temperature on the affected side was maintained at 35°C by a feed-back-controlled heat lamp to exclude temperature effects on the sensory receptor level. Activation of sympathetic neurons leads to a considerable increase of the area of allodynia in SMP patients indicating that in CRPS a pathologic coupling between sympathetic and nociceptive neurons does exist (from Janig and Baron 2003, Lancet with permission)

Several lines of evidence indicate that sympathetic activity and catecholamines influence activity of primary afferents after nerve damage (Figure 3). After *nerve transection* in experimental animals, surviving cutaneous afferents may develop noradrenergic sensitivity. Myelinated and unmyelinated afferents innervating the stump neuroma can be excited by adrenaline or by stimulation of sympathetic efferents that have regenerated into the neuroma [35, 36]. Within two weeks of a *partial nerve lesion*, electrical stimulation of the sympathetic trunk and injections of catecholamines can activate or sensitize C-nociceptors in the partially injured nerve [37]. As late as a year after complete section and re-anastomosis of peripheral nerves, electrical stimulation of the sympathetic trunk results in activation of regenerated C-fibers, probably nociceptors [38]. *In vitro* neurophysiological studies, using a primate skin-nerve preparation, have demonstrated that uninjured cutaneous C-fiber nociceptors that innervate skin partially denervated by a spinal nerve ligation have a higher incidence of adrenergic sensitivity than nociceptive afferents from normal skin [39]. Peripheral nerve injury in the rat leads to the development of a novel pattern of sympathetic fiber innervation of the skin [40]. Within a week after bilateral lesions of the mental nerve, sprouting of dopamine-beta-hydroxylase positive fibers is observed in the upper dermis, a region normally devoid of such fibers.

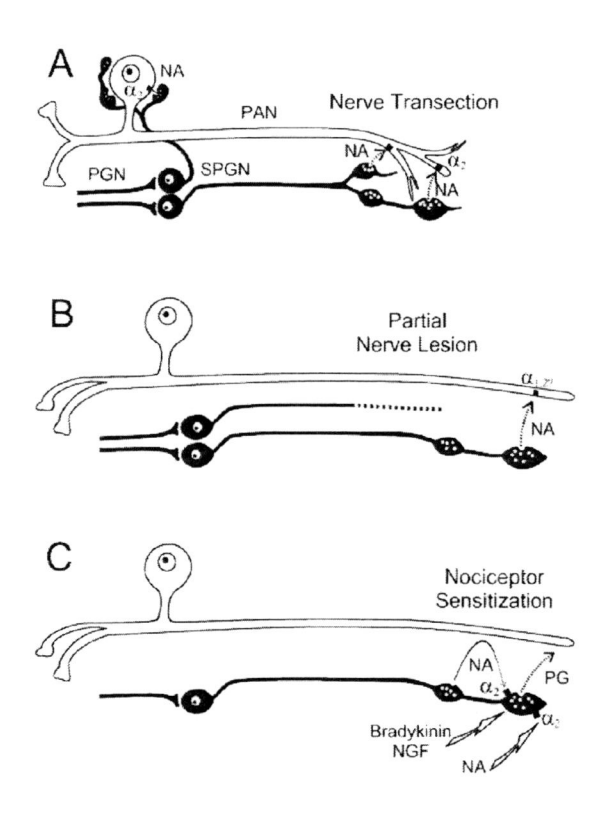

Figure 3. *Influence of sympathetic activity and catecholamines on primary afferent neurons (PAN).* A. Nerve transection. The interaction between the sympathetic efferent fibers and the sensory afferent fibers occurs in the neuroma and in the dorsal root ganglion. The coupling is mediated by norepinephrine (NA) released from sympathetic postganglionic neurons (SPGN) and α-adrenoreceptors expressed at the plasma membrane of afferent neurons. PGN, preganglionic neuron. B. Partial nerve lesion. Partial nerve injury results in a decrease of the sympathetic innervation density (stippled sympathetic postganglionic neuron). This denervation induces an up-regulation of functional α-adrenoceptors at the membrane of intact afferent fibers. C. After tissue inflammation intact but sensitized primary afferents acquire norepinephrine sensitivity. Norepinephrine acts indirectly on primary afferents by inducing the release of prostaglandins (PG) from sympathetic terminals that sensitize the afferents. Similarly, bradykinin and nerve growth factor (NGF) induced nociceptor sensitization is also mediated by the release of prostaglandins from sympathetic postganglionic neurons (from Baron 1999, Muscle and Nerve with permission)

In addition to the sympathetic-afferent interactions near the cutaneous receptors, sympathetic-sensory coupling might exist in the peripheral nerve at the site of injury, and the dorsal root ganglion where cell bodies of injured sensory nerves are located. After a complete nerve lesion, some DRG somata with Aβ-fibers and a few with C-fibers develop ectopic activity. Electrical stimulation of sympathetic efferents innervating the DRG may lead to an $\alpha_2$-adrenoceptor mediated increase of this spontaneous activity [41]. These physiological changes in adrenergic sensitivity are paralleled by anatomical changes within the DRG. After the nerve lesion, sympathetic postganglionic fibers that normally innervate blood vessels within the DRG sprout to form basket-like terminals around large primary afferent somata that project into the injured nerve [42, 43].

However, the relationship of this DRG sprouting to pain is uncertain as the sprouting of sympathetic terminals is largely around the somata of larger, presumably non-nociceptive primary afferents. In addition the time course of sprouting of sympathetic fibers does not correlate well with the time course of behavioral changes observed after partial nerve injuries (see Ref. 2 for further discussion).

A number of studies have attempted to examine the type of receptors that are involved in sympathetic-afferent coupling. $\alpha$-adrenoceptors have been suggested to mediate the excitation and depression of axotomized dorsal root ganglion cells and the excitation of afferent terminals in neuromas generated by activation of the sympathetic innervation. The cellular mechanisms underlying the increased sensitivity are unknown. A possible explanation is the novel expression or up-regulation of adrenoceptors. Alternatively, the receptors may normally be present on primary nociceptive afferents but not be functional; they may become uncovered and effective during the response to damage. The affinity for ligands or the effectiveness of the subsequent cellular transduction may change in injured nociceptive and non-nociceptive afferent neurons. These possibilities are not mutually exclusive and it is possible that several mechanisms contribute simultaneously to the expression of sympathetically mediated afferent excitation.

Perl and coworkers [37] suggest, on the basis of their experiments on polymodal nociceptors following partial nerve lesion, that the expression or up-regulation of adrenoceptors in primary afferent neurons is related to the sympathetic denervation of the target tissue, analogous to the development of the so-called denervation supersensitivity which is observed in effector tissues following their denervation. This is supported by their recent experimental observation that cutaneous nociceptive C-fibers in the rabbit ear may develop adrenoceptor sensitivity following surgical sympathectomy [44].

Knowledge about the subtypes of $\alpha$-adrenoreceptor(s) involved in the sympathetic-afferent coupling following nerve trauma is important for an understanding of the underlying neural mechanism, and may be useful in the design of more specific treatment modalities for neuropathic pain conditions involving sympathetic efferent activity. Sato and Perl [37] have shown that excitation and sensitization of polymodal nociceptors in the rabbit ear skin generated by electrical stimulation of the sympathetic supply or by norepinephrine after partial lesion of the auricular nerve, is largely mediated by $a_2$-adrenoceptors. Investigation of sympathetic-sensory coupling at the site of experimental nerve injury in neuromas and at the cell bodies of axotomized afferent neurons using type-selective agonists and antagonists has shown that this transmission is also largely mediated by $\alpha_2$-adrenoreceptors [45]. Recordings from primate cutaneous C-fiber nociceptors after an L6 spinal nerve ligation, however, showed a significantly higher incidence of response to the selective $\alpha_1$- and $\alpha_2$-adrenergic agonists, phenylephrine and brimonidine, respectively [39]. In normal (uninjured) DRG neurons mRNAs for $\alpha_{2A}$- and particularly $a_{2B}$-adrenoceptors are present whereas mRNAs for

$\alpha_1$-adrenoceptors are either absent or very low in level. After nerve lesion mRNA for $\alpha_{2A}$-adrenoceptors is clearly upregulated in DRG neurons [46].

Although most studies suggest a direct interaction of sympathetic and sensory fibers, the possibility for an indirect coupling between sympathetic and afferent nerve terminals should be considered. Changes in vascular perfusion of the micro-milieu surrounding the nociceptors occur after nerve trauma. These changes are a consequence of denervation and reinnervation by postganglionic vasoconstrictor neurons and afferent nociceptive neurons and the development of supersensitivity of blood vessels [47]. Whether these changes lead indirectly to sensitization of nociceptors awaits further studies.

The picture of SNS involvement in generation of pain is indeed a concept, but may not explain all features of CRPS. Inflammatory and central origin of pain in CRPS patients has been suggested and significant animal and human research support their contributions. It is also acknowledged that a subset of patients with CRPS has pain that is sympathetically independent (SIP). Moreover many other diseases have a component of SMP including, but not limited to, diabetic or other painful neuropathies, certain headaches and fibromyalgia. The sympathetic nervous system can be modulated at various levels to mange the SPM in these disorders. This concept will be discussed in the following section. In contrast to sympathetic nervous system, the parasympathetic nervous system has not been shown to have a clear association with pain disorders.

# Pharmacological Modulation of ANS

As previously discussed, autonomic nervous system comprises of two distinct outflow systems in the form of sympathetic and parasympathetic nervous system. Numerous pharmacological agents have been used to either increase or decrease this outflow or discharge of chemical transmitters.

## Systemic Sympatho-Modulatory Drugs

Many pain states have a component of 'SMP' that involves increased sensitivity of affected tissues to autonomic 'neurochemicals'. It is thus logical to assume that pharmacological inhibition of sympathetic discharge or opposition of peripheral effects of neurochemicals released during sympathetic stimulation will cause analgesia. The drugs that oppose the peripheral effects of impulses conveyed by postganglionic sympathetic fibers are called as Sympatholytic or antiadrenergic agents. These agents are further categorized as α-adrenergic receptor antagonists or β-adrenergic receptor antagonists based on their specificity to the receptor subtypes. There is an over-expression of α-adrenergic receptors in the peripheral painful extremity or neuromas in animal models of neuropathic pain. Clinically, α-1 adrenoceptor hyper-responsiveness has been observed in various neuropathic pain states like CRPS type 1 [29], diabetic peripheral neuropathic pain and central pain states following spinal cord injury. Other plausible theories of this increased responsiveness include increased concentrations of noradrenaline in the synaptic cleft and increased stimulation of otherwise normal alpha-1 adrenoceptors [48]. Corresponding clinical evidence suggest efficacy of α-adrenergic antagonists including imidazoline receptor drug (phentolamine), phenoxybenzomine and piperazinyl quinazoles (prazosin, terazosin) in SMP states [21, 49].

Intravenous alpha-adrenergic blockade with phentolamine (Phentolamine block, PhB) has been proposed as a safe and effective method of diagnosing SMP [21, 22]. Phentolamine is a short-acting and non-specific inhibitor of α-adrenoceptors. In their initial double-blinded study, Raja et al randomly assigned 20 patients to 25-35 mg of intravenous phentolamine or local anesthetic sympathetic block (LASB) with 0.25% bupivacaine. They observed similar pain relief response in both groups [21] despite differences in achieving 'true' sympathectomy in PhB group. Dellemijn et al later reproduced these findings and concluded that phentolamine infusion is less sensitive but more specific test of SMP than LASB [22]. In an attempt to find optimum test dose for PhB, Raja et al then compared the effect of two different doses of phentolamine (0.5 mg/kg and 1 mg/kg) on skin blood flow (using a laser Doppler blood flow monitor) and sympathetically mediated vasoconstrictor response (a reflex decrease in peripheral blood flow in response to deep inhalation) [7]. They concluded that the higher dose of phentolamine (1 mg/kg over 10 min) resulted in more complete adrenoceptor blockade. This high dose intravenous administration of phentolamine along with cutaneous temperature monitoring was thus proposed as an optimum way to evaluate the sympathetically mediated component in neuropathic pain states.

Prazosin, unlike phentolamine, is a specific α-1 adrenoceptor antagonist. It has been shown to attenuate cold induced allodynia in animal model of neuropathic pain in numerous studies [50, 51, 52, 53]. Terazosin, a similar agent, was suggested to have beneficial effects in SMP in a small study by Stevens et al. [54]. Terazosin is also suggested to have better compliance due its long elimination half-time and a long duration of action, hence requiring once a day dosing. Newer agents like doxazocin or tamsulosin have not been tested for their efficacy in SMP yet. Beyond α1-antagonists, α2 agonists are found to be efficacious in some neuropathic pain states. Their mechanism of action involves activation of α-2 receptors in dorsal horn of spinal cord. These receptors have an inhibitory role in the processing of descending sensory information via inhibitory neurotransmitter norepinephrine or acetylcholine [55, 56]. Specific α2 agonist drugs like clonidine, mivazerol, dexmedetomidine and fadolmidine, act via these central mechanisms for analgesia, although they also attenuate central sympathetic drive. There is also a peripheral α-2 adrenoceptor presynaptic dysfunction in neuropathic pain states causing diminished noradrenaline reuptake [48]. Activation of these peripheral α-2 adrenoceptors might reduce norepinephrine release and reducing α-1 adrenoceptor induced hyper-sensitivity [9].

## Regional Modulation of Sympathetic Activity

Numerous medications are used to attenuate regional sympathetic tone. The techniques involve intravenous infusion of drug in an extremity with restriction of blood flow using a tourniquet or injection of a local anesthetic in the vicinity at the level of the sympathetic ganglion or chain. The former technique is termed Intravenous Regional Sympathetic

Blockade (IRSB) and the latter Local Anesthetic Sympathetic Blocks (LASB) or just Regional Sympathetic Blocks.

### Intravenous Regional Sympathetic Blockade (IRSB)

Intravenous regional anesthesia is a technique that involves intravenous injection of a local anesthetic solution in a limb whose circulation isolated from the rest of the body by a tourniquet. It was initially described by August Bier in 1908. Hannington-Kiff modified this concept and proposed intravenous regional sympathetic blockade (IRSB) using guanethidine. Several other medications have since been used to perform this block including sympatholytics like reserpine, bretylium or clonidine; local anesthetics like prilocaine or lidocaine, and other drugs like ketanserin (5-HT2 antagonist). Performance of IRSBs does not require any special expertise. They are easier to perform and have better patient acceptance than LASB. These procedures have the risk of tourniquet related pain and significant side effects from the sudden release of high doses of medications in systemic circulation.

IRSBs were promoted as diagnostic tests for SMP but their utility for this purpose is limited. The ischemic tourniquet used during the procedure has been shown to relieve hyperalgesia in neuropathic pain patient [57] and can cause false positive results. Certain patients do not tolerate a tourniquet well. Guanethidine causes an initial release of norepinephrine before depletion of the catechol stores of sympathetic terminals and can exacerbate SMP. This medication is, therefore, often co-injected with local anesthetic agents to avoid any extremes of discomfort to the patient. Simultaneous analgesic effects of local anesthetics confound the results making this 'test' very non-specific to diagnose SMP. IRSBs have also been used for therapeutic purposes in SMP but their effectiveness is unclear. A meta-analysis by Perez et al [58] critically reviewing nine IVRB studies including six with the use of guanethidine showed no clinical long-term benefit of this technique. A randomized controlled trial of IVRB with guanethidine with prilocaine in 57 patients suffering from early CRPS type1 also failed to demonstrate any significant benefit [59]. Similar results have been reported in the past [60, 61] raising doubts on the efficacy of this technique. The use of other medications like clonidine, bretylium, ketorolac or ketanserin has shown marginal benefits in observational studies with a small number of patients, [60, 62, 63, 64] but their long term benefits are unproven at present.

### Local Anesthetic Sympathetic Block (LASB)

LASB is technically difficult procedures often done under fluoroscopic or CT guidance during which a needle is positioned in close proximity to the sympathetic ganglia and a local anesthetic solution is injected. They have the advantage of selectively blocking sympathetic ganglion and/or chain without concomitant blockade of sensory or motor fibers. Although numerous complications of LASB have been reported in the literature, these techniques are considered safe in experienced hands. Efficacy of the block is assessed by monitoring objective evidence of sympathetic blockade, e.g. cutaneous temperature monitoring or assessment of sympathetic function by sweat test [65] or skin conductance response. The patient is asked to report his or her pain intensity using a numeric pain score before and after sympathetic blockade and a positive response is usually considered as a 50% or greater improvement in pain scores in the light of adequate sympathectomy. A controlled study in patients with CRPS I has shown that immediately after the procedure, LASB with local anesthetic has the same magnitude of reduction in pain as a control injection with saline [66]. However, after 24 hours patients in the local anesthetic group continued to experience pain relief while the pain had returned to near baseline in the saline treated group. Thus, nonspecific effects of LASB are important in the immediate post-procedure period and that evaluating the efficacy of sympatholytic interventions is best done after 24 hours.

LASB has been considered as the 'gold standard' for diagnosing SMP in past [21, 22]. They can be used to halt efferent sympathetic signals at any ganglionic or trunk level like the thoracic sympathetic trunk, celiac plexus, superior hypogastric plexus and ganglion impar. A positive response to a temporary diagnostic local anesthetic block is reported to be a useful predictor of the success of subsequent sympathetectomy neuro-destructive procedures [67]. In order to reduce placebo responsiveness of LASB many physicians also perform PhB on a separate day. These two procedures provide complementary information and both may be needed to confirm the diagnosis of SMP [22].

Although the long-term efficacy of LASB remains unproven, LASB does provide short-term benefits in relieving spontaneous and evoked pain and reducing vasomotor symptoms. There is a relative paucity of randomized controlled trials to demonstrate the usefulness of LASB to treat SMP. Most of the trials have been done in CRPS patients (includes 'sympathetically independent pain or SIP' patients) and not specifically in SMP states. SIP patients are not expected to get any significant benefit from sympathetic blocks and their inclusion in the study biases the results. Recently, Cepeda et al [68] published a systematic review of randomized controlled trials of the effect of LASB in CRPS patients. The authors were unable to pool data from these studies due to significant differences in their design. They reviewed nonrandomized controlled studies, case series and randomized controlled trials with acceptable designs, published in English-language peer review journals from 1916 through 1999. Only 29 studies met the inclusion criteria of a sample size of at least 10 patients undergoing LASB with convincible evidence of CRPS. Interestingly, of these 29 studies, only 10 studies evaluated the technical success of block and only two of those assessed pain and outcome. Based on the data from 14 studies (454 patients) that quantified the magnitude of patient's responses and also reported the number of patients with different degrees of responses, the authors found that 29% patients undergoing LASB obtain full pain relief (>75% improvement) while 41% obtain partial relief (25-75% improvement). The authors concluded that less than one-third positive response ('full' pain relief) is consistent with 'placebo effect' and that the efficacy of sympathetic blocks for treatment of CRPS is inconclusive. These data are difficult to interpret as many of the 14 studies were published prior to 1960 and only two actually identified technical success of block and pain scores.

Conducting randomized controlled trials (RCTs) for LASB or IRSB for treatment of SMP is challenging due to some inherent difficulties in trial design. Randomization to placebo is almost impossible in these studies. Patients or physicians cannot be blinded as outcomes of adequate sympathectomy are obvious. Also, ethical issues might arise in performing technically challenging regional blocks with saline. Based on available data in literature, efficacy and duration of LASB is variable and indeed, unpredictable. Short duration of pain relief and reduction in vasomotor symptoms is often seen in clinical practice and should be utilized to improve mobility, range of motion and motor strength by physiotherapy. Repeated blocks are beneficial in selected patients with willingness to actively participate in physiotherapy and are showing signs of continuing improvement.

*Neuraxial Techniques*

Epidural or spinal modes can be used to deliver local anesthetic medications to achieve segmental sympathectomy. Moreover, other adjuvant agents can be added to enhance this effect. The epidural or spinal use of clonidine is such an example. In a randomized, blinded, placebo-controlled trial, Rauck et al showed efficacy of epidural clonidine infusion in patients with severe chronic pain from CRPS [69]. Following a positive initial response to a bolus of 300 to 700 micrograms of epidural clonidine, constant infusions significantly improved pain scores in almost 90% patients. Bolus clonidine was also shown to cause dose dependent side effects like sedation and decreased blood pressure and heart rate. One patient in this study developed meningitis. Catheter related infection is a realistic threat of long-term neuraxial infusion along with possibility of epidural hematoma formation. These risks can be reduced by use of internal pump-catheter delivery system although clinical studies are lacking in this respect.

# Sympathetic Denervation

## Chemical or Radiofrequency Sympathectomy

Radiofrequency denervation or chemical neurolytic destruction of sympathetic innervation is more interventional approaches to achieve long-term sympathectomy. The technique of radiofrequency denervation has been subjected to numerous amendments [70, 40]. Destruction of T2 and T3 ganglions is recommended for upper extremity SMP while guidelines for lower extremity involvement vary. Most authors suggest destruction of at least the first three ganglions (L1, L2, and L3); whereas others believe that the L4 and even L5 must be included for good long-term results. Complications of neurodestructive procedures include post-sympathectomy sympathalgia, compensatory hyperhidrosis, Horner's syndrome, wound infection, and spinal cord injury. There is a theoretical advantage of lesser incidence of post sympathetic neuralgia and more precise sympatholysis with radiofrequency technique in comparison to chemical neurolysis. Technical outcome data for these techniques vary. Wilkinson [71] reported almost 90% partial or complete evidence of sympathectomy for two years following radiofrequency denervation of T2 ganglion. Despite this high technical success, most authors report sustained pain relief in less than two thirds of patients at two years, and about one third at five years.

## Surgical Sympathectomy

Surgical sympathectomy has been used to treat hyperhidrosis, refractory angina and a variety of conditions involving over-active sympathetic nervous system including SMP states. They can be performed as open procedures or endoscopically. Krasna et al have suggested that endoscopic techniques are safe [72]. Post-operative morbidity from either open or endoscopic surgical procedures is likely to be more than the percutaneous techniques. Many surgeons prefer video assisted minimally invasive techniques instead of open sympathectomy to promote early postoperative recovery. In theory, similar results are expected as long as similar ganglionic destruction is achieved. Surgical techniques might have better outcomes due to the anatomic destruction following visualization of ganglionic structures. No comparative studies have been done as yet.

In a systematic review of the effects of percutaneous neuro-destructive procedures for neuropathic pain, Mailis et al [73] concluded that the practice of surgical and chemical sympathectomy is based on poor quality evidence, uncontrolled studies and personal experience. Therefore, more clinical trials of sympathectomy are required to establish the overall effectiveness and potential risks of this procedure. Because of the limited long-term outcomes, consideration should be given to neuromodulatory methods for SMP involving extremities. For other SMP syndromes, like visceral neuropathic pain in pancreatic cancer, chemical neurolysis continues to be the procedure of choice.

## Miscellaneous Techniques for ANS Modulation

Spinal cord stimulation (SCS) has gained acceptance for a wide variety of neuropathic pain syndromes. The technique involves insertion of a percutaneous lead in the epidural space that is connected to a battery implanted in a subcutaneous pocket. The percutaneous lead has four to eight compact electrodes close to its tip. Electrical stimulation is then used to stimulate the dorsal column of spinal cord, hence the name 'neurostimulation'. Apart from its effect on dorsal sensory nerve root fibers and descending spinal inhibitory pathways, neurostimulation may also modulate efferent sympathetic impulses. This is evident due to the improvement in microvascular blood flow and vasodilatation with dorsal column stimulation [74, 75]. Moreover, patients with good response to sympathetic blocks have been shown to have a likely long-term pain relief with SCS use [76]. A recent randomized control trial [77] and meta-analysis of literature [78, 79] showed that SCS results in a long-term pain reduction and health-related quality of life improvement, but no clinically important improvement of functional status, in chronic CRPS patients. The technique of neurostimulation has been shown to be more effective and less expensive than standard treatment protocol for the treatment of chronic CRPS [80].

Another novel technique recently used in pain population includes vagus nerve stimulation (VNS). It was previously used in the treatment for refractory epilepsy and has now shown some early benefits in management of resistant chronic headaches and migraines. Although most literature on its mechanism of action suggests that simulation of vagal afferents inhibits spinal nociceptive reflexes and transmission, these results are partly contradictory [81]. At present, this modality of modulation of autonomic nervous system should be considered as experimental and worthy of further studies.

## Conclusion

The sympathetic nervous system is involved in the generation or maintenance of pain in many disorders. Although the intricate mechanisms of the interactions of the sympathetic nervous system and the sensory nerves are not well understood, significant success has been achieved in controlling the pain in a subset of patients. Further research is needed in elucidating the alterations in central sympathetic modulation and the adrenoceptor pharmacology in patients with pain that is mediated or maintained by the sympathetic nervous system. Comparative studies in a randomized controlled fashion are warranted for the various subtype specific and non-specific alpha-adrenergic antagonists. Long-term benefits of sympathetic blocks need to be evaluated with controlled trials and further development of safer pharmacological derivatives may lead to improved outcomes in treating SMP in future. Neuromodulation techniques such as spinal cord stimulation have proven to be effective in providing long-term benefit and are cost effective in the treatment of CRPS.

## References

[1] Ganong, WF. The Autonomic Nervous System. In: Ganong WF, Ed. *Review of Medical Physiology*. McGraw-Hill Companies 20$^{th}$ Edition; 2001; Pp 217-23.

[2] Jänig, W; Baron, R. The role of the sympathetic nervous system in neuropathic pain: clinical observations and animal models. In: *Neuropathic Pain: Pathophysiology and Treatment*. Ed. by Hansson P, Fields HL, Hill RG, Marchettini P. Seattle: IASP Press; 2001; pp 125-49.

[3] Wasner, G; Schattschneider, J; Heckmann, K; Maier, C; Baron, R. Vascular abnormalities in reflex sympathetic dystrophy (CRPS I): mechanisms and diagnostic value. *Brain*. 2001 Mar;124(Pt 3):587-99.

[4] Kurvers, HA; Jacobs, MJ; Beuk, RJ; Van den Wildenberg, FA; Kitslaar, PJ; Slaaf, DW; Reneman RS. Reflex sympathetic dystrophy: evolution of microcirculatory disturbances in time. *Pain*. 1995 Mar;60(3):333-40.

[5] Drummond, PD; Finch, PM; Edvinsson, L; Goadsby, PJ. Plasma neuropeptide Y in the symptomatic limb of patients with causalgic pain. *Clin. Auton.Res*. 1994; 4: 113-6.

[6] Bruehl, S; Harden, RN; Galer, BS; Saltz, S; Backonja, M; Stanton-Hicks, M. Complex regional pain syndrome: are there distinct subtypes and sequential stages of the syndrome? *Pain*. 2002 Jan;95(1-2):119-24.

[7] Raja, SN; Choi, Y ; Asano, Y ; Holmes, C ; Goldstein, DS. Arteriovenous differences in plasma concentrations of catechols in rats with neuropathic pain. *Anesthesiology*. 1995 Nov;83(5):1000-8.

[8] Ali, Z; Raja, SN; Wesselmann, U; Fuchs, PN; Meyer, RA; Campbell, JN. Intradermal injection of norepinephrine evokes pain in patients with sympathetically maintained pain. *Pain*. 2000 Nov;88(2):161-8.

[9] Davis, KD; Treede, RD; Raja, SN; Meyer, RA; Campbell, JN. Topical application of clonidine relieves hyperalgesia in patients with sympathetically maintained pain. *Pain*. 1991 Dec;47(3):309-17.

[10] Drummond, PD. Noradrenaline increases hyperalgesia to heat in skin sensitized by capsaicin. *Pain* 1995; 60: 311-5.

[11] Liu, M; Parada, S; Rowan, JS; Bennett, GJ. The sympathetic nervous system contributes to capsaicin - evoked mechanical allodynia but not pinprick hyperalgesia in humans. *Journal of Neuroscience* 1996; 16: 7331-5

[12] Kinnman, E; Nygårds, EB; Hansson, P. Peripheral α-adrenoreceptors are involved in the development of capsaicin induced ongoing and stimulus evoked pain in humans. *Pain* 1997; 69: 79-85.

[13] Drummond, PD; Skipworth, S; Finch, PM. Alpha 1-adrenoceptors in normal and hyperalgesic human skin. *Clin.Sci.*(Colch.) 1996; 91: 73-7.

[14] Fuchs, PN; Meyer, RA; Raja, SN. Heat, but not mechanical hyperalgesia, following adrenergic injections in normal human skin. *Pain* 2001; 90: 15-23.

[15] Baron, R; Levine, JD; Fields, HL. Causalgia and reflex sympathetic dystrophy: does the sympathetic nervous system contribute to the generation of pain? *Muscle Nerve.* 1999; 22: 678-95

[16] Pedersen, JL; Rung, GW; Kehlet, H. Effects of sympathetic nerve block on acute inflammatory pain and hyperalgesia. *Anesthesiology* 1997; 86: 293-301.

[17] Levine, JD; Dardick, SJ; Roizen, MF; Helms, C; Basbaum, AI. Contribution of sensory afferents and sympathetic efferents to joint injury in experimental arthritis. *Journal of Neuroscience.* 1986; 6: 3423-9.

[18] Chabal, C; Jacobson, L; Russell, LC; Burchiel, KJ. Pain response to perineuromal injection of normal saline, epinephrine, and lidocaine in humans. *Pain.* 1992;49:9-12.

[19] Lin, EE; Horasek, S; Agarwal, S; Wu, CL; Raja, SN. Local administration of norepinephrine in the stump evokes dose-dependent pain in amputees. *Clin. J. Pain.* 2006.

[20] Arner, S. Intravenous phentolamine test: diagnostic and prognostic use in reflex sympathetic dystrophy. *Pain* 1991; 46: 17-22.

[21] Raja, SN; Treede, RD; Davis, KD; Campbell, JN. Systemic alpha-adrenergic blockade with phentolamine: a diagnostic test for sympathetically maintained pain. *Anesthesiology.* 1991 Apr;74(4):691-8.

[22] Dellemijn, PL; Fields, HL; Allen, RR; McKay, WR; Rowbotham, MC. The interpretation of pain relief and sensory changes following sympathetic blockade. *Brain.* 1994 Dec;117 (Pt 6):1475-87.

[23] Blaes, F; Schmitz, K; Tschernatsch, M; Kaps, M; Krasenbrink, I; Hempelmann, G; Brau, ME. Autoimmune etiology of complex regional pain syndrome (M. Sudeck). *Neurology.* 2004 Nov 9;63(9):1734-6.

[24] Torebjork, E; Wahren, L; Wallin, G; Hallin, R; Koltzenburg, M. Noradrenaline-evoked pain in neuralgia. *Pain.* 1995; 63: 11-20.

[25] Choi, B; Rowbotham, MC. Effect of adrenergic receptor activation on post-herpetic neuralgia pain and sensory disturbances. *Pain.* 1997; 69: 55-63.

[26] Baron, R; Schattschneider, J; Binder, A; Siebrecht, D; Wasner, G. Relation between sympathetic vasoconstrictor activity and pain and hyperalgesia in complex regional pain syndromes: a case-control study. *Lancet.* 2002 May 11;359(9318):1655-60.

[27] Drummond, PD; Finch, PM. Persistence of pain induced by startle and forehead cooling after sympathetic blockade in patients with complex regional pain syndrome. *J. Neurol. Neurosurg Psychiatry.* 2004 Jan;75(1):98-102.

[28] Jänig, W; Baron, R. Complex regional pain syndrome: mystery explained? *Lancet Neurol.* 2003; 2: 687-97.

[29] Arnold, JM; Teasell, RW; MacLeod, AP; Brown, JE; Carruthers, SG. Increased venous alpha-adrenoceptor responsiveness in patients with reflex sympathetic dystrophy. *Ann. Intern. Med.* 1993; 118: 619-21.

[30] Kim, SH; Na, HS; Sheen, K; Chung, JM. Effects of sympathectomy on a rat model of peripheral neuropathy. *Pain.* 1993; 55: 85-92.

[31] Ringkamp, M; Eschenfelder, S; Grethel, EJ; Häbler, HJ; Meyer, RA; Jänig, W; Raja, SN. Lumbar sympathectomy failed to reverse mechanical allodynia- and hyperalgesia-like behavior in rats with L5 spinal nerve injury. *Pain.* 1999; 79: 143-53.

[32] Yoon, YW; Lee, DH; Lee, BH; Chung, K; Chung, JM. Different strains and substrains of rats show different levels of neuropathic pain behaviors. *Experimental Brain Research.* 1999; 129: 167-71.

[33] Coderre, TJ; Xanthos, DN; Francis, L; Bennett, GJ. Chronic post-ischemia pain (CPIP): a novel animal model of complex regional pain syndrome-type I (CRPS-I; reflex sympathetic dystrophy) produced by prolonged hindpaw ischemia and reperfusion in the rat. *Pain.* 2004; 112: 94-105.

[34] Guo, TZ; Offley, SC; Boyd, EA; Jacobs, CR; Kingery, WS. Substance P signaling contributes to the vascular and nociceptive abnormalities observed in a tibial fracture rat model of complex regional pain syndrome type I. *Pain.* 2004;108:95-107.

[35] Blumberg, H; Jänig, W. Discharge pattern of afferent fibers from a neuroma. *Pain.* 1984; 20: 335-53.

[36] Burchiel, KJ. Spontaneous impulse generation in normal and denervated dorsal root ganglia: sensitivity to alpha-adrenergic stimulation and hypoxia. *Experimental Neurology.* 1984; 85: 257-72.

[37] Sato, J; Perl, ER. Adrenergic excitation of cutaneous pain receptors induced by peripheral nerve injury. *Science.* 1991; 251: 1608-10.

[38] Habler, HJ; Jänig, W; Koltzenburg, M. Activation of unmyelinated afferents in chronically lesioned nerves by adrenaline and excitation of sympathetic efferents in the cat. *Neurosci. Lett.* 1987; 82: 35-40.

[39] Ali, Z; Ringkamp, M; Hartke, TV; Chien, HF; Flavahan, NA; Campbell JN; Meyer RA. Uninjured C-fiber nociceptors develop spontaneous activity and alpha-adrenergic sensitivity following L6 spinal nerve ligation in monkey. *J. Neurophysiol.* 1999; 81: 455-66.

[40] Rocco, AG. Radiofrequency lumbar sympatholysis: The evolution of a technique for managing sympathetically maintained pain. *Reg. Anesth.* 1995; 20: 3-12.

[41] Michaelis, M; Devor, M; Jänig, W. Sympathetic modulation of activity in rat dorsal root ganglion neurons changes over time following peripheral nerve injury. *Journal of Neurophysiology.* 1996; 76: 753-63.

[42] McLachlan, EM; Jänig, W; Devor, M; Michaelis, M. Peripheral nerve injury triggers noradrenergic sprouting within dorsal root ganglia. *Nature.* 1993; 363: 543-6

[43] Chung, K; Yoon, YW; Chung, JM. Sprouting sympathetic fibers form synaptic varicosities in the dorsal root ganglion of the rat with neuropathic injury. *Brain Research.* 1997; 751: 275-80.

[44] Bossut, DF; Shea, VK; Perl, ER. Sympathectomy induces adrenergic excitability of cutaneous C-fiber nociceptors. *Journal of Neurophysiology.* 1996; 75: 514-7.

[45] Chen, Y; Michaelis, M; Jänig, W; Devor, M. Adrenoreceptor subtype mediating sympathetic-sensory coupling in injured sensory neurons. *J. Neurophysiol.* 1996; 76: 3721-30.

[46] Shi, TS; Winzer-Serhan, U; Leslie, F; Hökfelt, T. Distribution and regulation of alpha(2)-adrenoceptors in rat dorsal root ganglia. *Pain.* 2000; 84: 319-30.

[47] Koltzenburg, M; Häbler, H-J; Jänig, W. Functional Reinnervation of the Vasculature of the Adult Cat Paw Pad by Axons Originally Innervating Vessels in Hairy Skin. *Neuroscience.* 1995; 67: 245-52.

[48] Teasell, RW; Arnold, JM. Alpha-1 adrenoceptor hyperresponsiveness in three neuropathic pain states: complex regional pain syndrome 1, diabetic peripheral neuropathic pain and central pain states following spinal cord injury. *Pain Res. Man.* 2004 Summer;9(2):89-97.

[49] Muizelaar, JP; Kleyer, M; Hertogs, IA; DeLange, DC. Complex regional pain syndrome (reflex sympathetic dystrophy and causalgia): management with the calcium channel blocker nifedipine and/or the alpha-sympathetic blocker phenoxybenzamine in 59 patients. *Clin. Neurol. Neurosurg.* 1997; 99: 26-30.

[50] Kim, SK; Min, BI; Kim, JH; Hwang, BG; Yoo, GY; Park, DS; Na, HS. Effects of alpha1- and alpha2-adrenoreceptor antagonists on cold allodynia in a rat tail model of neuropathic pain. *Brain Res.* 2005 Mar 28;1039(1-2):207-10.

[51] Lee, YH; Ryu, TG; Park, SJ; Yang, EJ; Jeon, BH; Hur, GM; Kim, KJ. Alpha1-adrenoceptors involvement in painful diabetic neuropathy: a role in allodynia. *Neuroreport.* 2000 May 15;11(7):1417-20.

[52] Lee, DH; Liu, X; Kim, HT; Chung, K; Chung, JM. Receptor subtype mediating the adrenergic sensitivity of pain behavior and ectopic discharges in neuropathic Lewis rats. *J. Neurophysiol.* 1999 May;81(5):2226-33.

[53] Willenbring, S; DeLeo, JA; Coombs, DW. Sciatic cryoneurolysis in rats: a model of sympathetically independent pain. Part 2: Adrenergic pharmacology. *Anesth. Analg.* 1995 Sep;81(3):549-54.

[54] Stevens, DS; Robins, VF; Price, HM. Treatment of sympathetically maintained pain with terazosin. *Reg. Anesth.* 1993 Sep-Oct;18(5):318-21.

[55] Basbaum, AI; Fields HL. Endogenous pain control mechanisms: review and hypothesis. *Ann. Neurol.* 1978 Nov;4(5):451-62.

[56] Obata, H; Li, X; Eisenach, JC. alpha2-Adrenoceptor activation by clonidine enhances stimulation-evoked acetylcholine release from spinal cord tissue after nerve ligation in rats. *Anesthesiology.* 2005 Mar;102(3):657-62.

[57] Campbell, JN; Raja, SN; Meyer, RA; Mackinnon, SE. Myelinated afferents signal the hyperalgesia associated with nerve injury. *Pain.* 1988 Jan;32(1):89-94.

[58] Perez, RS; Kwakkel, G; Zuurmond, WW; de Lange, JJ. Treatment of reflex sympathetic dystrophy (CRPS type 1): a research synthesis of 21 randomized clinical trials. *J. Pain Symptom. Manage.* 2001 Jun;21(6):511-26.

[59] Livingstone, JA; Atkins, RM. Intravenous regional guanethidine blockade in the treatment of post-traumatic complex regional pain syndrome type 1 (algodystrophy) of the hand. *J. Bone Joint Surg. Br.* 2002 Apr;84(3):380-6.

[60] Jadad, AR; Carroll, D; Glynn, CJ; McQuay, HJ. Intravenous regional sympathetic blockade for pain relief in reflex sympathetic dystrophy: a systematic review and a randomized, double-blind crossover study. *J. Pain Symptom Manage.* 1995 Jan;10(1):13-20.

[61] Ramamurthy, S; Hoffman, J. Intravenous regional guanethidine in the treatment of reflex sympathetic dystrophy/causalgia: a randomized, double-blind study. Guanethidine Study Group. *Anesth. Analg.* 1995 Oct;81(4):718-23.

[62] Reuben, SS; Sklar, J. Intravenous regional anesthesia with clonidine in the management of complex regional pain syndrome of the knee. *J. Clin. Anesth.* 2002 Mar;14(2):87-91.

[63] Connelly, NR; Reuben, S; Brull, SJ. Intravenous regional anesthesia with ketorolac-lidocaine for the management of sympathetically-mediated pain. *Yale. J. Biol. Med.* 1995 May-Aug;68(3-4):95-9.

[64] Hord, AH; Rooks, MD; Stephens, BO; Rogers, HG; Fleming, LL. Intravenous regional bretylium and lidocaine for treatment of reflex sympathetic dystrophy: a randomized, double-blind study. *Anesth. Analg.* 1992 Jun;74(6):818-21.

[65] Stevens, RA; Stotz, A; Kao, TC; Powar, M; Burgess, S; Kleinman, B. The relative increase in skin temperature after stellate ganglion block is predictive of a complete sympathectomy of the hand. *Reg. Anesth. Pain Med.* 1998 May-Jun;23(3):266-70.

[66] Price, DD; Long, S; Wilsey, B; Rafii, A. Analysis of peak magnitude and duration of analgesia produced by local anesthetics injected into sympathetic ganglia of complex regional pain syndrome patients. *Clin. J. Pain* 1998; 14: 216-26.

[67] Bandyk, DF; Johnson, BL; Kirkpatrick, AF; Novotney, ML; Back, MR; Schmacht, DC. Surgical sympathectomy for reflex sympathetic dystrophy syndromes. *J. Vasc.Surg.* 2002; 35: 269-77.

[68] Cepeda, MS ; Lau, J ; Carr, DB. Defining the therapeutic role of local anesthetic sympathetic blockade in complex regional pain syndrome: a narrative and systematic review. *Clin. J. Pain.* 2002 Jul-Aug;18(4):216-33.

[69] Rauck, RL; Eisenach, JC; Jackson, K; Young, LD; Southern J. Epidural clonidine treatment for refractory reflex sympathetic dystrophy. *Anesthesiology.* 1993 Dec;79(6):1163-9.

[70] Noe, CE; Haynsworth, RF Jr. Lumbar radiofrequency sympatholysis. *J. Vasc. Surg.* 1993 Apr;17(4):801-6.

[71] Wilkinson, HA. Percutaneous radiofrequency upper thoracic sympathectomy. *Neurosurgery.* 1996 Apr;38(4):715-25.

[72] Krasna, MJ; Demmy, TL; McKenna, RJ; Mack, MJ. Thoracoscopic sympathectomy: the U.S. experience. *Eur. J. Surg. Suppl.* 1998;(580):19-21.

[73] Mailis, A; Furlan, A. Sympathectomy for neuropathic pain. *Cochrane Database Syst. Rev.* 2003;(2):CD002918.

[74] Jacobs, MJ; Jorning, PJ; Joshi, SR; Kitslaar, PJ; Slaaf, DW; Reneman, RS. Epidural spinal cord electrical stimulation improves microvascular blood flow in severe limb ischemia. *Ann. Surg.* 1988 Feb;207(2):179-83.

[75] Naver, H; Augustinsson, LE; Elam, M. The vasodilating effect of spinal dorsal column stimulation is mediated by sympathetic nerves. *Clin. Auton. Res.* 1992 Feb;2(1):41-5.

[76] Hord, ED; Cohen, SP; Cosgrove, GR; Ahmed, SU; Vallejo, R; Chang, Y; Stojanovic, MP. The predictive value of sympathetic block for the success of spinal cord stimulation. *Neurosurgery.* 2003 Sep;53(3):626-32; discussion 632-3.

[77] Kemler, MA; De Vet, HC; Barendse, GA; Van Den Wildenberg, FA; Van Kleef, M. The effect of spinal cord stimulation in patients with chronic reflex sympathetic dystrophy: two years' follow-up of the randomized controlled trial. *Ann. Neurol.* 2004 Jan;55(1):13-8.

[78] Grabow, TS; Tella, PK; Raja, SN. Spinal cord stimulation for complex regional pain syndrome: an evidence-based medicine review of the literature. *Clin. J. Pain.* 2003 Nov-Dec;19(6):371-83.

[79] Turner, JA; Loeser, JD; Deyo, RA; Sanders, SB. Spinal cord stimulation for patients with failed back surgery syndrome or complex regional pain syndrome: a systematic review of effectiveness and complications. *Pain.* 2004; 108: 137-47.

[80] Mekhail, NA; Aeschbach, A; Stanton-Hicks, M. Cost benefit analysis of neurostimulation for chronic pain. *Clin. J. Pain.* 2004 Nov-Dec;20(6):462-8.

[81] Multon, S; Schoenen, J. Pain control by vagus nerve stimulation: from animal to man...and back. *Acta. Neurol. Belg.* 2005 Jun;105(2):62-7.

*Chapter X*

# Mechanisms of Tricyclic Antidepressants in Pain Modulation

### *Peter Gerner and Ging Kuo Wang**

Department of Anesthesiology, Perioperative and Pain Medicine,
Harvard Medical School and Brigham and Women's Hospital,
Boston, MA. 02115

## Abstract

Tricyclic antidepressants (TCAs) have been the most commonly used drugs for patients with chronic pain since the 1960s. The antidepressive action of these drugs in CNS was the rationale behind their original uses, since many patients with such a pain syndrome are also depressed. Because TCAs have many recognized target sites in the CNS, PNS, and elsewhere, the underlying mechanisms of TCA efficacy in pain management have not yet been resolved. This chapter discusses a number of well-studied target sites and focuses on the *in vivo* and *in vitro* local anesthetic properties of TCAs as the underlying mechanism for their efficacy against pain. When injected intrathecally or at the rat sciatic notch, amitriptyline (a tertiary amine TCA) at 5 mM acts as a long-acting local anesthetic and is more potent than the local anesthetic bupivacaine at 15.4 mM (0.5%). At therapeutic plasma concentrations (~0.4-0.9 µM), amitriptyline preferentially blocks the open and inactivated $Na^+$ channels but has minimal effects on the resting $Na^+$ channels. This state-dependent binding of amitriptyline readily explains why amitriptyline elicits a profound use-dependent block of $Na^+$ currents during repetitive pulses. Such a use-dependent phenomenon will enable amitriptyline at the therapeutic plasma concentration to silence the ectopic discharge in damaged nerves but not the typical transmission of action potentials in normal nerves. Site-directed mutagenesis shows that the binding site for amitriptyline overlaps extensively with that for local anesthetics within the $Na^+$

---

*Correspondence to Dr. Ging Kuo Wang, Department of Anesthesiology, Perioperative and Pain Medicine, Brigham and Women's Hospital, 75 Francis St., Boston, MA 02115. Tel: 617732-6886. Fax: 617730-2801. email: wang@zeus.bwh.harvard.edu

channel. Together, these findings support the hypothesis that the voltage-gated Na$^+$ channel is one of the primary therapeutic targets of TCAs for chronic pain.

## Introduction

Tricyclic antidepressants (TCAs) were discovered fortuitously in 1950s for the treatment of major depressive illness, as well as for other psychiatric disorders such as anxiety, panic attacks, and insomnia [1]. The chemical structures of TCAs, such as amitriptyline and nortriptyline, contain a common tricyclic moiety and a tertiary amine or a secondary amine separated by an intermediate alkyl chain (Fig. 1). The tricyclic moiety of TCAs contributes most of the high hydrophobicity of these compounds, whereas the amine group is protonated in aqueous solution at neutral pH. Other types of antidepressants include selective serotonin-reuptake inhibitors (SSRI), monoamine oxidase inhibitors (MAOI), and atypical antidepressants. The sites and modes of action of various types of antidepressants for mood disorder are not completely understood but likely include pre- and postsynaptic neurons involving both adrenergic and serotonergic neurotransmitters.

Beside their common applications for major depressive illness, TCAs have also been used for the treatment of chronic pain since 1960s. To date, TCAs such as amitriptyline and nortriptyline remain the first choice of antidepressants for chronic pain [2]. SSRI and MAOI drugs may be useful when TCAs fail to provide pain relief or cause severe adverse effects. The underlying mechanisms for the analgesic efficacy of TCAs in chronic pain, however, have not been resolved. The original rationale for the use of TCAs in patients with chronic and often neuropathic pain was based on the premise that many patients with such pain syndromes are also depressed.

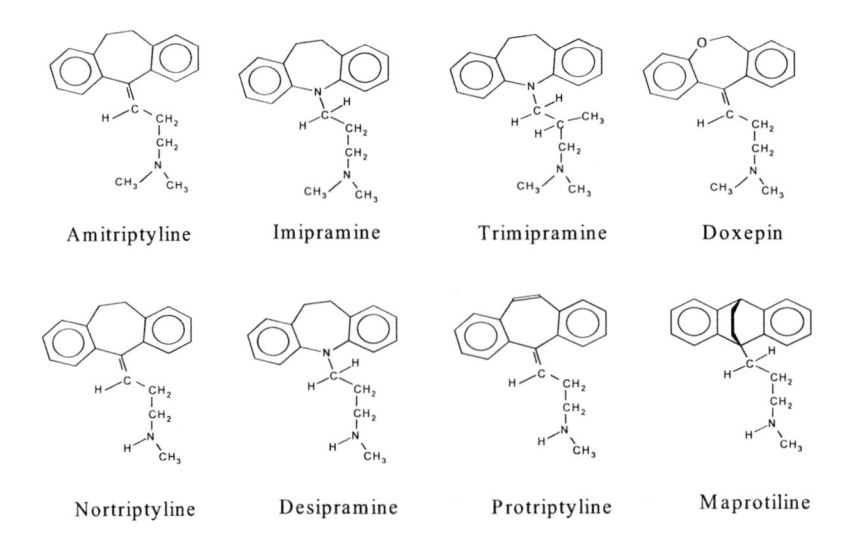

Figure 1. Chemical structures of tricyclic antidepressants. The first row shows tertiary amine TCAs, and the second row shows secondary amine TCAs. Imipramine, desipramine, and trimipramine contain a tricyclic moiety of dibenzocycloheptadienes; amitriptyline and nortriptyline contain a tricyclic dibenzoxepine; doxepin has a dibenzazepine; protriptyline has a dibenzocycloheptatriene; and maprotiline has an ethylene bridge across the central 6-carbon ring.

It is interesting to note that the clinical onset of analgesia with TCAs in chronic pain is more rapid than the usual onset of an antidepressant effect in depressed patients. Also, not all antidepressants are equally effective for chronic pain. Most controlled clinical trials with antidepressants such as citalopram, femoxetine, fluoxetine, trazodone, and zimelidine that are selectively serotonergic in their effects have shown that their analgesic effects are inferior to those of less selective antidepressants such as amitriptyline [3]. These observations have led to the suggestion that mechanisms in addition to the antidepressive action in the CNS are involved in the analgesic efficacy of TCAs in chronic pain. This chapter reviews the current hypotheses that explain the analgesic effect of TCAs for the treatment of chronic pain. We focus on the voltage-gated $Na^+$ channel as one of the primary targets for TCAs in pain therapy.

# Mechanisms for the Analgesic Efficacy of TCAs in Pain Management

TCAs produce a variety of pharmacologic actions in the CNS and PNS. Among them are three major modes of action (1): (a) *inhibition of noradrenaline and 5-hydroxytrptamine (5-HT; or serotonin) reuptake*; (b) *inhibition of N-methyl-D-aspartic acid (NMDA), nicotinic, histamine, and 5-HT receptors*; and (c) *block of voltage-gated ion channels including $Na^+$, $K^+$, and $Ca^{2+}$ channels*. Many of the side effects produced by TCAs are also the manifestations of these targets. Weakness, fatigue, confusion, and delirium are attributable to central effects of TCAs. Dry mouth, epigastric distress, constipation, palpitations, and urinary retention are due to adverse autonomic effects. Since the actions of TCAs in nervous systems are relatively broad and not at all specific, the mechanisms underlying their efficacy in pain management likely involve multiple routes both in the CNS and PNS. At least three hypotheses regarding the action of TCAs with respect to analgesic effects for chronic pain have been suggested.

## (i) Antidepressive Hypothesis in CNS

Our understanding of the central antidepressive effects of TCAs and its interpretation with respect to the underlying mechanism are limited by a lack of a compelling psychobiological theory of mood disorders. The same is also true for the etiology of many chronic pain syndromes. Thus, the antidepressive hypothesis for chronic pain will remain tentative. Additional experimental supports are needed to strengthen this hypothesis. Nevertheless, the analgesic effects of TCAs are likely due, at least in part, to their antidepressive action in the CNS. Chronic pain often associates with reactive depression, as noted by Paoli et al. [4] who first used imipramine to treat patients with chronic pain. In clinical trials, the majority of patients with coexisting chronic pain and depression obtained relief from both disorders when responding to MAOI or TCA therapy [2].

The analgesic and antidepressive action of TCAs could be caused by their action on central neurotransmitter functions, particularly those mediated by the catecholamine and indolamine systems [1]. TCAs increase synaptic levels of dopamine, norepinephrine, and serotonin. There are many other possible targets for TCAs in CNS. For example, TCAs clearly enhance opiate analgesia *in vivo* even in norepinephrine transporter knock-out mice [5]. Also, TCAs may bind directly to opiate receptors [6].

Analgesic effects of TCAs have also been attributed to nonspecific physiological effects such as sedation, diminished anxiety, muscle relaxation, and restored sleep cycles. Other specific TCA effects that have been invoked to explain their analgesic effects include central or peripheral histamine receptor blockade, inhibition of prostaglandin synthetase, and a calcium-channel blocking effect.

## (ii) Adenosine Hypothesis in CNS/PNS

The adenosine hypothesis for the peripheral action of TCAs in pain therapy has been summarized by Sawynok [7]. Clinical trials of topical amitriptyline with and without ketamine are based on this hypothesis [8]. Adenosine also displays a modest analgesic effect when applied intrathecally [9]. Tricyclic compounds appear to inhibit uptake of adenosine in the brain synaptosomal preparations, which leads to an increase in the amount of adenosine available for signaling. This notion is supported by the finding that caffeine (an adenosine-receptor blocker) partially reversed the antinociceptive effects of amitriptyline in the rat formalin test model. The hypothesis of an enhanced adenosine-signaling is further supported by the finding of inhibition by caffeine of the thermal antihyperalgesic effect of amitriptyline in a rat model of neuropathic pain.

Recently, uptake studies using cultured rat C6 glioma cells found that amitriptyline inhibited adenosine uptake by an adenosine transporter. In addition, in enzyme assays, amitriptyline had no effect on adenosine kinase or adenosine deaminase activity. Therefore, it was concluded that increased extracellular adenosine levels *in vivo* appear to be due in part to extracellular conversion of nucleotide and in part to inhibition of uptake [10].

## (iii) Sodium-Channel Hypothesis in CNS/PNS

Earlier reports showed that amitriptyline is a potent voltage-gated $Na^+$ channel blocker in guinea pig and rabbit cardiac myocytes [11,12]. Later experiments revealed that amitriptyline block of human cardiac $Na^+$ channels is also strongly state-dependent [13]. The blocking effects of cardiac $Na^+$ channels by amitryptyline were used as evidence to explain why overdoses of TCAs cause fatal arrhythmias [12,14].

Similar blocking effects by amitriptyline were found in neuronal $Na^+$ channels [15-17]. In particular, amitriptyline, like many local anesthetics, also elicits a profound use-dependent block of $Na^+$ currents. The similarities between amitriptyline and local anesthetics in blocking $Na^+$ channels have led to the hypothesis that amitriptyline acts as a local anesthetic for its efficacy in pain management. An extensive test of this hypothesis is to demonstrate that TCAs display local anesthetic properties *in vivo* and *in vitro,* as described next.

## TCAs Possess Local Anesthetic Properties

We will briefly outline the development of amitriptyline as a local anesthetic from basic electrophysiology experiments through the various developmental stages up to clinical experiments, although potential TCA neurotoxicity has so far prevented the application of TCAs as sole local anesthetic agents in humans [18].

*In vivo/preclinical evidence* When the blocking efficacy of TCAs was screened in a rat sciatic nerve block model, the duration of complete blockade of nociception and motor function by amitriptyline, doxepin, imipramine, trimipramine, and desipramine at 5 mM was approximately equal to or longer than that by bupivacaine at 0.5% (~15.4 mM) (Fig. 2A) [19]. However, nortriptyline and protriptyline produced only partial sciatic nerve blockade, whereas maprotiline failed to elicit even partial sciatic nerve blockade (Fig. 2B). TCAs are also effective in spinal anesthesia after intrathecal injection [20]. Custom-synthesized quaternary ammonium derivatives of amitriptyline, among them N-phenylethyl amitriptyline and N-methyl amitriptyline, were significantly more potent than bupivacaine, the latter even demonstrating differential block in a sheep spinal injection model [21,22]. Unfortunately, amitriptyline and particularly its quaternary ammonium derivatives appear to have a very narrow therapeutic window. For example, N-propyl amitriptyline at concentrations only several times higher than the minimal effective concentration produced severe axonal degeneration with corresponding sensory deficits [23].

Can the therapeutic ratio of amitriptyline be improved when tetrodotoxin (TTX) is co-injected? TTX is a naturally occurring $Na^+$ channel blocker from the puffer fish that lacks neurotoxicity even after prolonged application [24]. The use of hydrophilic TTX as a sole agent for peripheral nerve block appears to be limited, as the block is unreliable and minor in the majority of cases [25-27]. However, co-injection of TTX with the local anesthetic bupivacaine prolongs the block of both drugs extensively. Likewise, Barnett et al [27] recently showed that TTX and amitriptyline were significantly synergistic when co-administered in a percutaneous rat sciatic nerve block injection model. Their results suggest that co-injection of these two drugs may improve the therapeutic ratio of TCAs and their derivatives.

To understand the mechanism of this observed synergy; our group has shown that the synergistic action of amitriptyline and TTX is due both to pharmacodynamic synergism (different binding sites for amitriptyline and TTX) in the resting state (-150 mV) and to pharmacokinetic synergism (increased traversing of amitriptyline and/or TTX through nerve sheaths). This is evidenced *in vitro* by a modest (statistically significant) synergism when amitriptyline is co-infused with TTX at –150 mV in a culture dish containing single cells (bypassing the nerve sheath, endoneurium, and epineurium), where the single cell membrane is the only barrier between the drug and the local-anesthetic receptor (Gerner, P; unpublished observation).

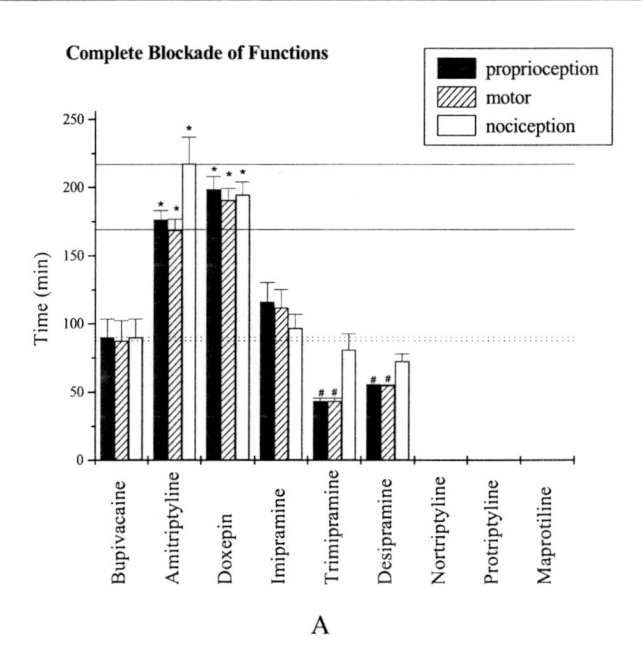

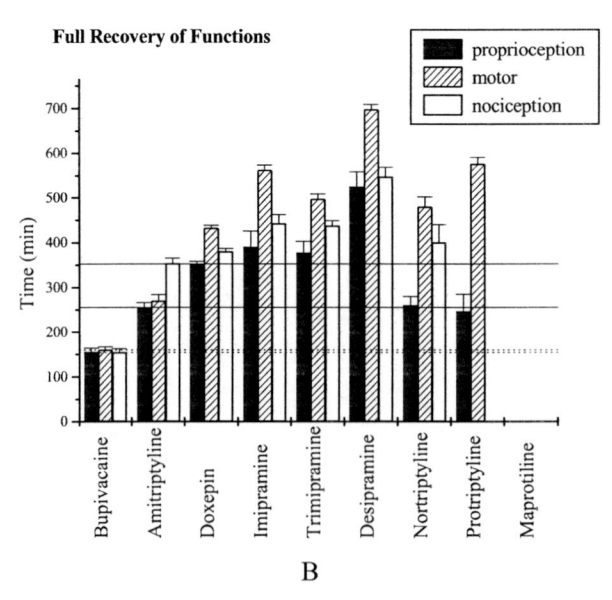

Figure 2. Duration of the complete blockade and the full recovery of rat sciatic nerve functions by various TCAs. (A) The duration of complete sciatic nerve blockade by bupivacaine at 15.4 mM and various TCAs at 5 mM was measured as described in Fig.2; data were averaged and plotted against each drug. Amitriptyline showed the longest complete blockade of nociception. Solid and dotted lines across the data indicate the range of the duration of complete sciatic nerve blockade by amitriptyline and bupivacaine, respectively. Symbols (*, #) indicate $P < 0.05$ when compared with bupivacaine data. (B) The duration to reach the full recovery of sciatic nerve functions after the injection of bupivacaine at 15.4 mM and various TCAs at 5 mM was measured as described in Fig. 2; data were averaged and plotted against each drug. Solid and dotted lines across the data indicate the range of the duration to reach the full recovery of sciatic nerve functions after the injection of amitriptyline and bupivacaine, respectively. The number of rats used in these experiments was 6 for bupivacaine, trimipramine and nortriptyline; 8 for amitriptyline, imipramine, and maprotiline; 12 for doxepin; 5 for protriptyline; and 7 for desipramine.

On the basis of *in vivo* studies by Barnett et al. [27], which demonstrate highly pronounced synergism (indicated by the greatly prolonged duration of blockade) of amitriptyline combined with TTX, we suggest that pharmacokinetic synergism is the major mechanism for the strong synergism of amitriptyline combined with TTX injected subfascially for sciatic nerve block in rats. The 50% effective dose of amitriptyline alone was 6.1 mM but dramatically decreased to only 0.3 mM when co-injected with TTX at a concentration of 20 µM (Gerner, P; unpublished observation), indicating that the combination of a very hydrophobic drug (amitriptyline) with a very hydrophilic drug (TTX) is useful clinically as a means of increasing permeability across nerve sheaths. Although it is usually assumed that hydrophobic local anesthetics penetrate more easily through nerve membranes, extremely hydrophobic drugs such as amitriptyline do not follow this logic, probably because these drugs may be 'too' hydrophobic and may get 'stuck' in the respective membranes. The strong synergism also occurs in the co-application of N-propyl-amitriptyline and TTX (Fig. 3) [23], indicating the existence of the phenomenon of synergistic action for TCAs and their derivatives when co-injected with TTX.

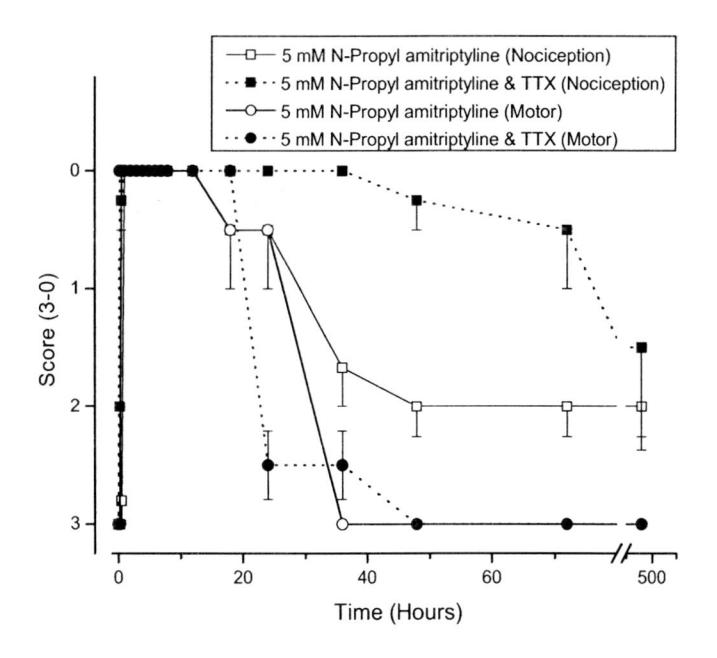

Figure 3. Sciatic nerve block with 0.2 ml of N-propyl amitriptyline at 5 mM. Statistically significant differential block was present with or without the addition of TTX (0= full block, 3= no block).

*In vitro structure/activity relationship* The finding that not all TCAs are equally potent as local anesthetics in the rat sciatic nerve model suggests that pharmacological or physicochemical properties of TCAs may affect their local anesthetic potency *in vivo*. Analogous to the discussion above for the synergistic action of TTX and amitriptyline, this apparent inequality in TCA potency could be at the binding site with the Na$^+$ channel (e.g., binding affinity) or at the membrane barrier sites (e.g., nerve sheath permeability). To distinguish these two possibilities, we measured dose-response block of hNav1.5 Na$^+$

channels by TCAs [19]. Figure 4 gives an example of these measurements with a conditioning pulse at −140 mV for the resting block and at −70 mV for the inactivated block.

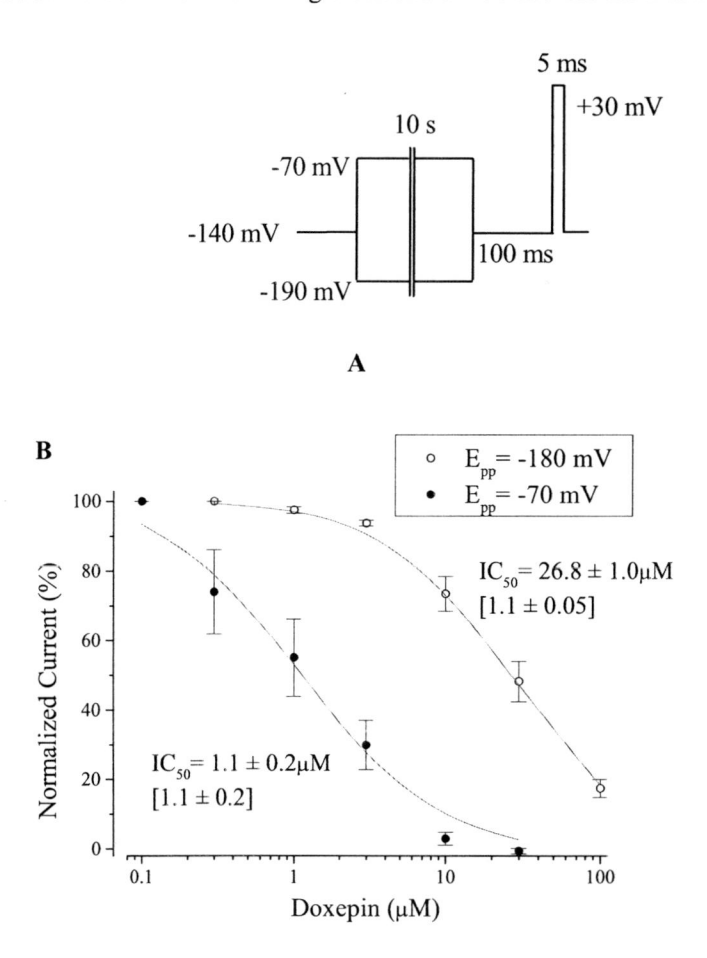

Figure 4. Dose-response block of hNav1.5 Na$^+$ channels by doxepin. (A) Superimposed traces of Na$^+$ currents expressed in the presence of 10 μM doxepin at prepulse voltages of −180 mV and −70 mV for 10 s. Without drug, the difference in outward peak current elicited by the test pulse was slight. With 10 μM doxepin present, the difference between the two prepulse voltages was large. (B) The resting and inactivated affinities for doxepin in hH1 wild type were measured (see A, inset) with prepulses of −180 mV (open circles) or −70 mV (solid circles), respectively, at various drug concentrations. The data were normalized with respect to the peak current of the lowest drug concentration and fitted with the Hill equation (solid lines). The IC$_{50}$ values for both resting and inactivated channels are given. Hill coefficients are in brackets.

The conditioning pulse was set for 10 s to allow the slow binding between doxepin and the inactivated channel to reach steady state. The resting block was ~24 times less potent than the inactivated block by doxepin. Figure 5 summarizes the results of all TCAs tested. We found that, despite the absence of *in vivo* block by maprotiline, this antidepressant retained its potency in blocking Na$^+$ channels *in vitro*. This finding leads us to conclude that the lack of potency in the sciatic nerve model is due to the inability of maprotiline to penetrate various membrane barriers rapidly [19].

*In vivo/clinical evidence* Before clinical studies were contemplated, a number of pilot studies with high-dose and/or repeat applications of amitriptyline using topical and nerve block models were performed in rats and sheep, e.g., prolonged topical (cutaneous) application of up to 6% amitriptyline did not result in significant side effects, and rat sciatic nerve blockade with high doses did not reveal neurobehavioral deficits or detectable histopathological toxicity.

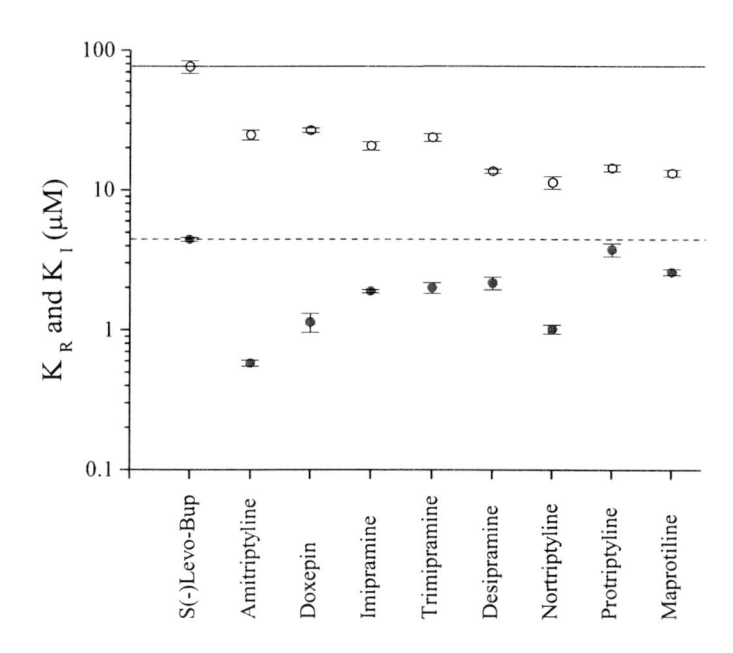

Figure 5. Resting and inactivated affinities of various TCAs. The binding affinities of the TCAs are given in terms of $K_R$ and $K_I$, which are defined as the $IC_{50}$ values for resting and inactivated hNav1.5 channels, respectively. $K_R$ (open circles) and $K_I$ (closed circles) values are plotted for each TCA and were determined in an identical manner to those of doxepin (see Fig 3B) with n = 5-7. The solid and dotted lines indicate the $K_R$ and $K_I$ values for (S)-bupicacaine, respectively.

Furthermore, the dose necessary to produce onset of seizure, apnea, and toxicity was higher for i.v. amitriptyline than for i.v. bupivacaine or levobupivacaine (Fig. 6), suggesting that the systemic toxicity of amitriptyline is less than that of the conventional local anesthetic, bupivacaine [28]. Therefore, a clinical trial of TCA appeared justified.

In healthy human volunteers, topical application of amitriptyline was significantly more effective than placebo (Fig. 7) [29]. Although no comparison was done with EMLA cream or the 5% Lidoderm patch in that study, transdermal amitriptyline appeared to be quite effective, as several subjects had complete analgesia that lasted for several hours in the respective test area. However, concentration-dependent redness of the skin might be indicative of a toxic response. Recently, a double-blind, randomized, placebo-controlled 3-week study evaluated the efficacy of topical 2% amitriptyline, 1% ketamine, and a combination of the two in treating patients with neuropathic pain revealed no significant difference in efficacy between groups [8]. Of note, the plasma level of amitriptyline appeared to be in the nontoxic range when applied as directed (4 ml of cream to the site of maximum pain three times per day for 3 weeks).

When amitriptyline was evaluated for ulnar nerve blockade in a pilot study with healthy human volunteers [30], it was less effective than bupivacaine—contrary to all animal studies.

This might be due to the nerve sheaths in humans being thicker than those in rats. Meanwhile, additional animal studies using a more sensitive method suggested severe neurotoxic potential. As a result, further clinical exploration of amitriptyline as a local anesthetic was abandoned. Currently, co-injection of amitriptyline along with neurotoxicity-preventing agents is being investigated.

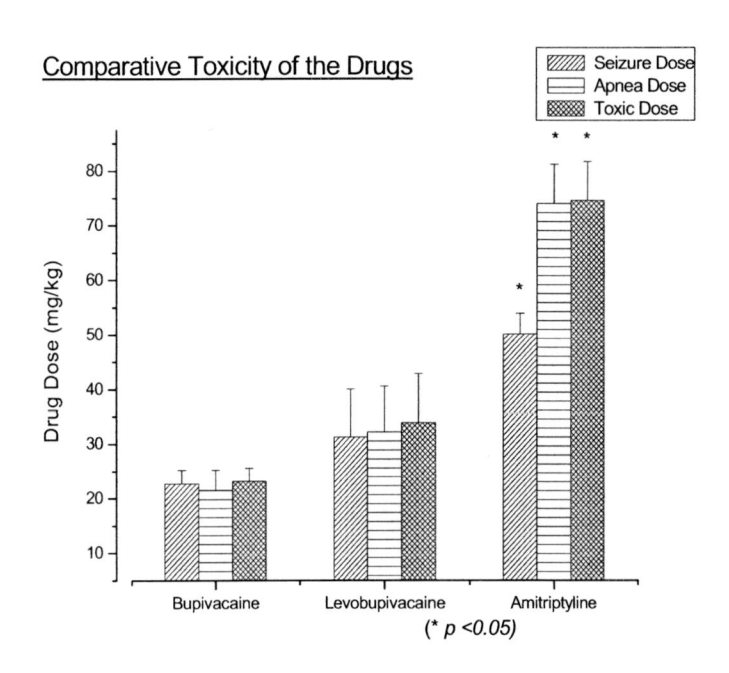

Figure 6. Cumulative dose of drugs at the onset of seizure, apnea, and toxic dose (heart rate of 50 beats/min or respiratory arrest for 30 seconds). Dose required to cause the toxic symptoms were significantly higher in the amitriptyline group (n=10) when compared to bupivacaine (n=7) and levobupivacaine (n=6); (P < 0.05). In the bupivacaine and levobupivacaine groups, the toxic symptoms occurred fairly rapidly in succession when compared with the occurrence in animals in the amitriptyline group.

Although it seems clear that amitriptyline, the most studied TCA, will not find clinical use as a sole agent for regional anesthesia because of its neurotoxic potential, it is also clear that $Na^+$ channel blockade is an intrinsic property of all TCAs and that this property also plays a major role in the efficacy of oral TCA for chronic pain. It is not yet known if amitriptyline will play a role in managing acute pain and preventing chronic pain, respective studies are currently under way in several centers and should clarify the role of TCAs beyond the therapy for chronic pain.

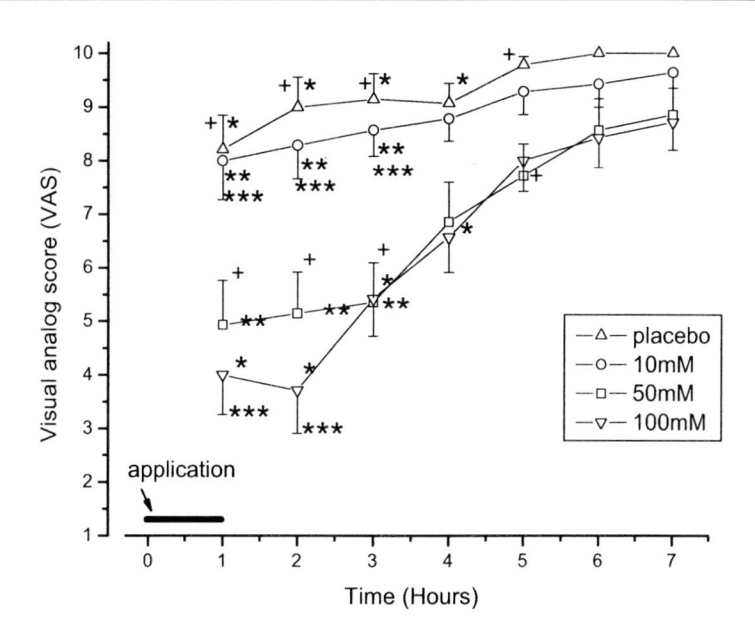

Figure 7. Analgesia after patch removal for placebo (vehicle only) and amitriptyline at various concentrations. Application time was 1 hour (arrow). Following removal of the patch, blinded subjects were 'poked' each hour with a blunt needle at a designated test area vs. a control area and the respective visual analog score (VAS) was reported to the blinded experimenter. Data are presented as mean ± SEM. Overall significance was determined by ANOVA for repeated measurements, Post-hoc analysis (pairwise comparison of different concentrations and/or placebo at each time point) was done by Scheffe's method. $p<0.05$ for *(placebo vs. 100 mM), ** (10 vs. 50 mM), *** (10 vs. 100 mM) and + (placebo vs. 50 mM amitriptyline).

# Effect of Tricyclic Antidepressants on Neural Discharge and High-Frequency Firing via the Sodium-Channel Route

The following discussion focuses on the $Na^+$-channel hypothesis for TCA efficacy in patients with neuropathic pain. Ectopic discharge originating in injured peripheral nerves will feed into the CNS, providing a primary neuropathic signal and maintaining a diseased state by central amplification [31]. We will use this pain pathway as an example to illustrate how TCAs may modulate pain sensation. Figure 8 shows a simplified flow chart for this signaling pathway. The flow chart starts from the origin of nociception (or triggering point) to relay circuits and finally to pain sensation. Neural discharges occur in discrete neurons at the origin of nociception that transmit the noxious information toward relay circuits. Subsequent neural discharges via relay circuits may transmit the encoded information for pain sensation in the CNS.

```
┌─────────────────┐     ┌─────────────────┐     ┌─────────────────┐
│  Origin of Pain │────▶│ Relay circuitry │────▶│  Pain sensation │
└─────────────────┘     └─────────────────┘     └─────────────────┘
          │    ┌──────────────┐     │    ┌──────────────┐
          └───▶│Ectopic neural│     └───▶│Ectopic neural│
               │  discharge   │          │  discharge   │
               └──────┬───────┘          └──────┬───────┘
                       ⚡                        ⚡
                  ┌──────────────────────────────────────────┐
                  │ TCAs may alleviate pain by blocking high-│
                  │ frequency action potentials but leave the│
                  │ normal impulses intact                   │
                  └──────────────────────────────────────────┘
```

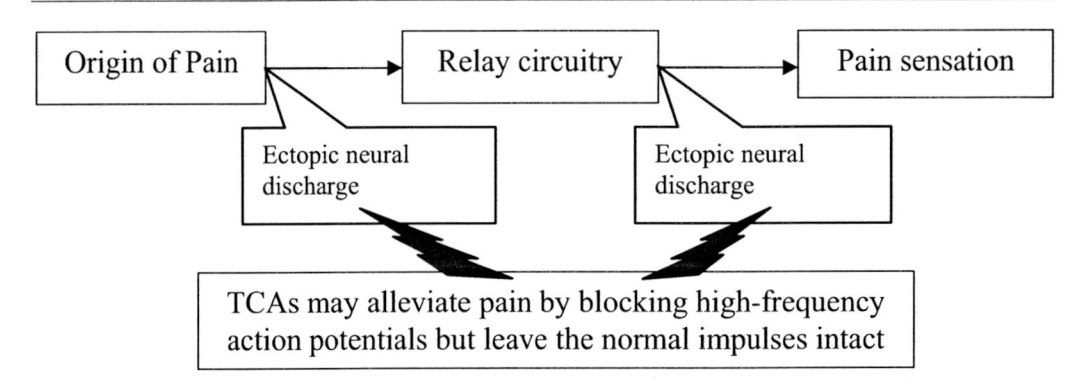

Figure 8. How do TCAs silence ectopic neural discharge and high-frequency firing via the sodium-channel route? Painful nociceptive states that originate in the PNS and CNS because of nerve injury may initiate ectopic discharge (left box). Such discharge is processed and integrated by the relay circuits as a sensitized state, and the nociceptive information is eventually transmitted to the CNS and causes pain sensation. This pain pathway requires voltage-gated $Na^+$ channels, which are responsible for the generation of action potentials and ectopic neural discharges. At the therapeutic plasma concentrations, TCAs potently block the open $Na^+$ channels during high-frequency firing. Normal impulse transmission may not be affected since resting $Na^+$ channels are not sensitive to TCAs at this plasma concentration range and since $Na^+$ channels do not open frequently without ectopic discharge. This hypothesis is likely also applicable to the efficacy of lidocaine in neuropathic pain at the low concentration reported by Boas et al. [31].

How do TCAs alleviate pain at the cellular and molecular levels? As illustrated at the bottom of the diagram, one likely action of TCAs is to block abnormal neural discharges at critical signaling areas, such as at the origin of nociception, in nerve trunks, at relay circuits, and in CNS pain perception. Such an action of TCAs at therapeutic plasma concentrations can be achieved by blocking the $Na^+$ channels that open frequently during repetitive neural discharge. The profound use-dependent block of $Na^+$ currents elicited by amtriptyline during repetitive pulses [12] is consistent with this explanation. However, what is unclear is why TCAs do not block most of normal impulses at their therapeutic plasma concentrations.

This paradox is in fact similar to the classic mystery of the effectiveness of lidocaine for neuropathic pain at low concentrations [32]. Devor et al. [33] reported that lidocaine at relatively low concentrations is effective in silencing the ectopic repetitive firing in injured peripheral nerves. Low doses of lidocaine effective at blocking ectopic discharge, however, fail to block the initiation or propagation of impulses by electrical stimulation. This mystery may be resolved if we assume that lidocaine preferentially blocks the open and inactivated states of $Na^+$ channels during ectopic discharge, which makes $Na^+$ channels repetitively cycle through state transitions. Normal initiation and propagation of impulses probably require less frequent opening of $Na^+$ channels because of their lower frequency of action-potential firing. Recently, lidocaine was found to block the open $Na^+$ channels with a high affinity at ~20 μM [34], which is within the therapeutic plasma concentration range reported for its antiarrhythmic action [35] and for its treatment of neuropathic pain [32]. The resting block by lidocaine ($IC_{50}$ = 314 μM), in contrast, is 15-fold weaker than that of the open-channel block. Such high potency of lidocaine toward the open $Na^+$ channel implies that ectopic hyperexcitability found under pathological conditions is susceptible to lidocaine open-channel block. The inactivated state also displays a high affinity toward lidocaine (~10 μM for cardiac channels) [36]. However, local anesthetics generally have a larger on-rate with the open state than with the inactivated state. Therefore, the inactivated block of Na⁺ channels may play a secondary role in blocking the ecotopic neural discharge.

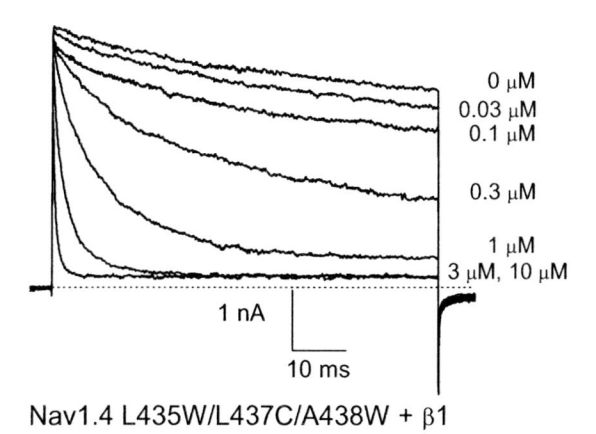

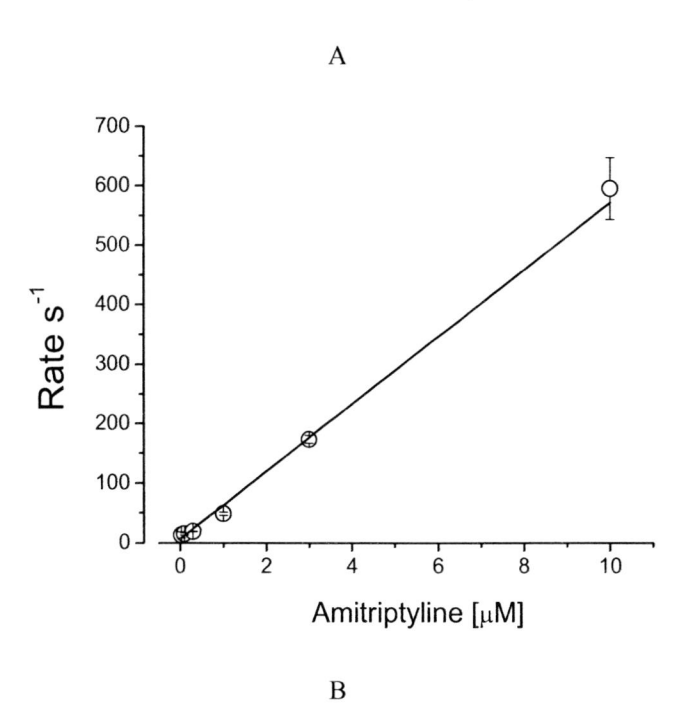

Figure 9. Open-channel block of inactivation-deficient mutant Na⁺ channels by amitriptyline. (A) Superimposed mutant Na⁺ currents (Nav1.4-L435W/L437C/A438W + β1 subunit) were recorded at various concentrations of amitriptyline. The Na⁺ currents were evoked by a 140-ms test pulse to +30 mV every 30 s. A steady state at each drug concentration was established before application of the next concentrated solution. (B) The decaying phase of the normalized relative Na⁺ current was fitted with a single exponential function, and the corresponding τ value (time constant) was inverted and plotted against the corresponding amitriptyline concentration. Data were fitted with a linear regression, y = 56.5x + 6.93. The on-rate ($k_{on}$) corresponded to the slope of the fitted line (56.5 µM⁻¹s⁻¹) and the off-rate ($k_{off}$) corresponded to the y-intercept (6.93 s⁻¹). The dissociation constant was determined by the equation $K_D = k_{off}/k_{on}$ and equaled 0.12 µM. Another linear regression, y = 36x + 11.1, could be fitted when the data points of 3 and 10 µM were excluded.

Like the local anesthetic lidocaine, TCAs appear to preferentially target the open and the inactivated states of $Na^+$ channels for their efficacy in neuropathic pain. Figure 9A illustrates the time-dependent block of the persistent late $Na^+$ currents by amitriptyline at various concentrations ranging from 0.03 µM to 10 µM. Figure 10 shows the dose-response curves for the resting and open $Na^+$ channel block by amitriptyline. The $IC_{50}$ for the open state is 0.26 µM (37), which is at the therapeutic plasma concentration for amitriptyline (~0.30–0.90 µM) (1). The potency ratio for open vs. resting state is >100-fold ($IC_{50}$; 0.26 µM vs. 33 µM). The estimated on-rate and off-rate for the open-channel block at +50 mV are 56.5 $µM^{-1}s^{-1}$ and 6.93 $s^{-1}$, respectively (Fig. 9B). The $IC_{50}$ for the inactivated $Na^+$ channel is 0.51 µM, which is only twofold less potent than the open $Na^+$ channel (see Fig. 4). This result again suggests that TCAs block open and inactivated $Na^+$ channels effectively. It is therefore likely that the open-channel block by TCAs plays a dominant role in blocking the ectopic discharge because of their fast on-rate kinetics, in a manner similar to that by lidocaine. In fact, based on their unpublished observations Devor and Seltzer [31] wrote that amitriptyline "suppresses ectopic neuroma discharge." In contrast, most resting channels are not affected by TCAs at their therapeutic plasma concentration.

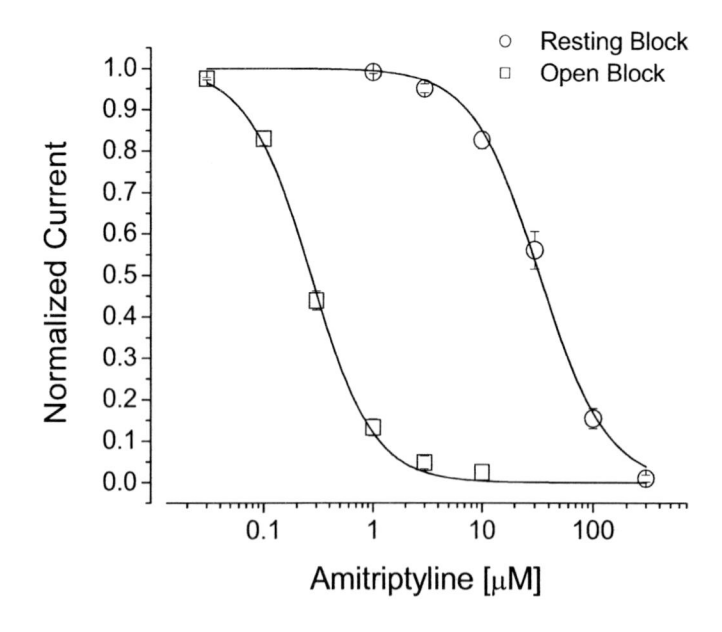

Figure 10. Dose-response curves for amitriptyline block of inactivation-deficient mutant $Na^+$ channels. Dose-response curves for open-channel block and resting-channel block. All pulses were delivered at 30-s intervals. Solid lines represent fits to the data with the Hill equation. $IC_{50}$ values ± S.E. [Hill coefficients ± S.E.] are 0.26 ± 0.01 µM [1.5 ± 0.09] for open-channel block (open square, n = 5) and 33.0 ± 1.8 µM [1.4 ± 0.1] for resting-channel block (open circle, n = 5). For detailed methods see reference [33].

Like lidocaine, TCAs also interact with $Na^+$ channels within the inner cavity of the $Na^+$ channel. The α-subunit of the $Na^+$ channel protein alone forms a function channel and contains four repeated domains (D1-D4), each with six transmembrane segments (S1-S6). The receptor for local anesthetics has been mapped within multiple S6 segments, which encircle the inner cavity of the $Na^+$ channels [38, 39]. Site-directed mutagenesis showed that the receptor for TCAs overlaps the receptor for the local anesthetic receptor extensively. Mutations that affect lidocaine binding also affect amitritpyline binding in a comparable, although not identical, manner [37]. This observation leads to the suggestion that TCAs and local anesthetics block the ectopic neural discharge within the inner cavity of the $Na^+$ channel. This conclusion and the preferential block of the open and inactivated states of $Na^+$ channels adequately explain why both lidocaine and amitriptyline are effective for neuropathic pain.

## Future Directions

Up to date, we are still in need of a clear understanding of the mechanisms that cause chronic pain and its associated depression. Without such knowledge, it is unlikely that rational treatments of diverse pain symptoms would be achieved. However, pain sensation often requires high-frequency action potential discharges. Such discharges are due to frequent openings of voltage-gated $Na^+$ channels. Indeed, pain sensation (nociception) could be caused by mutation of the voltage-gated $Na^+$ channel alone, as demonstrated recently in patients with familial erythromelalgia, familial hemiplegic migraine, and generalized epilepsy [40]. During the last decade, it has become increasingly evident that genetic defects in voltage-gated $Na^+$ channels cause a variety of diseases, such as long QT and Brugada syndromes, paramyotonia congenital, hyperkalemic periodic paralysis, and hypokalemic periodic paralysis. We anticipate that many more $Na^+$ channel defects contributing to abnormal nociceptive transmission responsible for the development and maintenance of central and local pain would be discovered in the future.

In theory, targeting abnormal/persistent openings of $Na^+$ channels would be beneficial for treating both chronic and acute pain as well as a variety of genetic diseases mentioned above, which will require finding novel open–$Na^+$ channel blockers that are more potent and more selective than drugs currently available for chronic pain management [41]. In this regard, there are a number of approaches to finding selective open-channel blockers that target the abnormal firings of action potentials. The first approach is to screen drugs that may have high potency toward the open $Na^+$ channel using inactivation-deficient mutant $Na^+$ channels as a tool (e.g., Fig. 9A). Existing compounds that display local anesthetic properties could be screened using a high throughput assay system. Drugs selected with high affinities toward the open state of $Na^+$ channels could be potentially beneficial for patients with chronic pain. The second is to synthesize additional novel drugs that display high affinities toward the $Na^+$ channel. Initial attempts using this approach have shown its feasibility [22]. The receptor-based drug design will be possible in the future when the three-dimensional structure of the local anesthetic docking site is resolved (e.g., reference 42). The third approach is to optimize the bioavailability of drugs that have high potency toward the open $Na^+$ channel but fail to penetrate the neural sheaths/membranes efficiently. This may be achieved by using drug carriers or a drug delivery system that minimizes the drug barriers. The fourth is to reduce adverse side effects by combining amitriptyline with other classes of channel blockers, such as tetrodotoxin, that also have a high affinity toward the $Na^+$ channel (27).

## Conclusion

Intended or otherwise, TCAs have many potential target sites in the CNS, PNS, and elsewhere. As a result, TCAs have both beneficial and adverse effects for patients with major depressive disorders or chronic pain. At therapeutic plasma concentrations, TCAs are potent $Na^+$ channel blockers that preferentially interact with the open and inactivated states of $Na^+$ channels. Such state-dependent binding of TCAs explains their efficacy in blocking ectopic discharge and their minimal effects on normal impulses. By single injections, TCAs also act as long-acting local anesthetics when tested in a rat sciatic nerve model or in a rat spinal model. These *in vivo* observations further support the hypothesis that the voltage-gated $Na^+$ channel may be one of the primary targets of TCAs related to the clinical pain management. Site-directed mutagenesis of $Na^+$ channels shows that the binding sites for TCAs and for local anesthetics overlap extensively. In light of the frequent use of TCAs in clinical pain management, further development of oral, topical, and/or injectable TCAs or their derivatives that selectively target the open state of voltage-gated $Na^+$ channels with high affinities may have a direct impact on clinical pain management in the future.

## References

[1] Baldessarini RJ. Drugs and the treatment of psychiatric disorders: depression and anxiety disorders. In: Hardman JG, Limbird L E, Gilman A G, eds. *The pharmacological basis of therapeutics*. New York: The McGraw-Hill Companies, Inc., 2001:447-84.

[2] Monks R, Merskey H. Psychotropic drugs. In: Wall PD, Melzack R, eds. *Textbook of pain*. New York: Churchill Livingstone, 1999:1155-86.

[3] McQuay HJ, Tramer M, Nye BA, et al. A systematic review of antidepressants in neuropathic pain. *Pain* 1996;68:217-27.

[4] Paoli F, Darcourt G, Cossa P. [Preliminary note on the action of imipramine in painful states.]. *Rev. Neurol.* (Paris) 1960;102:503-4.

[5] Bohn LM, Xu F, Gainetdinov RR, Caron MG. Potentiated opioid analgesia in norepinephrine transporter knock-out mice. *J. Neurosci.* 2000;20:9040-5.

[6] Biegon A, Samuel D. Interaction of tricyclic antidepressants with opiate receptors. *Biochem. Pharmacol.* 1980;29:460-2.

[7] Sawynok J. Topical and peripherally acting analgesics. *Pharmacol. Rev.* 2003; 55:1-20.

[8] Lynch ME, Clark AJ, Sawynok J. A pilot study examining topical amitriptyline, ketamine, and a combination of both in the treatment of neuropathic pain. *Clin. J. Pain.* 2003;19:323-8.

[9] Eisenach JC, Rauck RL, Curry R. Intrathecal, but not intravenous adenosine reduces allodynia in patients with neuropathic pain. *Pain.* 2003;105:65-70.

[10] Sawynok J, Reid AR, Liu XJ, Parkinson FE. Amitriptyline enhances extracellular tissue levels of adenosine in the rat hindpaw and inhibits adenosine uptake. *Eur. J. Pharmacol.* 2005;518:116-22.

[11] Ogata N, Narahashi T. Block of sodium channels by psychotropic drugs in single guinea-pig cardiac myocytes. *Br. J. Pharmacol.* 1989;97:905-13.

[12] Barber MJ, Starmer CF, Grant AO. Blockade of cardiac sodium channels by amitriptyline and diphenylhydantoin: Evidence for two use-dependent binding sites. *Circulation Research.* 1991;69:677-96.

[13] Nau C, Seaver M, Wang S-Y, Wang GK. Block of human heart hH1 sodium channels by amitriptyline. *J. Pharmacol. Exp. Ther.* 2000;292:1015-23.

[14] Nattel S. Frequency-dependent effects of amitriptyline on ventricular conduction and cardiac rhythm in dogs. *Circulation.* 1985;72:898-906.

[15] Pancrazio JJ, Kamatchi GL, Roscoe AK, Lynch C. Inhibition of neuronal $Na^+$ channels by antidepressant drugs. *J. Pharmac. Exp. Ther.* 1998;284:208-14.

[16] Gerner P, Mujtaba M, Sonnott CJ, Wang GK. Amitriptyline versus bupivacaine in rat sciatic nerve blockade. *Anesthesiology.* 2001;94:661-7.

[17] Brau ME, Dreimann M, Olschewski A, et al. Effects of drugs used for neuropathic pain management on tetradotoxin-resistant $Na^+$ currents in rat sensory neurons. *Anesthesiology.* 2001;94:137-44.

[18] Gerner P. Tricyclic antidepressants and their local anesthetic properties: from bench to bedside and back again. *Reg. Anesth. Pain. Med.* 2004;29:286-9.

[19] Sudoh Y, Cahoon EE, Gerner P, Wang GK. Tricyclic antidepressants as long-acting local anesthetics. *Pain.* 2003;103:49-55.

[20] Chen YW, Huang KL, Liu SY, et al. Intrathecal tri-cyclic antidepressants produce spinal anesthesia. *Pain.* 2004;112:106-12.

[21] Gerner P, Mujtaba M, Khan MA, et al. N-Phenylethyl amitriptyline in rat sciatic nerve blockade. *Anesthesiology.* 2002;96:1435-42.

[22] Gerner P, Haderer AE, Mujtaba M, et al. Assessment of differential blockade by amitriptyline and its N-methyl derivative in different species by different routes. *Anesthesiology.* 2003;98:1484-90.

[23] Gerner P, Luo SH, Zhuang ZY, et al. Differential block of N-propyl derivatives of amitriptyline and doxepin for sciatic nerve block in rats. *Reg. Anesth. Pain Med.* 2005;30:344-50.

[24] Sakura S, Bollen AW, Ciriales R, Drasner K. Local anesthetic neurotoxicity does not result from blockade of voltage-gated sodium channels. *Anesth. Analg.* 1995;81:338-46.

[25] Kohane DS, Yieh J, Lu NT, et al. A re-examination of tetrodotoxin for prolonged duration local anesthesia. *Anesthesiology.* 1998;89:119-31.

[26] Kohane DS, Smith SE, Louis DN, et al. Prolonged duration local anesthesia from tetrodotoxin-enhanced local anesthetic microspheres. *Pain.* 2003;104:415-21.

[27] Barnet CS, Tse JY, Kohane DS. Site 1 sodium channel blockers prolong the duration of sciatic nerve blockade from tricyclic antidepressants. *Pain.* 2004;110:432-8.

[28] Srinivasa V, Gerner P, Haderer A, et al. The relative toxicity of amitriptyline, bupivacaine, and levobupivacaine administered as rapid infusions in rats. *Anesth. Analg.* 2003;97:91-5.

[29] Gerner P, Kao G, Srinivasa V, et al. Topical amitriptyline in healthy volunteers. *Reg Anesth Pain Med* 2003;28:289-93.

[30] Fridrich P, Eappen S, Jaeger W, et al. Phase Ia and Ib study of amitriptyline for ulnar nerve block in humans: side effects and efficacy. *Anesthesiology.* 2004;100:1511-8.

[31] Devor M, Seltzer Z. Pathphysiology of damaged nerves in relation to chronic pain. In: Wall PD, Melzack R, eds. *Textbook of Pain.* New York: Churchill Livingstong, 1999:129-64.

[32] Boas RA, Covino BG, Shahnarian A. Analgesic responses to I.V. lignocaine. *Br. J. Anaesth.* 1982;54:501-5.

[33] Devor M, Wall PD, Catalan N. Systemic lidocaine silences ectopic neuroma and DRG discharge without blocking nerve conduction. *Pain.* 1992;48:261-8.

[34] Wang S-Y, Mitchell J, Moczydlowski E, Wang GK. Block of inactivation-deficient Na$^+$ channels by local anesthetics in stably transfected mammalian cells: Evidence for drug binding along the activation pathway. *J. Gen. Physiol.* 2004;124:691-701.

[35] Roden DM. Antiarrhythmic drugs. In: Hardman JG, Limbird L E, Molinoff P B, Ruddon R W, Gilman A G, eds. Goodman and Gilman's *The Pharmacological Basis of Therapeutics.* New York: Macmillan Publishing Company, 2001:933-70.

[36] Bean BP, Cohen CJ, Tsien RW. Lidocaine block of cardiac sodium channels. *J. Gen. Physiol.* 1983;81:613-42.

[37] Wang GK, Russell C, Wang SY. State-dependent block of voltage-gated Na$^+$ channels by amitriptyline via the local anesthetic receptor and its implication for neuropathic pain. *Pain.* 2004;110:166-74.

[38] Catterall WA, Mackie K. Local anesthetics. In: Hardman JG, Limbird L E, Molinoff P B, Ruddon R W, Gilman A G, eds. Goodman and Gilman's *The Pharmacological Basis of Therapeutics.* New York: Macmillan Publishing Company, 2001:367-84.

[39] Nau C, Wang GK. Interactions of local anesthetics with voltage-gated Na$^+$ channels. *J. Membr. Biol.* 2004;201:1-8.

[40] Strupp M. Mutations in voltage-gated sodium channels in familial hemiplegic migraine, erythromelalgia, and other disorders. *J. Neurol.* 2005;252:1139-41.

[41] Wang GK, Strichartz GR. Therapeutic Na$^+$ channel blockers beneficial for pain syndromes. *Drug Development Research* 2002;54:154-8.

[42] Lipkind GM, Fozzard HA. Molecular Modeling of Local Anesthetic Drug Binding by Voltage-Gated Na Channels. *Mol. Pharmacol.* 2005;68:1611-22.

*Chapter XI*

# Antidepressant Medication in Clinical Pain Management

### *Donna Greenberg*[*]
Department of Psychiatry, MGH Cancer Center,
Dana Farber/Partners Cancer Care
Associate Professor of Psychiatry, Harvard Medical School,
Boston MA02114

## Abstract

Pain perception depends on parallel, somewhat independent, sensory and affective neural pain processing networks. Depressive disorder and depressive symptoms color pain via brain areas associated with emotional integration more than sensory perception. Patients with major depressive disorder often have more than one painful symptom in a context of hopelessness about relief. Both depression and anxiety disorders act to perpetuate pain symptoms, and clinical depression is common among chronic pain patients.

Antidepressant medications are evidence-based treatments for major depressive disorder, anxiety disorder, and mixed anxiety-depressive syndromes. In patients with pain, enhanced management of major depressive disorder reduces disability when emphasis is placed on medication adherence and graded improvements in cognitive-behavioral and physical function. Antidepressant medications with combined serotonergic-noradrenergic mechanisms also treat the sensory dimension of neuropathic pain independent of the treatment of depression. Patients with chronic pain should be defined in dimensions that consider the presence of 1) major depressive disorder, 2) anxiety disorder, 3) known somatic disease pathology or pathophysiology, 4) health beliefs, 5) illness behavior, and 6) social factors like the effect of the condition on employment or financial benefits. The judgment of what works depends strongly on a case mix: severity, chronicity, and comorbidity. Antidepressant medication trials in patients with pain should employ state-of-the-art treatments of depressive and anxiety disorders, characterize patients on

---

[*]WRN 605 Massachusetts General Hospital, 55 Fruit St. Boston, Ma 02114.Tel: 617 726 2984

multiple dimensions, make head-to-head drug comparisons, and combine drug treatment with physical and cognitive-behavioral programs that emphasize function.

# Introduction

"Punishing, grueling, cruel, vicious, killing, annoying, troublesome, miserable, intense, unbearable, sickening, suffocating, fearful, frightful, terrifying, agonizing, dreadful, and torturing" are affective words that describe pain. Melzack used these words to capture pain's emotional tone and significance independent of the sensory features of the pain. Recent functional magnetic resonance imaging and pain threshold reports have supported the theory that sensory and affective components of pain depend on parallel, somewhat independent neural pain processing networks [1, 2].

In patients with chronic pain, depressed mood may not actually change the sensory threshold to pain. The relationship between depression and pain was examined in one sample of patients with the chronic pain of fibromyalgia, using quantitative sensory testing, neural responses to painful pressure, and functional magnetic resonance imaging. Neither the level of depressive symptoms nor the presence of comorbid major depressive disorder correlated to sensory testing results or to the magnitude of neuronal activation in the primary and secondary somatosensory cortices. Clinical pain was only related weakly to sensory testing. Clinical pain was more directly related to integrated processing of affect and pain, the magnitude of neuronal activation in insula bilaterally, contralateral anterior cingulate cortex, and prefrontal cortex. Depressive symptoms or major depressive disorder were linked to the motivational-affective dimension, neuronal activation in the amydalae and anterior insula [3].

Recurrent pain brings on vigilance, stress, and chronic anxiety. Patients with more severe refractory pain and worse function tend to have more depressive symptoms, lower quality of life, less ability to work, and more use of health care. Continued pain and the setbacks of disability serve as a stressor promoting the risk of depressive disorder. A review by Fishbain judged the prevalence of major depressive disorder to be 54% in chronic pain patients [4].

## Depression and Pain Comorbidity

In primary care and medical specialty settings, sixty percent of patients with major depressive disorder report pain [5,6,7]. Compared to patients with chronic medical illness, patients with major depressive disorder perceive their general health as poorer and have more physical, social, and vocational limitations. They also have more pain complaints than those with chronic medical illness [8]. Patients with clinical depression often have more than one pain complaint. Reviewing1000 patients from a health maintenance organization, Dworkin et al [9] found that patients with one pain complaint were no more depressed than controls; however, patients with two pain complaints were six times more likely and patients with three pain complaints eight times more likely to have a clinical depression.

The tendency to express psychological distress with somatic symptoms and without reference to depressed mood has been thought to vary from culture to culture; however, a large study of somatic symptoms in patients with depressive disorder in 16 primary care centers in 14 countries did not show cultural variability. Of those patients who presented with somatic symptoms of depression, 60 percent acknowledged psychological symptoms when asked [10]. Only 11 percent denied them. One half of the depressed patients also had multiple unexplained symptoms. Across cultures, if patients already had a relationship with the primary care physician, they were more apt to report the psychological symptoms associated with somatic symptoms.

Clinical depression may be viewed as a psychobiological factor that perpetuates chronic somatic pain symptoms and their negative meaning [11]. In the setting of depression, patients are pessimistic and worried. They are easily irritated and tend to interpret symptoms with negativity and hopelessness. Concentration is poor. They often cannot sleep. Any pain bearable with daylight, piece of mind, concentration, and optimism becomes malignant, dreadful, and hopeless in the wee hours of the night. Patients presume catastrophe and may assume that any pain is a sign of cancer. Sleep architecture is disrupted during major depressive disorder, so those who wake frequently during the night because of depression take note of pains that might not normally awaken them.

In *Darkness Visible* [12], Styron eloquently describes his own experience with the anguish and pain of major depressive disorder (p.62):

"In depression, faith in deliverance, in ultimate restoration, is absent. The pain is unrelenting, and what makes the condition intolerable is the foreknowledge that no remedy will come—not in a day, an hour, a month, or a minute. If there is mild relief, one knows that it is only temporary; more pain will follow. It is hopelessness even more than pain that crushes the soul. So the decision-making of daily life involves not, as in normal affairs, shifting from one annoying situation to another less annoying—or from discomfort to relative comfort, or from boredom to activity—but moving from pain to pain. One does not abandon, even briefly, one's bed of nails, but is attached to it wherever one goes...the sufferer from depression... like the walking wounded...therefore finds himself, like a waling casualty of war, thrust into the most intolerable social and family situations."

## Major Depressive Disorder

How then do antidepressant medications benefit the patient in pain? Although some medications in this pharmacological class relieve neuropathic pain, antidepressants as a drug class have been developed and promoted primarily to treat major depressive disorder. In order to discuss the role of these medications in the treatment of pain, we must clarify the nature of major depressive disorder.

Major depressive disorder is a relapsing syndrome with significant morbidity and mortality, and complications of suicide, inanition, and significant functional impairment.[8] Much like asthma, major depressive disorder has a genetic predisposition and environmental triggers. Because its clinical presentation varies, and no consistent laboratory abnormalities are known, diagnosis of the syndrome for research consensus has been based on established criteria of symptoms and signs. The lifetime prevalence of major depressive disorder is

16.2% and the 12-month prevalence is 6.6% in adults [13]. Major depressive disorder is more common in women than men, with a risk-ratio of 1.7 to 1.0 over a lifetime and 1.4 to 1.0 for 12 months. Risk factors are personal or family history of depressive disorder, prior suicide attempts, female gender, lack of social supports, stressful life events, and current substance abuse. More than 50% of those who have one episode have another. The second episode is often within 2 years, but the majority (75%) of recurrences occur within 10 years [14,15].

The diagnostic criteria for a major depressive episode define the core features of the disorder, a change from previous functioning, not due to a general medical condition, and not including mood-incongruent delusions or hallucinations. The episode must cause clinically significant distress or impairment in social or occupational functioning, and not be better accounted for by bereavement. In the American Psychiatric Association Diagnostic and Statistical Manual of Mental Disorders, 4$^{th}$ edition, Text Revision (DSM-IV-TR) published in 2000, the criteria include five or more symptoms present over 2 weeks with at least one of the symptoms noted to be either depressed mood or loss of interest or pleasure. (1) Depressed mood typically occurs most of the day, nearly every day by the patient's report or the observation of tearfulness. (2) Interest in what is normally interesting is diminished in all or almost all activities most of the day, nearly every day. (3) Another symptom is loss of appetite nearly every day, or a significant weight loss when not dieting, or a significant weight gain like 5% of body weight in a month. (4) Insomnia or hypersomnia nearly every day is another symptom as is (5) fatigue or loss of energy nearly every day. (6) The patient may report or others may observe indecisiveness or diminished ability to think or concentrate. (7) Feelings of worthlessness or excessive or inappropriate guilt, which may be delusional, must occur nearly every day. (8) Recurrent thoughts of death, recurrent suicidal ideation without a specific plan, a suicide attempt, or a specific plan for committing suicide may be noted as another symptom. (9) The one physical sign rather than symptom is psychomotor agitation or retardation nearly every day. This is an observed sign and not just the patient's subjective feeling of restlessness or being slowed down [16].

Depression may be a stronger determinant of disability than is stable chronic medical illness. Mortality rates are higher in patients with medical illness and major depressive disorder or even sub-threshold depression. Medical illness, past depression, and present depression are a predictive triad for in-hospital mortality [17,18]. However, medical morbidity and the associated disorders of an older population do not prevent treatment response [19,20]. With the initiation of antidepressant treatment, 200 patients with ischemic heart disease, diabetes, and obstructive lung disease and co-morbid depression showed significant improvements in mood, social and emotional functioning, and disability [21].

Since the 1950s, multiple medications synthesized to treat this condition have been tested in systematic placebo-controlled, randomized studies. A Cochrane evidence-based report finds that medical patients with depression are more likely to improve with antidepressants than with placebo [22]. Overall, antidepressants had been thought to have a clinical response rate of 65%, half of that a partial response [23]. To claim a clinical response the researcher must find at least 50% reduction in symptoms. The further challenge of full remission implies that patients no longer meet criteria for the syndrome [24].

Although there are many different antidepressant medications in different classes, most antidepressant medications have similar rate and tempo of effectiveness. Finding the right drug for a given patient means watching for benefit over 4 to 8 weeks and taking note of side effects. A recent study of effectiveness in a multi-center "real world" trial using citalopram up to 60 mg. in 2876 outpatients found a remission rate around 30%; the overall response rate was 47%. Most had shown this improvement by 8 weeks, and the outcome was similar to that seen in 8-week antidepressant trials [25]. In eight-week efficacy trials, remission rates were noted to be 35-40% and response rates 50-55 percent [26]. When the patients who did not achieve remission on citalopram were switched to buproprion sustained-release up to 400 mg, sertraline up to 200 mg, or venlafaxine extended release up to 375 mg, another one quarter of patients achieved remission in a study of 727 adult outpatients lasting 14 weeks. Any of the medications were judged to be reasonable second steps [26].

The methodology for these psychopharmacologic studies include diagnosis by a structured interview that assesses current symptoms, lifetime diagnosis, and comorbid psychiatric diagnoses Drug response is typically assessed by a validated provider-measured scale [27]. The Hamilton Depression Scale, one of the most widely used scales, has a factor for somatic symptoms. The presence of heaviness in limbs, back or head, backaches, headache, muscle aches, loss of energy and fatiguability are graded as "1", and any clear-cut symptom is graded as "2". An item for somatic symptoms of anxiety includes gas, indigestion, diarrhea, cramps, belching among others. It is graded "0-4" depending on severity. Often somatic painful symptoms improve more rapidly than core emotional symptoms [27-29].

A minimum course of six months of treatment with antidepressant medication reduces the risk of relapse [30]. Long-term antidepressant therapy seems to have a prophylactic effect. For patients with two or more serious recurrences in five years or three serious lifetime recurrences, long-term antidepressant treatment is recommended. However, antidepressant treatment is often discontinued; in one study of more than 800 patients treated between 1996 and 2001, only 28 percent of patients continued antidepressant therapy for more than 90 days [31].

Better adherence to antidepressant medication makes a difference. When care for major depressive disorder is enhanced, even in the primary care setting, depressive disorder is more likely to improve, and so is the pain and function of patients with a painful comorbid condition like arthritis [32]. A randomized controlled trial of 1801 depressed older adults in 18 primary care clinics led to benefits that extended to decreased pain, improved function, and quality of life. The year-long intervention included antidepressant medication prescribed by primary care physicians and 6-8 sessions of a problem solving treatment given by a depression care manager. A stepped care algorithm guided acute and follow-up care over 12 months. Intervention patients were twice as likely to have marked reduction in depressive symptoms and to no longer meet criteria for major depressive disorder. The intervention did not systematically focus on arthritis. Half of the comparison usual care patients used antidepressant medication, but antidepressant use in the enhanced care intervention increased from 43 to 66 percent at 12 months.

The diagnosis of major depressive disorder relies on the presence of specific symptoms, but some of these symptoms may also be caused by chronic pain. Wilson et al tackled the dilemma of how to place the symptoms that could be related either to depression or pain by using a semi-structured interview (Schedule for Affective Disorders and Schizophrenia-

SADS) in 129 patients with chronic pain in a tertiary care center. The researchers defined major depressive disorder by the inclusive method, using all somatic symptoms; by the Endicott criteria that reduced the importance of somatic symptoms; and by patients' attribution of the symptoms to pain, an etiologic approach to diagnosis [33]. The most overlap occurred with the symptoms of insomnia, fatigue, and difficulty concentrating. These symptoms occurred in 34-53% of the non-depressed group with pain. However, they occurred at a higher rate, 85-94%, of the depressed group with pain.

When patients were asked why they thought that they had these symptoms, many attributed the symptoms to pain. If those symptoms attributed to pain were excluded from criteria for major depressive disorder, 45% no longer met criteria for major depressive disorder. Judging from other measures, the false negative rate was too high if this method were used. Patients likely to respond to an antidepressant may miss the opportunity to be treated. The authors detail reasons why patients attribute somatic symptoms to pain: the belief that pain is the root of their problem or patient discomfort with the stigma of acknowledging psychological symptoms. The conclusion is that all somatic symptoms present in the patient with chronic pain should be included in the diagnostic assessment of depression whether the patient attributes them to pain or not.

## Anxiety and Anxiety Disorders

Anxiety is a common element of the affective experience of pain and another factor that perpetuates symptoms. The patient in pain becomes aware of a threat. When the threat from the body or the environment reaches the central limbic system, vigilance progresses to hypervigilance and panic [34]. Anxiety, for instance, conditioned by the painful experience of repeat dressing changes, comes to be associated with the cues of dressing changes and anticipation of pain. Anticipation of pain is associated with increased activity in the prefrontal cortex [35]. On the other hand, when the patient anticipates pain relief, the beliefs and expectations associated with a placebo may produce analgesia. Placebos alter the experience of pain, decreasing brain activity in pain-sensitive brain regions including the thalamus, insula, and anterior cingulate cortex. Factors that reduce anxiety or are believed to reduce anxiety should add to that benefit.

A history of anxiety disorder is common in patients with major depressive disorder, and depressive disorder is common in patients with pain. In The US National Comorbidity Survey, anxiety disorder occurred in 58% of depressed patients, and 67% of those with generalized anxiety disorder had a lifetime history of comorbid unipolar depressive disorder.[36] Multiple anxiety disorders increase the risk of depression [37]. Patients with subsyndromal anxiety and subsyndromal major depressive disorder are as common in general medicine as those who meet criteria for one disorder [38]. Those who do not meet criteria for an anxiety disorder or depressive disorder may be diagnosed as having a mixed anxiety-depressive disorder if they have at least one month of persistent or recurrent dysphoric mood accompanied by four or more of the following symptoms: difficulty concentrating, sleep disturbance, fatigue or low energy, irritability, worry, easily moved to tears, hypervigilance, anticipating the worst, hopelessness, low self esteem, or feelings of worthlessness.

Antidepressant medications have shown benefit for panic disorder, particularly for spontaneous panic attacks [39,40], for generalized anxiety disorder [41], for obsessive-compulsive disorder, and for mixed anxiety-depressive disorder[38]. Patients with hypochondriasis have a preoccupation with fear of having a serious disease; reassurance does not relieve the doubt that a serious ailment is present. These patients come to attention in physician offices because of their hyperfocus on somatic symptoms including pain. Forty-five percent of those with persistent hypochondriasis after a year also meet criteria for anxiety or depressive disorders [42].

## The Pain Complaint Described on Multiple Relevant Dimensions May Clarify the Role of Major Depressive Disorder

The patients with chronic pain, some known medical diagnoses, and heterogeneous behavioral issues who come to pain clinics present challenges beyond the effort to diagnose comorbid major depressive disorder or anxiety disorder. In their hope for a revised taxonomy of somatoform disorders, Mayou et al have suggested that complex patients with pain disorder should be described on multiple dimensions [43]. The presence of psychiatric diagnoses like anxiety disorder and depressive disorder should be documented. Furthermore, other distinct dimensions should be clearly stated like1) known somatic disease pathology or pathophysiology, 2) health beliefs, 3) illness behavior, and 4) social factors like the effect of the condition on employment or financial benefits. Pain could be characterized by its course (acute, chronic, or recurrent), and by the number of other pains or other symptoms present.

Abnormal illness behavior means the way the individual patient thinks about, perceives, and behaves because of his illness [44]. Patients may continue in a sick role because of socioeconomic or cultural incentives. Models of parental illness behavior and family environment affect how patients respond to physical concerns. Patients with childhood adversity frequently consult doctors about medically unexplained symptoms; both depression and patients' particular attributions have been shown to mediate the link between childhood adversity and frequent consultations for somatic symptoms [45]. The cognitive tendency to catastrophic thinking is associated with more pain and more disability, and the tendency to feel helpless adds to the severity of pain [46]. Illness worry, denial, and disease conviction vary across a spectrum. The diagnosis of depression with features of hopelessness, pessimism, and somatic symptoms may be the context for illness behavior. While antidepressant medication treats major depressive disorder, specific cognitive and behavioral treatments may be important to enhance the treatment depending on the patient's health beliefs and illness behavior.

To judge the potential benefit of antidepressant medication for pain, the first question in practice is whether this patient has major depressive disorder as a primary diagnosis. The diagnosis of the disorder by diagnostic criteria is bolstered clinically by a past history of the disorder, a family history, previous suicide attempts, and female gender. In many cases, depressive disorder predated the pain complaint; interview assessments include queries about lifetime history of depressive disorder. Validated patient or provider instruments may be used to follow the patient's clinical course. Since depressive disorder is a relapsing disease with more risk of relapse when medication is stopped, it is helpful to know whether a patient has taken antidepressant medication and whether it was effective. Relapse may occur any time after the cessation of an antidepressant medication. In complex pain patients, historical details of timing and treatments may be especially important. For instance, has antidepressant medication been discontinued recently?

The antidepressant of choice is the antidepressant that has the best side effect profile for a given patient. Most are well tolerated and take several weeks to lead to a response. The dose is increased if there is no response and side effects are tolerated.

## The Role of Antidepressant Medications for Neuropathic Pain

Certain antidepressant medications have a long track record for analgesia in neuropathic pain even when patients do not have major depressive disorder; however, the mechanism is still not entirely clear. Amitriptyline, imipramine, and desipramine, of the tricyclic antidepressants, which have both serotonergic and noradrenergic activity, are highly effective at relatively low dose. Maprotiline, a tricyclic relatively selective for norepinephrine, was not as effective as tricyclic antidepressant medication but performed better than serotonin reuptake inhibitors [47-50]. *Tricyclic antidepressants*, the first widely used antidepressants, are not used as commonly now for treatment of depressive disorder because of the side effect profile and the lethality of overdose. They are anticholinergic, causing dry mouth, grogginess, urinary retention, constipation and cognitive impairment. They are similar to quinidine with the possibility of increasing bundle branch block. Postural hypotension is a side effect. The dose effective for neuralgic pain, for instance, 50-75 mg amitriptyline, is a relatively low dose compared to doses used to treat major depressive disorder.

*The serotonin reuptake inhibitors* did not perform as well as tricyclic antidepressants for neuropathic pain. In practice, serotonin reuptake inhibitors, have a more favorable safety and adverse effect profile. They are widely used for major depressive disorder and less dangerous in overdose.

*Venlafaxine extended release*, a serotonin-norepinephrine reuptake inhibitor, is effective for neuropathic pain, particularly at doses of 150 mg extended release or higher, when the noradrenergic component plays a larger role. Venlafaxine extended release was studied in a double blind, randomized, placebo-controlled study of efficacy, safety, and tolerability for patients with diabetic peripheral neuropathy [51]. None of the patients were depressed at the start of the study by self-report on the Beck Depression Inventory. A response represented a 50% reduction in pain. In each patient group, high dose, low dose, and placebo, there were more than 60 patients. The higher dose of venlafaxine ER 150 mg to 225 mg/day was significantly more effective than placebo and better than 75 mg at week six. The lower dose, 75 mg, was not better than placebo. Mild to moderate nausea, dyspepsia, sweating, somnolence, and insomnia were adverse effects.

Venlafaxine was similarly but not quite as effective for neuropathic pain as tricyclic medications. The number needed to treat was 4.5 after six weeks of treatment, slightly higher than that reported for tricyclic antidepressants, 2.6 patients. The lower dose of 75 mg venlafaxine is more purely serotonergic; the higher dose, 150 mg to 225 mg, is associated with a progressive increase in noradrenergic effect but no further increase in serotonin reuptake blockade. It was not clear whether the improved effect was related to the presence of norepinephrine blockade or to the changing balance of serotonin and noradrenalin. In a randomized, controlled trial of venlafaxine versus imipramine in painful polyneuropathy, venlafaxine had shown similar effectiveness, with a number needed to treat of 5.2 compared to 2.7 for imipramine [52, 53]. The elimination half-life of venlafaxine's active metabolite is 11 hours. It should not be used in patients with narrow angle glaucoma.

*Duloxitene*, also a noradrenergic-serotonergic agent, has an indication for treatment of diabetic peripheral neuropathy. The benefit was noted as 30% reduction of pain in 50% of those treated compared to 34 percent with placebo in two controlled studies of more than one thousand patients. All patients could use acetomenophen. The drug-related adverse events were nausea, dry mouth, constipation, diarrhea, fatigue, dizziness, somnolence, sweating, insomnia, urinary and erectile dysfunction [54].

Duloxitene is a strong inhibitor of cytochrome P450 2D6. This cytochrome facilitates the metabolism of some pain medications: hydrocodone to hydromorphone, codeine to morphine, and tramadol to n-desmethyl tramadol, the active metabolite. The half-life is 16 hours, ranging from 12 to 21. Hypertension and narrow angle glaucoma are precautions. These enteric-coated pills may be poorly absorbed with co-administration of drugs that block acid production or that delay stomach emptying [55].

Both venlafaxine and duloxetine are widely used for major depressive disorder and have similar response, remission, and adverse effects. Direct comparisons of these drugs would be valuable [56]. Both venlafaxine and duloxetine, because of short half-lives, can be associated with a withdrawal syndrome characterized by dizziness, nausea, headache, paresthesia, irritability, and nightmares.

*Bupropion sustained release*, a distinct antidepressant with a dopaminergic/noradrenergic action, has also been shown to improve neuropathic pain in patients who are not depressed. The improvement was noted in a double blind, randomized, placebo-controlled crossover trial. Patients began to show benefit at 2 weeks and that improvement continued through 3 and 6 weeks in 73 percent of 41 patients [57].

## Conclusion

The serotonergic-noradrenergic antidepressant medications: tricyclic antidepressants, venlafaxine, and duloxitene, have a benefit for neuropathic pain, but the newer agents have not been compared head-to-head in controlled studies. Major depressive disorder should be diagnosed and treated with state-of-the-art standards in chronic pain patients. If possible, enhanced interventions that augment medication adherence and cognitive-behavioral treatments should be included. The direct benefit of antidepressant medication in patients with non-neuropathic syndromes depends directly on whether they have depressive disorder, anxiety disorder, or mixed-anxiety disorder, and whether dose is adjusted for benefit and side effects. Adherence facilitates outcome, and a key measure of outcome is function. Patients with chronic pain should be defined in dimensions that consider the presence of 1) major depressive disorder, 2) anxiety disorder, 3) known somatic disease pathology or pathophysiology, 4) health beliefs, 5) illness behavior, and 6) social factors like the effect of the condition on employment or financial benefits. The interpretation of studies in these patients will be very much related to the case mix of severity, chronicity, and comorbidity of illness. Antidepressant medication trials in patients with pain should characterize the patients in these dimensions, make drug-to-drug comparisons, and combine drug treatment with physical and cognitive programs that emphasize function.

# References

[1] Melzack R, Wall PD. Pain mechanisms: a new theory. *Science. 1*965; 150: 971-979.
[2] Melzack R, Casey KL. Sensory, motivational, and central control determinants of pain: a new conceptual model. In: Kenshalo D, editor. *The skin senses*. Springfield (IL): Chas C. Thomas; 1968. P. 423-443.
[3] Giesecke T, Gracely RH, Williams DA, Geisser ME, Apetzke FW, Clauw DJ. The relationship between depression, clinical pain, and experimental pain in a chronic pain cohort. *Arthritis and Rheumatism*. 2005;52: 1577-1584.
[4] Fishbain D: Evidence-based data on pain relief with antidepressants *Ann. Med.* 2000;32:305-316.
[5] Lindsay PG, Wyckoff M. The depression-pain syndrome and its response to antidepressants. *Psychosomatics*. 1981;22:571-7.
[6] Magni G, Schifano F de Leo D. Pain as a symptom in elderly depressed patients: relationship to diagnostic subgroups. *Arch. Psychiatr. Neurol. Sci.* 1985;235:143-5.
[7] Von Knorring L, Perris C, Eisemann M, Eriksson U, Perris H. Pain as a symptom in depressive disorders: I. Relationship to diagnostic subgroup and depressive symptomatology. *Pain.* 1983; 15:19-26.
[8] Wells KB, Stewart A, Hays RD, Burnam MA Rogers W Daniels M Berry S Greenfield S Ware J. The functioning and well-being of depressed patients: results from the Medical Outcomes Study. *JAMA* 1989; 262:914-9.
[9] Dworkin SF, von Korff MR, Le Resche L.Multiple pains and psychiatric disturbance: an epidemiologic investigation. *Arch. Gen. Psychiatry.* 1990; 47: 239-44.
[10] Simon GE, von Korff M, Piccinelli M et al. An international study of the relation between somatic symptoms and depression. *N. Engl. J. Med.* 1999; 341:1329.
[11] Mayou R, Bass C, Sharpe M. Overview of epidemiology, classification, and aetiology. In *Treatment of Functional Somatic Symptoms*. eds. Mayou R, Bass C, Sharpe M. New York, Oxford University Press, 1995, pp.42-65, fig. 3.3 p. 59.
[12] Styron W. *Darkness Visible*. New York, Vintage Books, 1992 P.62.
[13] Kessler RC, Berglund P, Bemler O, Jin R, Koretz D, Merikangas KR, et al. The epidemiology of major depressive disorder. *JAMA.* 2003;289:3095-3105.

[14] Depression Guideline Panel. Depression in Primary Care: Volume 1. *Detection and Diagnosis.* Clinical Practice Guideline, Number 5. Rockville, MD. US Department of Health and Human Services, Public Health Service, Agency for Health Care Policy and Research; 1993.

[15] Glick ID, Suppes T, DeBattista C, Hu RJ, Marder S. Psychopharmacologic treatment strategies for depression, bipolar disorder, and schizophrenia. *Ann. Intern. Med.* 2001; 134:47-60.

[16] American Psychiatric Association Diagnostic and Statistical Manual of Mental Disorders, 4$^{th}$ edition, *Text Revision* (DSM-IV-TR). Washington, D.C.. American Psychiatric Association Press. 2000.

[17] Cavanaugh SA, Furlanetto LM, Creech SD, Powell LH. Medical illness, past depression, and present depression: a predictive triad for in-hospital mortality. *Am. J. Psychiatry.* 2001;158: 43-48.

[18] Roach MJ, Connors AF, Dawson NV, et al. Depressed mood and survival in seriously ill hospitalized adults. *Arch. Intern. Med.* 1998; 158:397-404.

[19] Krishnan KRR. Comorbidity and depression treatment. *Biol. Psychiatry.* 2003;53:701-706.

[20] Krishnan KRR, Delong M, Kraemer H, Carney R, Spiegel D, Gordon C, et al. Comorbidity of depression with other medical diseases in the elderly. *Biol. Psychiatry.* 2002;52:559-588.

[21] Simon GE, von Korff M, Lin E. Clinical and functional outcomes of depression treatment in patients with and without chronic medical illness. *Psychological Medicine* 2005; 35:271-279.

[22] Gill D, Hartcher S. Antidepressants for depression in medical illness. *Cochrane. Database Syst. Rev.* 2003; 4:CD 001312.

[23] Frank E, Karp JF, Rush AJ. Efficacy of treatments for major depression. *Psychopharm. Bull.* 1993;29:457-475.

[24] Keller MB. Past, present, and future directions for defining optimal treatment outcome in depression – remission and beyond. *JAMA* 2003; 289: 3152-3160.

[25] Trivedi MH, Rush AJ, Wisniewski SR, Nierenberg AA. Evaluation of outcomes with citalopram for depression using measurement-based care in STAR*D: implications for clinical practice. *Am. J. Psychiatry.* 2006; 163:28-40.

[26] Rush AJ, Trivedi MH, Wisniewski SR, Stewart JW, Nierenberg AA. Bupropion-SR, sertraline, or venlafaxine-XR after failure of SSRIs for depression. *New. Engl. J. Med.* 2006;354:1231-1242.

[27] Hamilton M. Rating scale for depression. *J. Neurol. Neurosurg. Psychiatr.* 1960;23:56-62.

[28] Barkin RL, Barkin S. The role of venlafaxine and duloxetine in the treatment of depression with decremental changes in somatic symptoms of pain, chronic pain, and the pharmacokinetics and clinical considerations of duloxetine pharmacotherapy. *Amer. J. Therapeutics.* 2005;12, 431-438.

[29] Denninger JW, Mahal Y, Merens W et al. *The relationship between somatic symptoms and depression.* Presented at the 155th annual meeting of the American Psychiatic Association, Phil May 21, 2002 (abst NR251:68).

[30] Practice guideline for major depressive disorder in adults. American Psychiatric Association. *Am. J. Psychiatry.* 1993;150 (4 suppl): 1-26.
[31] Olfson M, Marcus SC, Tedeschi M, Wan GJ. Continuity of antidepressant treatment for adults with depression in the United States. *Am. J. Psychiatry.* 2006;163:101-108.
[32] Lin EHB. Katon W, Von Korff M, Tang L, Williams JW, Kroenke K et al. Effect of improving depression care on pain and functional outcomes among older adults with arthritis, a randomized controlled trial. *J. Amer. Med. Assoc.* 2003;290:2428-2434.
[33] Wilson KG, Mikail SF, D'Eon JL. Minns JE. Alternative diagnostic criteria for major depressive disorder in patients with chronic pain. *Pain.* 2001;91:227-234.
[34] Chapman CR. The emotional aspect of pain. *Current and Emerging Issues in Cancer Pain: Research and Practice,* ed. CR Chapman and KM Foley. Raven Press, Ltd., NY 1993 pp.83-98
[35] Wager TD, Rilling JK, Smith EE, Sokolik A, Casey KL, Davidson RJ, Kosslyn SM, Rose RM Cohen JD. Placebo-induced changes in fMRI in the anticipation and experience of pain. *Science.* 2004; 303:1162-1167.
[36] Kessler RC, Nelson CB, McGonagle KA et al. Comorbidity of DSM IIIR major depressive disorder in the general population: results from the US National Comorbidity Survey. *Br. J. Psychiatry Suppl.* 1996;30;17-30.
[37] Judd LL, Kessler RC, Paulus MP et al. Comorbidity as a fundamental feature of generalized anxiety disorders: results from the National Comorbidity Study (NCS) *Acta Psychiatr. Scand. Suppl.* 1998;393:6-11.
[38] Pollack MH. Comorbid anxiety and depression. *J. Clin. Psychiatry.* 2005; 66 supp 8 22-29.
[39] Uhlenhuth EH, Martuzas W, Warner TD, Paine S, Lydiard RB, Pollack MH. Do antidepressants selectively suppress spontaneous (unexpected) panic attacks? A replication. *J. Clin. Psychopharmacol.* 2000; 20: 622-627.
[40] Rapaport MH, Wolkow R, Rubin A, Hackett E, Pollack M. Ota KY. Sertraline treatment of panic disorder: results of a long-term study. *Acta Psychiatr. Scand.* 2001; 104:289-298
[41] Pollack MH, Meoin P, Otto MW, Hackett D. Predictors of outcome following venlafaxine extended-release treatment of DSM-IV generalized anxiety disorder: a pooled analysis of short- and long-term studies. *J. Clin. Psychopharmacology.* 2003; 23:250-259.
[42] Simon GE. Gureje O, Fullerton C. Course of hypochondriasis in an international primary care study. *Gen. Hosp. Psychiatry.* 2001; 23:51-55.
[43] 43 Mayou R, Kirmayer L, Simon G, Kroenke K, Sharpe M. Somatoform disorders: time for a new approach in DSM V. *Am. J. Psychiatry.* 2005;162:847-855.
[44] Kirmayer LJ, Looper KJ. Abnormal illness behavior. *Curr. Opinion in Psychiatry.* 2006;19:54-60.
[45] Fiddler M, Jackson J, Kapur N, Wells A, Creed F.. Childhood adversity and frequent medical consultations. *Gen. Hosp. Psychiatry.* 2004;26:367-377.
[46] Sullivan MJ, Lynch Me, Clark AJ. Dimensions of catastrophic thinking associated with pain experience and disability in patients with neuropathic pain conditions. *Pain* 2005;113:310-315.

[47] Max MB. Antidepressants as analgesics In: Fields HL, Liebeskind JC ed. *Progress in Pain Research and Management.* Seattle, WA: IASP Press; 1994, p.229-446.

[48] Max MB, Kishore-Kumar R, Schafer SC, Meister B, Gracely RH, Smuller B, Dubner R. Efficacy of desipramine in painful diabetic neuropathy: a placebo-controlled trial. *Pain.* 1991;45:3-9.

[49] Max MB, Lynch SA, Muir J, Shoaf SE, Smoller B, Dubner R. Effects of desipramine, amitriptyline, and fluoxetine on pain in diabetic neuropathy a placebo-controlled trial. *New Engl. J. Med.* 1992;326:1250-6.

[50] Watson CP, Chipman M, Reed K, Evans RJ, Birkett N. Amitriptyline versus maprotiline in postherpetic neuralgia: a randomized, double-blind, crossover trial. *Pain.* 1992;48:29-36.

[51] Rowbotham MC, Goli V, Kunz NR, Lei D. Venlafaxine extended release in the treatment of painful diabetic neuropathy: a double-blind, placebo-controlled study. *Pain.* 2004;110:697-706.

[52] Sindrup SH, Bach FW, Madsen C, Gram LF, Jensen Ts. Venlafaxine versus imipramine in painful polyneuropathy: a randomized, controlled trial. *Neurology.* 2003;60:1284-9.

[53] Bradley RH, Barkin RL, Jerome J, DeYoung K, Dodge CW. Efficacy of venlafaxine for the long term treatment of chronic pain with associated major depressive disorder. *Amer. J. Therapeutics.* 2003;10:318-323.

[54] Goldstein DJ, Lu Y, Detke MJ, Lee TC, Iyengar S. Duloxetine vs. placebo in patients with painful diabetic neuropathy. *Pain.* 2004:116: 109-18.

[55] Preskorn SH. Duloxetine. *J. Psychiatric Practice.* 2004;10:375-385.

[56] Peter MJV, van Baardewijk M, Einarson TR. Duloxetine and venlafaxine-XR in the treatment of major depressive disorder: a meta-analysis of randomized clinical trials. *Ann. Pharmacother.* 2005;39:1798-807.

[57] Semenchuck MR, Sherman S, Davis B. Double-blind, randomized trial of bupropion SR for the treatment of neuropathic pain. *Neurology.* 2001;57:1583-1588.

*Chapter XII*

# Developing Pain Pathways and Analgesic Mechanisms – Towards Translational Studies

### *Maria Fitzgerald*[*]

Professor of Developmental Neurobiology, UCL Department of Anatomy and
Developmental Biology, University College London,
Gower Street, London WC1E 6BT

## Abstract

Key features of the development of nociceptive and pain processing that may impact upon clinical care of infants and children in pain are reviewed. The postnatal maturation of pain behaviour is described as the imprecise and poorly directed nociceptive reflexes of the neonate gradually become refined due to the development of excitatory and inhibitory synaptic connections within nociceptive circuits. In addition, the influence of higher brain centres over nociceptive reflex circuits matures postnatally, altering the ability of higher centres in the brain to modulate pain. Evidence that nociceptive circuit maturation is influenced by exposure to sensory stimulation is reviewed and the possibility that excessive handling or tissue damage and inflammation may change the normal pain responses in later life discussed. Developmental mechanisms of peripheral and central sensitization that underlie hyperalgesia and prolonged pain states are highlighted along with recent insights into developmental analgesia in animal models. Higher level and cortical responses to noxious stimulation in infants is discussed.

---

[*]Tel: +44 (0)20 7679 1303 Fax: +44 (0)20 7383 0929 www.wprc.ucl.ac.uk e-mail: m.fitzgerald@ucl.ac.uk

## Introduction

Research into the developmental neurobiology of somatosensory processing and pain pathways has increased considerably in recent years, leading to a greater understanding of the underlying synaptic development and plasticity of nociceptive systems over the postnatal period [1-4]. At the same time clinicians responsible for the treatment of infant and childhood pain are emphasising the need for a specialised approach to paediatric pain management and lamenting the paucity of well-designed clinical analgesic trials [5-10]. The aim of this chapter is to begin to form a link between these two endeavours. While clinical analgesic trials in children face substantial ethical and co-morbidity challenges, equally important is an understanding the developmental mechanisms underlying the pain itself.

The difficulty of measuring pain in infants is acknowledged by all. The most commonly used infant clinical pain scoring system, the premature infant pain profile (PIPP) ascribes a value to a variety of infant behaviours such as sleep state, crying and facial expression then adds an arbitrary weighting for postmenstrual age and from this produces a composite score [11, 12]. While this has been a useful research tool, its interpretation in younger infants is limited by an inadequate appreciation of underlying developmental changes in sensory and motor physiology. In addition, analgesic efficacy in infants is not only influenced by immature pharmacokinetics and drug metabolism but also by the developmental structural and functional regulation of receptor mechanisms in the maturing nervous system [2, 13]. As a result, strong conclusions drawn in some trials of infant analgesics should be viewed with caution [14].

This chapter discusses some of recent advances in the basic science of developmental pain and analgesia that may be translated into a better understanding of the human pain experience and help in the design and interpretation of future clinical investigations and trials. Observations made at the single cell level on, for instance, synaptic inhibitory currents in the rat spinal cord, may not be instantly translatable to the pain experienced by a newborn infant but an appreciation of the contribution that such studies make to the understanding of nociceptive circuits within the whole organism are essential if we are going to go beyond simplistic behavioural observations of infants and truly understand the mechanisms of action of analgesic agents and the impact of tissue injury upon developing sensory circuits.

Translating results from the laboratory to the clinic raises the difficult problem of comparisons between species. A rat is born at a relatively immature stage of development. With respect to spinal cord sensory pathways, we have argued that at birth, the newborn rat is similar to a human infant at the end of the second trimester or, more accurately since it is no longer in a uterine environment, to an extremely preterm infant (25-30 weeks). However, the postnatal development of a rat is highly accelerated compared to a human, reaching adulthood by 6 weeks. As a result it becomes increasingly problematic to ascribe a particular age in rats, e.g. 21 days old to a particular age in human childhood. It is preferable to interpret rat ages in terms of zones; the first 2 weeks as infancy- young childhood, the 3rd and 4th week as young childhood to puberty and 4-6 weeks as adolescence. The increasing dominance of the cortex over human sensation and behaviour with increasing maturity also adds to the difficulty. Nevertheless, the underlying synaptic and cellular maturation is likely to be the same in both species.

# I. Newborn Nociceptive Reflexes Are Imprecise and Poorly Directed

Spinally mediated nociceptive reflexes are exaggerated in magnitude and duration compared to the adult but they lack functional precision. Considerable fine-tuning occurs over the postnatal period. As a result, they cannot be interpreted in exactly the same way at each stage of development. A noxious prick on the foot of a very young rat pup or human infant can cause movements of the whole body and simultaneous responses from all four limbs, but these gradually mature into the restricted limb or foot movements over the postnatal period. This is because neonatal spinal withdrawal reflexes have lower cutaneous thresholds, are easily sensitized by repeated stimulation and consist of more synchronized and prolonged muscle contractions than those of adults. Furthermore, reflex receptive fields are large and disorganised such that the withdrawal itself can be evoked from a wider area of the limb and is not always appropriate to the stimulus [15]. For the first 10 days after birth, rat pups have a 75% error rate in the direction of a tail flick on noxious stimulation of the tail and this gradually improves to the adult rate of less than 10% by postnatal day 21 [16]. Preterm human infant limb and abdominal withdrawal reflexes show analogous lack of tuning [17, 18].

This increased excitability and lack of focussed, directed response to a noxious stimulus in the newborn can be explained by the different sensory circuit properties in the infant spinal cord and brainstem. At birth, cutaneous receptive fields of spinal cord dorsal horn cells, particularly those in the deep dorsal horn, are relatively larger than those in adults and decrease rapidly in size over the first two postnatal weeks. Noxious stimulation of the skin at early postnatal ages (P0-P3) often results in a prolonged afterdischarge of action potentials (lasting 30-90 sec following termination of the stimulus), again an effect that decreases in amplitude and duration with age [19, 20].

# II. The Reflex Behaviour Reflects Changes in the Underlying Nociceptive Circuitry

The changing nature of nociceptive circuitry over the postnatal period is incompletely understood but is related to rapid synaptic growth and organisation. Large myelinated A fibre sensory afferents, conveying a sense of touch and pressure from the skin and other peripheral tissues form connections in the CNS earlier than the unmyelinated C fibre nociceptive afferents do [21]. In addition, they terminate over a wider dorso-ventral extent from lamina II-V in the neonatal cord, only gradually withdrawing to deeper laminae after 3 weeks [22]. The earlier maturation and widespread presence of functional A fibre terminals in the first weeks of life has a major influence upon the physiological responses of dorsal horn neurons and spinal cord neuronal activity and gene activation which, in the adult is only triggered by nociceptive C fibre inputs, can also be activated by A fibres in young spinal cord [23, 24]. As C fibre inputs proliferate and strengthen, over the postnatal period [25], the influence of A fibres over nociceptive circuits declines through what appears to be a competitive mechanism [22].

Important also is the maturation of excitatory synaptic signalling in immature reflex circuits. Synaptic inputs from nociceptive fibres are not simply getting stronger over the postnatal period and are changing their signalling properties. The major excitatory neurotransmitter is glutamate and its receptors (AMPA, NMDA, kainate and metabotropic receptors) are made up of subunits that are all developmentally regulated over the postnatal period in the sensory circuits of the spinal cord dorsal horn. Overall glutamatergic activity in the newborn seems to lead to longer channel opening times and greater $Ca^{2+}$ influx than in adults, properties that are thought to be critical for growth and synaptogenesis but will also impact upon nociceptive transmission. One example is the lower ratio of GluR2 to GluR 1, 3 and 4 subunits in the AMPA receptor (responsible for fast excitatory transmission) in a young spinal cord [26]. The GluR2 subunit is important because it reduces the $Ca^{2+}$-permeability of AMPA receptors so the lower levels in spinal neurons during the early postnatal period will mean a greater $Ca^{2+}$ influx into neurons every time AMPA receptors are excited. These $Ca^{2+}$-permeable AMPA receptors have been demonstrated in both GABAergic (inhibitory) and NK1 positive (excitatory) interneurons in the neonatal spinal cord dorsal horn [27]. NMDA receptor concentration and subunit composition also change with age and neonatal spinal cord dorsal horn NMDA receptors have an unusually high $Mg^{2+}$ sensitivity [28] and, like AMPA receptors, allow greater $Ca^{2+}$ influx than mature neurons [29].

As important as the excitatory input is the development of inhibitory connections. The increased excitability and lack of precision of neonatal nociceptive reflexes could arise from immature inhibitory synapses. The main inhibitory neurotransmitters, GABA and glycine and their receptors (GABAR and GlyR) are also postnatally regulated in the postnatal spinal cord dorsal horn. Initially, virtually all the inhibitory activity in the newborn spinal cord dorsal horn is mediated by GABA, and there is little or no glycinergic activity, despite the presence of functional GlyR [30]. Since glycinergic inputs mediate fast inhibitory events, their slow maturation relative to GABA inputs will affect the timing and synchronization of inhibition. The early GABAergic currents are also four times slower in their decay time than in adults, a property that interestingly appears to be maintained by the high levels of circulating neurosteroids in the immature CNS [31].

A feature of $GABA_AR$ activation in the developing CNS is that it can be excitatory rather than inhibitory, as the high intracellular $Cl^-$ concentrations $[Cl]_i$ in immature neurons result in a reversal potential for $Cl^-$ ions ($E_{Cl}$) that is more positive than both the resting potential and action potential threshold. The onset of expression of the $K^+$-$Cl^-$ co-transporter KCC2, decreases $[Cl]_i$ over the postnatal period, leading to a negative shift in $E_{Cl}$, such that GABA become progressively inhibitory [32]. From the point of view of nociceptive circuits, GABA excitation is likely to be more important in early development where there is little or no glutamate excitatory input but it is still evident in the very newborn spinal cord, where some superficial dorsal horn neurons in spinal cord slices depolarize in response to $GABA_AR$ activation with the response becoming exclusively hyperpolarizing by P6-P7 [30]. However it is important to note that even then, $E_{Cl}$ was always more negative than action potential threshold so that depolarizing GABA responses will still inhibit the firing of newborn superficial dorsal horn neurons. Indeed, dorsal horn neurons in a young spinal cord are strongly disinhibited by GABA antagonists, demonstrating the presence of a tonic GABAergic inhibition [33]. It has been argued, however, that under conditions of excessive GABAergic activity and build-up of chloride ions, immature neurons may fail to pump out chloride fast enough, leading to a prolonged depolarization and $Ca^{2+}$ entry [34].

## III. The Influence of Higher Brain Centres over Nociceptive Reflex Circuits Matures Postnatally

A further factor contributing to excitation and inhibition in spinal nociceptive circuits is the descending activity from the brainstem. The brainstem is known to exert powerful descending control over spinal nociceptive processing in adults. The spinal cord is normally under tonic inhibitory control from higher centres such that spinalization leads to an increased excitability. The key brainstem areas involved are the rostroventral medulla (RVM) and the periaqueductal grey (PAG) [35, 36]. The PAG receives inputs from the dorsal horn, and a wide range of higher centres including the amygdala and cortex. The PAG projects to the RVM, which in turn sends descending projections to the dorsal horn, many of which contain serotonin (5-HT) as a neurotransmitter. There has been considerable research on these areas in relation to nociceptive processing in the adult and the physiological properties of the cells, their projections and interconnections, neurotransmitter and receptor expression and sensitivity to pharmacological agents have been well described. Recent literature has also emphasised descending excitatory pathways as well as inhibitory ones, depending upon which precise pathways are activated [37]. The brainstem therefore appears to influence spinal nociceptive behaviour by controlling the balance of excitation and inhibition over the dorsal horn.

Spinal transection before P15 has markedly less impact on spinal sensory circuits than transection at older ages [38] due to the prolonged postnatal maturation of descending fibre systems. Brainstem serotonergic fibres invade the grey matter around birth but the adult termination pattern and density is not achieved until P21 in the lumbar spinal cord [39, 40]. Although descending inputs to the mature spinal cord can clearly produce both excitatory and inhibitory effects on nociceptive processing, the role of this system in modulating spinal sensory processing in the neonate is less clear. The fact that electrical activation of the periacqueductal gray (PAG) region does not produce analgesia until P21 [41] and stimulating the dorsolateral funiculus is unable to inhibit the firing of dorsal horn neurons until at least P10 [42, 43], strongly suggests that descending inhibition has little functional impact on the neonatal spinal cord dorsal horn. In support of this, the classic biphasic behavioural response to formalin, thought to arise from descending inhibition, is also not apparent in the rat pup until 2 weeks of age [44]. The delayed postnatal functional maturation of descending inhibition is likely to be due to low levels of serotonin in synaptic terminals during the early postnatal period, as application of D-amphetamine at doses sufficient to enhance monoamine release does not affect pain behaviour before P10 [45] and intrathecal 5-HT3 agonist does not depress the formalin test response until P10 [46]. While the low 5-HT levels may limit synaptic transmission, they may still influence synaptic maturation as exposure to 5-HT causes rapid insertion of AMPARs into the synaptic membrane of neonatal spinal SG neurons

[47]. Recently it has become evident that while descending inhibition over noxious evoked responses is more or less absent in the newborn, there are powerful supraspinal influences over $GABA_A$ receptor signalling as young as P3 [48] although the source of this control is not yet known.

## IV. Nociceptive Circuit Maturation Is Influenced by Exposure to Sensory Stimulation

There is increasing evidence that the normal maturation of nociceptive systems is influenced by exposure of the infant to sensory stimulation. Sensory activity could arise from nociceptive or non-nociceptive afferents but under normal physiological circumstances nociceptor activation would be rare in the first postnatal weeks while tactile stimulation would be considerable. While daily noxious stimulation does not affect postnatal tuning of the nociceptive tail reflex, blocking low intensity tactile inputs from the tail with local anaesthetic, during the critical 10-day period, prevents it. Regular tactile input can arise from spontaneous twitching during sleep in both rats and human infants and this has been proposed to be responsible for shaping nociceptive circuits in early life [16, 49].

There is also evidence that C fibre activity influences the synaptic organization of lamina II. Neonatal destruction of C fibres by systemic administration of the neurotoxin capsaicin, prevents or delays the development of a number of synaptic processes. Capsaicin treatment delays the postnatal reduction in spinal cord dorsal horn cell NMDA-evoked calcium influx [29], prevents the withdrawal of A fibre synaptic from lamina II [50, 51], prevents the organisation of NK1-R expression patterns [52] and leads to abnormal maturation of GABAergic and descending inhibition [53, 54] and disorganized receptive fields [55]. The mechanism underlying these effects are not known but are likely to involve pre- and post-synaptice spike timing mechanisms as described in the developing hippocampus [56] involving NMDA receptor activation [22].

An important question is whether the reverse is true, i.e. can increased C fibre input early in development alter the normal development of nociceptive circuits? The well-documented numerous invasive procedures that preterm infants undergo in intensive care, where it is not always possible to achieve adequate levels of analgesia, could produce increased C fibre activity, which in turn could alter the subsequent development of the nervous system. This is currently an area of considerable research, and there is evidence of long lasting changes induced by early injury in animal models [1]. Neonatal hindpaw inflammation, for example, has a pronounced effect on the central terminal fields of C fibres and the spinal cord dorsal horn cell response to a second inflammatory challenge is increased well into adulthood [57-59]. Skin wounds in the newborn also have prolonged effect long after the wound has healed and the skin remains hypersensitive and dorsal horn receptive field (RF) sizes are still expanded for at least six weeks [60, 61].

While the mechanisms underlying these long-term alterations in pain behaviours are not known, consideration of the changing synaptic connectivity and signalling in postnatal nociceptive pathways and the balance of inhibition versus excitation raises a number of possibilities [2]. Long term reduction in sensory and pain perception have also been reported over the whole body, probably due to an alteration or resetting of the stress response since exposure to stress during the perinatal period is known to influence adult nociceptive behavior [57,62]. This could be viewed as a useful adaptive response in response to early trauma. Any long term sensitization occurring at segmental level could be masked so that a strong stimulus such as re-inflammation is required to uncover it. This is an area that requires more research before firm conclusions can be drawn.

## V. The Development of Peripheral and Central Sensitization Mechanisms Are Important in Pediatric Pain

While it is important to understand the development of nociception, most clinical pain involves hyperalgesia, arising from both peripheral and central sensitization. Tissue injury and inflammation can lead to persistent pain and hyperalgesia that lasts for days, weeks or months. This is due to increased spike activity from sensitization of peripheral nociceptor terminals in the injured area which also triggers changes in gene expression in sensory central neurons resulting in central sensitisation [63]. The extent to which this happens in the immature system is still under investigation.

Hyperalgesic behaviour can be produced from experimental inflammation in newborn animals but the effect is not as great as in adults [64-67]. This is backed up by electrophysiological studies showing that sensitisation of spinal cord dorsal horn cells after inflammation of the hindpaw occurs at all postnatal ages although the exact pattern of effects is age-dependent [20]. Hypersensitivity to tissue damage can also be measured in human infants, where 'tenderness' or a fall in reflex thresholds is established for days and weeks in the presence of local skin or deep visceral tissue injury [17, 68, 69]. The effect is small in the youngest infant and increases with age and in both rats and man. Secondary hyperalgesia, which spreads into an area surrounding the original injury, appears to develop later than primary hyperalgesia in newborn rats [86]. Skin wounding leads to long lasting increases in mechanical sensitivity in the damaged region, long after the skin has healed and this is accompanied by expanded receptive fields in dorsal horn cells [70, 71].

The maturation of primary hyperalgesia will reflect peripheral nociceptor terminal maturity. C fibres are capable of peripheral sensitisation from before birth but peripheral C fibre terminals do not release sufficient substance P to produce neurogenic extravasation until postnatal day 10 [72, 73]. Neonatal injuries release much higher concentrations of growth factors into the damaged tissue than similar injuries in adults, but interestingly NGF is not able to directly sensitize C fibre terminals in the newborn until 10 days of life [74]. Nevertheless exposure of neonatal C fibre terminals to inflammatory mediators accelerates their phenotypic development and increases their terminal density of nociceptors in the injured region [75-77]. Immature cutaneous nociceptor terminals are also normally restricted in their ability to penetrate into the most superficial layers of the skin by the molecule ephrin A4, which is downregulated by skin injury permitting long lasting hyperinnervation of the injured region [78].

The postnatal maturation of hyperalgesia may relate to the development of substance P (SP) signalling which is known to have a key role in this form of central sensitization. C fibre afferent evoked SP signalling is likely to be low in the neonate and their receptors (NK1), although functional in the newborn spinal cord, undergo substantial postnatal reorganisation [79]. In slice preparations, NMDA dependent C-fibre evoked depolarization of spinal cord cells and 'wind-up' of cells to repeated C-fibre stimulation has been demonstrated in the young (8-14 day) spinal cord but it is not clear that it occurs earlier than that [80]. In any event, it is evident that different protein kinase C mediated pathways are triggered in the dorsal horn of young versus old rats by inflammation [81]. Recently the role of descending brainstem excitatory pathways in maintaining persistent pain has been emphasised [35] but the developmental regulation of this system has not been investigated (see section iii). One central component of inflammatory pain, namely the disinhibition of dorsal horn neurons, is thought to occur through the depression of glycinergic neurotransmission by the inflammatory mediator prostaglandin $E_2$ ($PGE_2$) thus the lack of glycinergic signalling in immature spinal cord may be a limiting factor to the development of hyperalgesia [82].

## VI. Our Knowledge of the Maturation of Nociceptive Processing at Higher Levels of the CNS Is Limited

Very little is known about the development of higher pain processing in man. The strong responses to noxious stimulation observed in the preterm infants, could be entirely mediated at the spinal or brainstem level with little or no cortical involvement. Indeed, below 32 weeks of postconceptional age, several key behavioural and autonomic pain responses are the same in normal infants and infants with brain injury associated with white matter damage [83]. It is possible, therefore, that despite some anatomical evidence of thalamocortical projections in the human brain from 24 weeks [84] functional nociceptive connections with cortical cells and circuits are not formed until much later. Since the true experience of pain includes emotional and affective components, which require a higher level cortical processing, knowledge of the maturation of infant cortical responses to noxious stimulation would be a major step towards understanding the infant pain experience.

Following integration in the spinal cord dorsal horn, sensory and nociceptive information is conducted to supraspinal centres via ascending tracts to targets in the brainstem, mid-brain, hypothalamus, thalamus and amygdala. A key ascending pathway involved in pain and hyperalgesia arises from lamina I of the spinal cord dorsal horn, particularly NK1-expressing neurons receiving Aδ and C fibre nociceptive inputs, which project to the parabrachial area of the brainstem. These neurones then project to the amygdala (affective components of pain) and the hypothalamus (autonomic functions such as changes in heart rate and blood pressure). Outputs from these structures are passed via the periaqueductal grey (PAG), which in turn sends descending projections back to the spinal cord dorsal horn in a spino-bulbar-spinal loop. Descending projections to the dorsal horn arise from the brainstem nuclei, including nucleus raphe magnus (NRM), raphe dorsalis, reticularis, paragigantocellularis

(NRPG), as well as locus coeruleus, periaqueductal grey and mesencephalic reticular formation [85]. Very little is known about the maturation of these regions [86].

Recently, some insight has been gained into central pain processing in human infants by measuring changes in cerebral oxygenation over the somatosensory cortex response to noxious stimulation using real time near-infrared spectroscopy in infants between 25 and 45 weeks of postmenstrual age [87]. Interestingly, noxious stimulation produced a clear cortical response, measured as an increase in [HbT] in the contralateral somatosensory cortex, from 25 weeks. Cortical responses were significantly greater in awake compared to sleeping infants and in awake infants the response increased with age. The response was modality specific in that no response was detected following non-noxious stimulation of the heel, even when accompanied by reflex withdrawal of the foot. This study concluded that noxious information is transmitted to the preterm infant cortex from 25 weeks and that consequently there is the potential for both higher-level pain processing and nociceptive activity dependent changes in the human brain from a very early age [87].

## VII. Developmental Pharmacology Research Has Provided Insights into Immature Analgesic Mechanisms

A number of reviews have summarized the clinical pharmacology and clinical outcomes of commonly used analgesics and anaesthetics in paediatrics [7]. Examination of the developmental neurobiology of receptor expression and function can provide additional insight into the mechanism of analgesic action in the developing nervous system and how efficacy may be determined by the developmental state of pain pathways.

### (a) Opioids

The actions of opioids in the immature nervous system are especially interesting since they are increasingly used in neonates and children and they have been the subject of a number of recent clinical investigations [88, 90]. In rat pups, the analgesic potency of systemic and epidural morphine to noxious mechanical stimulation is significantly greater in the neonate and declines with postnatal age [65, 89, 90]. This may well be related to the postnatal regulation of mu opioid receptor (MOR) function. MOR expression and calcium imaging following MOR activation in rat dorsal root ganglia show that a significantly greater number of neonatal DRG neurons express functional MOR compared to adult. This exuberant expression is confined to the large, neurofilament positive A fibre sensory neurons, while expression in small, C nociceptive, neurofilament negative neurons remains unchanged. The MOR expressed on large DRG neurons in neonates are functional and are subject to postnatal developmental regulation [91, 92]. Morphine analgesic potency in thermal nociceptive tests either remains unchanged or increases with age depending on the test used.

Within the CNS, mu and kappa opioid receptor binding-sites are spread relatively diffusely throughout the spinal cord at birth in the rat. Overall binding peaks at P7 and subsequently decreases to adult levels with the mu opioid receptor binding sites becoming denser in the superficial dorsal horn. C-fibre evoked dorsal horn neuronal responses recorded from anaesthetized rat pups were more sensitive to spinal morphine at P21 than at P14 despite the fact that mu receptor binding was greater at P14, indicating the importance of other factors, such as coupling of the receptors in opioid function [93]. Morphine also acts at the level of the brainstem and an important central mechanism of opioid analgesia is through activation of descending monoamine-mediated inhibition from the rostroventral medulla. This pathway is known to undergo marked postnatal development, as described in section (iii), and this will have an impact on analgesia. Morphine- and glutamate-induced analgesia mediated by the PAG are developmentally regulated [94].

Codeine analgesia is known to be dependent on metabolism to morphine, but studies in rat pups in two strains, Sprague-Dawley and Dark Agouti that model human metabolic phenotypes because of marked differences in enzyme activity, have shown that codeine analgesia is also developmentally regulated with low efficacy in the early postnatal period. Analgesic effects in the adult rat are not predictive of efficacy in development in either strain, which has important implications for further study and, possibly, for clinical use [95].

## (b) Sedative-Hypnotics

Sedatives such as benzodiazepines act upon $GABA_A$ receptors, which are mainly expressed in the thalamus, cortex and spinal cord through a specialised site on the alpha1 subunit [96]. Alpha subunits exhibit age dependent expression throughout several areas of the brain, in general, and the density of immunoreactive product for alpha1 is greatest in the adult brain, while alpha2 is highest in younger tissue [97]. Intrathecal administration of midazolam produces analgesia and diminishes $A\delta$- and C-fiber evoked polysynaptic excitatory postsynaptic currents dorsal horn neurons suggesting that midazolam modulates the benzodiazepine site on GABAergic interneurons in the spinal cord dorsal horn [98], but the effects upon the immature spinal cord remain unknown. The developmental regulation of potassium chloride pump discussed in section (ii) may be also important here.

## (c) Nonsteroidal Anti-Inflammatory Drugs

The basic mechanism of analgesic actions of nonsteroidal anti-inflammatory drugs (NSAIDs) results from the inhibition of prostaglandin synthesis (prostacyclin or PGE2), thus preventing nociceptor sensitization. However, it is also clear that NSAIDs exert their analgesic effect through a variety of other peripheral and central mechanisms [99]. The analgesic action of paracetamol (aminocetophen) is likely to be mediated in the CNS, where it inhibits activation of nociceptive systems by excitatory neurotransmitters such as glutamate and substance P, possibly through cyclo-oxygenase (cox) or neuronal nitric oxide synthase (nNOS) inhibition. Paracetamol is thought to inhibit the prostaglandin production, by action on cyclo-oxygenases related to cox 1 and cox 2. Ketorolac, a potent NSAID, has been reported to be ineffective as either an anti-inflammatory or analgesic agent in the neonatal rat formalin model, but is effective by 3 weeks of age [100]. The effects of cox-1 inhibitors on rat models of postoperative pain also depend on postnatal age [101].

## (d) Local Anesthetics

Local anaesthetics are known to act upon $Na^+$ channels. Of particular interest for analgesia is their use-dependent block. Upon prolonged depolarizations, voltage-dependent $Na^+$ channels open and subsequently inactivate, involving both fast and slow inactivated conformational states. Slow inactivation is thought to be accompanied by rearrangement of the channel pore and local anaesthetics that elicits depolarization-dependent ('use-dependent') $Na^+$ channel block modulate the kinetics of slow inactivated states [102].

These actions will be influenced by the developmental regulation of $Na^+$ channels [103]. Inflammatory hypersensitivity is selectively attenuated by very low doses of bupivacaine which do not affect the sensory threshold in the contralateral uninflamed limb and this effect is age-related, with younger rats being more sensitive than older rats [104].

## (e) Alpha2-Agonists

Spinally mediated selective reversal of inflammatory hyperalgesia by epidural dexmedetomidine can be achieved at all ages; relatively lower doses are effective in early life, but the therapeutic window is narrow. These data have implications for the use and dosing of epidural alpha2 agonists in neonates and infants [105].

# Conclusion

In this chapter, I have reviewed some key features of the development of nociceptive and pain processing that may impact upon clinical care of infants and children in pain. The first point was to emphasize that nociceptive reflex behaviour is imprecise and poorly directed and that it changes markedly with age. This is due to the development of excitatory and inhibitory synaptic connections in nociceptive circuits. Pain assessment in young infants must take this into account. In addition, the influence of higher brain centres over nociceptive reflex circuits matures postnatally, so that in young infants the ability of higher centres in the brain to modulate pain is different from that in older patients. Importantly there is evidence that nociceptive circuit maturation is influenced by exposure to sensory stimulation. Thus excessive handling or tissue damage and inflammation may change the normal pain responses in later life although this has yet to be confirmed in human subjects.

It is pointed out that increased understanding of the developmental mechanisms underlying the peripheral and central sensitization mechanisms that produce hyperalgesia and prolonged pain states are important for a better treatment of pediatric pain, but the study of developmental pharmacology has provided insights into immature analgesic mechanisms. Our knowledge of the maturation of nociceptive processing at higher levels of the CNS is limited but cortical responses to noxious stimulation have been recorded in the youngest preterm infant, opening the door for further study in this area.

# References

[2] Baccei, M.L. and Fitzgerald, M. The Development of Pain Pathways and Mechanisms in *The Textbook of Pain* (eds. McMahon,S.B. and Koltzenburg,M.) Elsevier, 2005.
[3] Fitzgerald, M. The development of nociceptive circuits. *Nat. Rev. Neurosci.* 6, 507-520 (2005).
[4] Fitzgerald, M. and McDermott, A.in *The Neurobiology of Pain* (eds. Hunt,S. and Koltzenburg,M.), OUP, 2006.
[5] Fitzgerald, M. and Hathway, G. The Development of Nociceptive Systems in *Handbook of the Senses, Pain (*eds Basbaum,A. and Bushnell,C.*)* Academic Press 2006.
[6] Anand, K.J. *et al.* Analgesia and local anesthesia during invasive procedures in the neonate *Clin. Ther.* 27, 844-876 (2005).
[7] Anand, K.J. *et al.* Analgesia and anesthesia for neonates: study design and ethical issues *Clin. Ther.* 27, 814-843 (2005).
[8] Berde, C.B. and Sethna,N.F. Analgesics for the treatment of pain in children *N. Engl. J. Med.* 347, 1094-1103 (2002).
[9] Berde, C.B. *et al.* Anesthesia and analgesia during and after surgery in neonates. *Clin. Ther.* 27, 900-921 (2005).
[10] Howard,R.F. Current status of pain management in children *JAMA* 290, 2464-2469 (2003).
[11] Tibboel, D., Anand, K.J., and van den Anker, J.N. The pharmacological treatment of neonatal pain *Semin. Fetal Neonatal. Med.* 10, 195-205 (2005).
[12] Ballantyne, M., Stevens, B., McAllister, M., Dionne, K., and Jack, A. Validation of the premature infant pain profile in the clinical setting. *Clin. J. Pain* 15, 297-303 (1999).
[13] McNair, C., Ballantyne, M., Dionne, K., Stephens, D., and Stevens, B. Postoperative pain assessment in the neonatal intensive care unit. *Arch. Dis. Child Fetal Neonatal Ed.* 89, F537-F541 (2004).
[14] Pattinson, D. and Fitzgerald, M. The neurobiology of infant pain: development of excitatory and inhibitory neurotransmission in the spinal dorsal horn *Reg. Anesth. Pain Med.* 29, 36-44 (2004).
[15] Carbajal, R. *et al.* Morphine does not provide adequate analgesia for acute procedural pain among preterm neonates *Pediatrics* 115, 1494-1500 (2005).
[16] Schouenborg, J. Somatosensory imprinting in spinal reflex modules *J. Rehabil. Med.*73-80 (2003).
[17] Waldenstrom, A., Thelin, J., Thimansson, E., Levinsson, A., and Schouenborg, J. Developmental learning in a pain-related system: evidence for a cross-modality mechanism. *J. Neurosci.* 23, 7719-7725 (2003).

[18] Andrews, K. and Fitzgerald, M. Cutaneous flexion reflex in human neonates: a quantitative study of threshold and stimulus-response characteristics after single and repeated stimuli *Dev. Med. Child Neurol.* 41, 696-703 (1999).

[19] Andrews, K.A., Desai, D., Dhillon, H.K., Wilcox, D.T., and Fitzgerald, M. Abdominal sensitivity in the first year of life: comparison of infants with and without prenatally diagnosed unilateral hydronephrosis *Pain.* 100, 35-46 (2002).

[20] Fitzgerald, M. and Jennings, E. The postnatal development of spinal sensory processing. *Proc. Natl. Acad. Sci. U. S. A* 96, 7719-7722 (1999).

[21] Torsney, C. and Fitzgerald, M. Age-dependent effects of peripheral inflammation on the electrophysiological properties of neonatal rat dorsal horn neurons. *J. Neurophysiol.* 87, 1311-1317 (2002).

[22] Nakatsuka, T., Ataka, T., Kumamoto, E., Tamaki, T., and Yoshimura, M. Alteration in synaptic inputs through C-afferent fibers to substantia gelatinosa neurons of the rat spinal dorsal horn during postnatal development. *Neuroscience.* 99, 549-556 (2000).

[23] Beggs, S., Torsney, C., Drew, L.J., and Fitzgerald, M. The postnatal reorganization of primary afferent input and dorsal horn cell receptive fields in the rat spinal cord is an activity-dependent process. *Eur. J. Neurosci.* 16, 1249-1258 (2002).

[24] Jennings, E. and Fitzgerald, M. C-fos can be induced in the neonatal rat spinal cord by both noxious and innocuous peripheral stimulation. *Pain.* 68, 301-306 (1996).

[25] Jennings, E. and Fitzgerald, M. Postnatal changes in responses of rat dorsal horn cells to afferent stimulation: a fibre-induced sensitization. *J. Physiol.* 509, 859-868 (1998).

[26] Baccei, M.L., Bardoni, R., and Fitzgerald, M. Development of nociceptive synaptic inputs to the neonatal rat dorsal horn: glutamate release by capsaicin and menthol. *J. Physiol.* 549, 231-242 (2003).

[27] Jakowec, M.W., Fox, A.J., Martin, L.J., and Kalb, R.G. Quantitative and qualitative changes in AMPA receptor expression during spinal cord development 2. *Neuroscience.* 67, 893-907 (1995).

[28] Engelman, H.S., Allen, T.B., and MacDermott, A.B. The distribution of neurons expressing calcium-permeable AMPA receptors in the superficial laminae of the spinal cord dorsal horn. *J. Neurosci.* 19, 2081-2089 (1999).

[29] Green, G.M. and Gibb, A.J. Characterization of the single-channel properties of NMDA receptors in laminae I and II of the dorsal horn of neonatal rat spinal cord. *Eur. J. Neurosci.* 14, 1590-1602 (2001).

[30] Hori, Y. and Kanda, K. Developmental alterations in NMDA receptor-mediated [Ca2+]i elevation in substantia gelatinosa neurons of neonatal rat spinal cord. *Brain Res. Dev. Brain Res.* 80, 141-148 (1994).

[31] Baccei, M.L. and Fitzgerald, M. Development of GABAergic and glycinergic transmission in the neonatal rat dorsal horn. *J. Neurosci.* 24, 4749-4757 (2004).

[32] Keller, A.F., Breton, J.D., Schlichter, R., and Poisbeau, P. Production of 5alpha-reduced neurosteroids is developmentally regulated and shapes GABA(A) miniature IPSCs in lamina II of the spinal cord. *J. Neurosci.* 24, 907-915 (2004).

[33] Ben Ari,Y. Excitatory actions of gaba during development: the nature of the nurture. *Nat. Rev. Neurosci.* 3, 728-739 (2002).

[34] Bremner, L., Fitzgerald, M., and Baccei, M. Functional $GABA_A$ receptor-mediated inhibition in the neonatal dorsal horn *J.Neurophysiol.in press* (2006).

[35] Cordero-Erausquin, M., Coull, J.A., Boudreau, D., Rolland, M., and De,Koninck, Y. Differential maturation of GABA action and anion reversal potential in spinal lamina I neurons: impact of chloride extrusion capacity. *J. Neurosci.* 25, 9613-9623 (2005).

[36] Gebhart, G.F. Descending modulation of pain. *Neurosci Biobehav. Rev.* 27, 729-737 (2004).

[37] Ren, K. and Dubner, R. Descending modulation in persistent pain: an update *Pain* 100, 1-6 (2002).

[38] Suzuki, R., Rygh, L.J., and Dickenson, A.H. Bad news from the brain: descending 5-HT pathways that control spinal pain processing. *Trends Pharmacol. Sci.* 25, 613-617 (2004).

[39] Weber, E.D. and Stelzner, D.J. Behavioral effects of spinal cord transection in the developing rat *Brain Res.* 125, 241-255 (1977).

[40] Bregman, B.S. Development of serotonin immunoreactivity in the rat spinal cord and its plasticity after neonatal spinal cord lesions. *Brain Res.* 431, 245-263 (1987).

[41] Rajaofetra, N., Sandillon, F., Geffard, M., and Privat,A. Pre- and post-natal ontogeny of serotonergic projections to the rat spinal cord *J. Neurosci. Res.* 22, 305-321 (1989).

[42] van Praag, H. and Frenk, H. The development of stimulation-produced analgesia (SPA) in the rat. *Brain Res. Dev. Brain Res.* 64, 71-76 (1991).

[43] Boucher, T., Jennings, E., and Fitzgerald, M. The onset of diffuse noxious inhibitory controls in postnatal rat pups: a C-Fos study. *Neurosci. Lett.* 257, 9-12 (1998).

[44] Fitzgerald, M. and Koltzenburg, M. The functional development of descending inhibitory pathways in the dorsolateral funiculus of the newborn rat spinal cord. *Brain Res.* 389, 261-270 (1986).

[45] Guy, E.R. and Abbott, F.V. The behavioral response to formalin in preweanling rats *Pain* 51, 81-90 (1992).

[46] Giordano, J. Antinociceptive effects of intrathecally administered 2-methylserotonin in developing rats *Brain Res. Dev. Brain Res.* 98, 142-144 (1997).

[47] Abbott, F.V. and Guy, E.R. Effects of morphine, pentobarbital and amphetamine on formalin-induced behaviours in infant rats: sedation versus specific suppression of pain. *Pain* 62, 303-312 (1995).

[48] Li, P. and Zhuo, M. Silent glutamatergic synapses and nociception in mammalian spinal cord. *Nature* 393, 695-698 (1998).

[49] Hathway, G. *et al.* A postnatal switch in GABAergic control of spinal cutaneous reflexes. *Eur. J. Neurosci.* 23, 112-118 (2006).

[50] Petersson, P., Waldenstrom, A., Fahraeus, C., and Schouenborg, J. Spontaneous muscle twitches during sleep guide spinal self-organization *Nature.* 424, 72-75 (2003).

[51] Shortland, P., Molander, C., Woolf, C.J., and Fitzgerald, M. Neonatal capsaicin treatment induces invasion of the substantia gelatinosa by the terminal arborizations of hair follicle afferents in the rat dorsal horn. *J. Comp. Neurol.* 296, 23-31 (1990).

[52] Yang, K., Furue, H., Fujita, T., Kumamoto, E., and Yoshimura, M. Alterations in primary afferent input to substantia gelatinosa of adult rat spinal cord after neonatal capsaicin treatment *J. Neurosci. Res.* 74, 928-933 (2003).

[53] Ohtori, S. et al. Neonatal capsaicin treatment decreased substance P receptor immunoreactivity in lamina III neurons of the dorsal horn. *Neurosci. Res.* 38, 147-154 (2000).

[54] Cervero, F. and Plenderleith, M.B. C-fibre excitation and tonic descending inhibition of dorsal horn neurones in adult rats treated at birth with capsaicin. *J. Physiol* 365, 223-237 (1985).

[55] Chiang, C.Y., Hu, J.W., and Sessle, B.J. NMDA receptor involvement in neuroplastic changes induced by neonatal capsaicin treatment in trigeminal nociceptive neurons. *J. Neurophysiol.* 78, 2799-2803 (1997).

[56] Wall, P.D., Fitzgerald, M., and Woolf, C.J. Effects of capsaicin on receptive fields and on inhibitions in rat spinal cord. *Exp. Neurol.* 78, 425-436 (1982).

[57] Bi, G. and Poo, M. Synaptic modification by correlated activity: Hebb's postulate revisited. *Annu. Rev. Neurosci.* 24, 139-166 (2001).

[58] Ren, K. et al. Characterization of basal and re-inflammation-associated long-term alteration in pain responsivity following short-lasting neonatal local inflammatory insult *Pain.* 110, 588-596 (2004).

[59] Ruda, M.A., Ling, Q.D., Hohmann, A.G., Peng, Y.B., and Tachibana, T. Altered nociceptive neuronal circuits after neonatal peripheral inflammation *Science.* 289, 628-631 (2000).

[60] Tachibana, T., Ling, Q.D., and Ruda, M.A. Increased Fos induction in adult rats that experienced neonatal peripheral inflammation *Neuroreport.* 12, 925-927 (2001).

[61] Reynolds, M.L. and Fitzgerald, M. Long-term sensory hyperinnervation following neonatal skin wounds *J. Comp Neurol.* 358, 487-498 (1995).

[62] Torsney, C. and Fitzgerald, M. Spinal dorsal horn cell receptive field size is increased in adult rats following neonatal hindpaw skin injury. *J. Physiol.* 550, 255-261 (2003).

[63] Ren, K., Novikova, S.I., He, F., Dubner, R. and Lidow, M.S. Neonatal local noxious insult affects gene expression in the spinal dorsal horn of adult rats. *Mol. Pain.* 22;1-27 (2005)

[64] Woolf, C.J. and Salter, M.W. Neuronal plasticity: increasing the gain in pain. *Science.* 288, 1765-1769 (2000).

[65] Jiang, M.C. and Gebhart, G.F. Development of mustard oil-induced hyperalgesia in rats. *Pain.* 77, 305-313 (1998).

[66] Marsh, D., Dickenson, A., Hatch, D., and Fitzgerald, M. Epidural opioid analgesia in infant rats II: responses to carrageenan and capsaicin *Pain.* 82, 33-38 (1999).

[67] Yi, D.K. and Barr, G.A. The induction of Fos-like immunoreactivity by noxious thermal, mechanical and chemical stimuli in the lumbar spinal cord of infant rats. *Pain.* 60, 257-265 (1995).

[68] Howard, R.F., Hatch, D.J., Cole, T.J., and Fitzgerald, M. Inflammatory pain and hypersensitivity are selectively reversed by epidural bupivacaine and are developmentally regulated *Anesthesiology.* 95, 421-427 (2001).

[69] Andrews, K. and Fitzgerald, M. Wound sensitivity as a measure of analgesic effects following surgery in human neonates and infants *Pain.* 99, 185-195 (2002).

[70] Andrews, K.A., Desai, D., Dhillon, H.K., Wilcox, D.T., and Fitzgerald, M. Abdominal sensitivity in the first year of life: comparison of infants with and without prenatally diagnosed unilateral hydronephrosis *Pain.* 100, 35-46 (2002).

[71] Torsney, C. and Fitzgerald, M. Spinal dorsal horn cell receptive field size is increased in adult rats following neonatal hindpaw skin injury. *J. Physiol.* 550, 255-261 (2003).

[72] Reynolds, M.L. and Fitzgerald, M. Long-term sensory hyperinnervation following neonatal skin wounds *J. Comp Neurol.* 358, 487-498 (1995).

[73] Fitzgerald, M. and Gibson, S. The postnatal physiological and neurochemical development of peripheral sensory C fibres. *Neuroscience.* 13, 933-944 (1984).

[74] Koltzenburg, M. and Lewin, G.R. Receptive properties of embryonic chick sensory neurons innervating skin *J. Neurophysiol.* 78, 2560-2568 (1997).

[75] Zhu, W., Galoyan, S.M., Petruska, J.C., Oxford, G.S., and Mendell, L.M. A developmental switch in acute sensitization of small dorsal root ganglion (DRG) neurons to capsaicin or noxious heating by NGF. *J. Neurophysiol.* 92, 3148-3152 (2004).

[76] Lewin, G.R. Neurotrophins and the specification of neuronal phenotype. *Philos. Trans. R. Soc. Lond. B. Biol. Sci.* 351, 405-411 (1996).

[77] Beland, B. and Fitzgerald, M. Influence of peripheral inflammation on the postnatal maturation of primary sensory neuron phenotype in rats. *J. Pain.* 2, 36-45 (2001).

[78] Reynolds, M.L. and Fitzgerald, M. Long-term sensory hyperinnervation following neonatal skin wounds *J. Comp. Neurol.* 358, 487-498 (1995).

[79] Moss, A. *et al.* Ephrin-A4 inhibits sensory neurite outgrowth and is regulated by neonatal skin wounding. *Eur. J. Neurosci.* 22, 2413-2421 (2006).

[80] Kar, S. and Quirion, R. Neuropeptide receptors in developing and adult rat spinal cord: an in vitro quantitative autoradiography study of calcitonin gene-related peptide, neurokinins, mu-opioid, galanin, somatostatin, neurotensin and vasoactive intestinal polypeptide receptors. *J. Comp. Neurol.* 354, 253-281 (1995).

[81] Sivilotti, L.G., Thompson, S.W., and Woolf, C.J. Rate of rise of the cumulative depolarization evoked by repetitive stimulation of small-caliber afferents is a predictor of action potential windup in rat spinal neurons in vitro. *J. Neurophysiol.* 69, 1621-1631 (1993).

[82] Sweitzer, S.M. *et al.* Protein kinase C epsilon and gamma: involvement in formalin-induced nociception in neonatal Rats. *J. Pharmacol. Exp. Ther.* 309, 616-625 (2004).

[83] Zeilhofer, H.U. The glycinergic control of spinal pain processing. *Cell. Mol. Life Sci.* 62, 2027-2035 (2006).

[84] Oberlander, T.F., Grunau, R.E., Fitzgerald, C., and Whitfield, M.F. Does parenchymal brain injury affect biobehavioral pain responses in very low birth weight infants at 32 weeks' postconceptional age? *Pediatrics.* 110, 570-576 (2002).

[85] Lee, S.J., Ralston, H.J., Drey, E.A., Partridge, J.C., and Rosen, M.A. Fetal pain: a systematic multidisciplinary review of the evidence *JAMA* 294, 947-954 (2005).

[86] Mantyh, P.W. and Hunt, S.P. Setting the tone: superficial dorsal horn projection neurons regulate pain sensitivity, *Trends Neurosci.* 27, 582-584 (2004).

[87] Walker, S.M., Meredith-Middleton, J., Lickiss, T., Moss, A., Fitzgerald, M. Primary and secondary hyperalgesia can be differentiated by postnatal age and ERK activation in the spinal dorsal horn of the rat pup.*Pain* (under review)

[88] Slater, R. *et al.* Cortical responses to noxious stimulation in preterm infants. *J. Neurosci.* 26, 3662-6 (2006).

[89] Marsh DF, Hatch, DJ, Fitzgerald M, Opioid systems and the newborn. *Brit. J. Anaesth.* 79:787-795 (1997)

[90] Marsh, D., Dickenson, A., Hatch, D., and Fitzgerald, M. Epidural opioid analgesia in infant rats I: mechanical and heat responses *Pain.* 82, 23-32 (1999).

[91] Nandi, R. and Fitzgerald, M. Opioid analgesia in the newborn *Eur. J. Pain* 9, 105-108 (2005).

[92] Beland, B. and Fitzgerald, M. Mu- and delta-opioid receptors are downregulated in the largest diameter primary sensory neurons during postnatal development in rats *Pain.* 90, 143-150 (2001).

[93] Nandi, R. *et al.* The functional expression of mu opioid receptors on sensory neurons is developmentally regulated; morphine analgesia is less selective in the neonate *Pain.* 111, 38-50 (2004).

[94] Rahman, W., Dashwood, M.R., Fitzgerald, M., Aynsley-Green, A., and Dickenson, A.H. Postnatal development of multiple opioid receptors in the spinal cord and development of spinal morphine analgesia *Brain Res. Dev. Brain Res.* 108, 239-254 (1998).

[95] Tive, L.A. and Barr, G.A. Analgesia from the periaqueductal gray in the developing rat: focal injections of morphine or glutamate and effects of intrathecal injection of methysergide or phentolamine. *Brain Res.* 584, 92-109 (1992).

[96] Williams, D.G., Dickenson, A., Fitzgerald, M., and Howard, R.F. Developmental regulation of codeine analgesia in the rat. *Anesthesiology.* 100, 92-97 (2004).

[97] Mohler, H., Crestani, F., and Rudolph, U. GABA(A)-receptor subtypes: a new pharmacology. *Curr. Opin. Pharmacol.* 1, 22-25 (2001).

[98] Paysan, J. and Fritschy, J.M. GABAA-receptor subtypes in developing brain. Actors or spectators? *Perspect. Dev. Neurobiol.* 5, 179-192 (1998).

[99] Kohno, T. *et al.* Actions of midazolam on excitatory transmission in dorsal horn neurons of adult rat spinal cord. *Anesthesiology.* 104, 338-343 (2006).

[100] Graham, G.G. and Scott,K.F. Mechanism of action of paracetamol. *Am. J. Ther.* 12, 46-55 (2005).

[101] Gupta, A., Cheng, J., Wang, S., and Barr, G.A. Analgesic efficacy of ketorolac and morphine in neonatal rats *Pharmacol. Biochem. Behav.* 68, 635-640 (2001).

[102] Ririe, D.G., Prout, H.M., and Eisenach, J.C. Effect of cyclooxygenase-1 inhibition in postoperative pain is developmentally regulated. *Anesthesiology.* 101, 1031-1035 (2004).

[103] Lai, J., Porreca,F., Hunter, J.C., and Gold, M.S. Voltage-gated sodium channels and hyperalgesia. *Annu. Rev. Pharmacol. Toxicol.* 44, 371-397 (2004).

[104] Benn, S.C., Costigan, M., Tate, S., Fitzgerald, M., and Woolf, C.J. Developmental expression of the TTX-resistant voltage-gated sodium channels Nav1.8 (SNS) and Nav1.9 (SNS2) in primary sensory neurons. *J. Neurosci.* 21, 6077-6085 (2001).

[105] Howard, R.F., Hatch, D.J., Cole, T.J., and Fitzgerald, M. Inflammatory pain and hypersensitivity are selectively reversed by epidural bupivacaine and are developmentally regulated *Anesthesiology.* 95, 421-427 (2001).

[106] Walker, S.M., Howard, R.H., Keay, K.A., and Fitzgerald, M. Developmental age influences the effect of epidural dexmedetomidine on inflammatory hyperalgesia in the rat pup. *Anesthesiology.* 102, 1226-34 (2005).

*Chapter XIII*

# Pediatric Pain Management: In Translation

*Allyssa LeBel*

Children's Hospital, Harvard Medical School, Boston

## Abstract

Age-dependent differences in pain physiology and pharmacology and heritability of nociception and antinociception are now established in animal species. Such research supports and provokes human investigations of the ontogeny, variability, and plasticity of pain sensitivity and analgesia in the developing organism. As well, timely US Federal Government mandates to study pediatric pharmaceutical use contribute to current scientific efforts in this vulnerable population. Pediatric pain researchers are now primed to translate the basic animal literature into well-designed human trials. Recent research has been especially productive in the study of neonatal pain, neuropathic pain disorders, pediatric opioid metabolism and efficacy, and pharmacogenetics.

## Introduction

Despite increasing efforts in translational research, the current treatment of clinical pain, especially chronic pain, does not yet readily benefit from recent advances in experimental neuroscience. Children with pain are notable and compelling examples of this dilemma. For the most part, the smaller number of informative pediatric clinical trials is due to unique challenges in this patient population [1]. These include pain assessment in a developing and sometimes non-verbal individual, necessary parental input on behalf of the child complicating ethical consent, lower frequency of some pain disorders in children (sometimes due to under-recognition) compared with adults, and inappropriate assumptions that pediatric patients should respond in the same way to interventions as adults. Such issues have particularly affected pharmaceutical use, with both under and overuse practice and "off-label "designations for 50-75% of agents used in pediatrics [2]. Gratefully, this international problem is currently being addressed by new well-controlled drug trials. For example, in the United States, the Food and Drug Administration Modernization Act (FDAMA) was enacted in November 1997. Between July 1998 and January 2003, following more than 50 pediatric studies and clinical investigations, data analyzed resulted in 49 new pediatric drug labels with revised dosing and safety information [3]. Such efforts to increase well-controlled studies involving children are welcome and dovetail with current National Institutes of Health (NIH) initiatives to translate biomedical laboratory information into bedside medicine. Few areas of clinical need are more fundamental and valid than the alleviation of pain in children. This chapter presents some developments in the nascent field of translational pediatric pain. The specific topics are, as follows:

(1) neonatal nociception and implications for treatment and the development of pain sensitivity;
(2) pediatric neuroplasticity and neuropathic pain;
(3) opioids in the developing organism; and
(4) pharmacogenetics and analgesia, considerations for the future.

## Pain and the Neonate

In a separate chapter in this volume by Dr. Fitzgerald, the detailed discussion is provided regarding different developmental stages of pain and pain pathways. The following discussion provides a brief summary of several important issues related to clinical pediatric pain.

Although newborns were historically considered to have an immature nervous system, incapable of pain transmission, neurobiologic studies since the1980's now support *increased* perinatal sensitivity to pain. As early as 1967, Paul Yakolev, defined the development of human myelin with light microspopy and myelin staining of whole brain and spinal cord anatomic sections [4]. This technique was further refined by electron microscopy and most recently confirmed by structural magnetic resonance imaging (MRI) [5]. In the central nervous system, the full complement of cortical neurons, approximately 1000 million, are present at 20 weeks gestation. Pain transmission pathways complete myelination in the spine and brainstem between 22 and 30 weeks gestation. Myelination extends up to the thalamus by 30 weeks, and to the cortex by 37 weeks or term. Cortical descending inhibition develops post-term. Connections between the periphery and primary cortices develop before associatve cortical pathways, and the fastest myelination occurs during the first eight months post-term. Of note, in contrast to the peripheral nervous system, myelination in central sensory systems appears earlier than in motor systems [6-8]. Therefore, anatomically, the nociceptive pathways for pain transmission are active before development of modulatory neural systems.

Regarding peripheral nociception, cutaneous sensory nerve terminals are present in the perioral region at 7 weeks gestation and spread to all body areas by 20 weeks gestation. Nerve growth factors regulate the extension of peripheral nociceptive fibers into the dorsal spinal cord, with the larger A fibers entering prior to the C fibers, at 8-12 weeks. At birth, A and C fiber territories overlap in the developing substantia gelatinosa [9]. Neonatal maturation of low-threshold mechanoreceptors innervating the "hairy" skin of newborn mice per histological examination follows this pattern in neonatal mice [10]. Therefore, the neonatal response to a non-specific sensory stimulus is low threshold, non-specific, and poorly organized. Noxious and non-noxious stimuli produce similar physiologic and behavioral infant responses, complicating an accurate assessment of pain.

Excititory and inhibitory neurotransmitters and neuromodulators related to pain are present in the fetus, with the balance favoring excitation. Calcitonin gene-related peptide (CGRP), substance P, and the glutamate-NMDA systems are present at 8-10 weeks gestation. Enkephalin and vasoactive intestinal peptide (VIP) appear at 10 to 14 weeks. Catecholamines are present in late gestation, and, serotonin, at 6 weeks post-natal. Of note, the receptors for excitatory neurotransmitters are numerous and widely distributed in the neonate, regressing toward and adult system in the post-natal months. As well, in the developing nervous system, inhibitory chemicals, such as gamma- amino butyric acid (GABA) and glycine, may act as excitatory transmitters [11,12]. In an experimental murine model, the spinal cord concentration of NMDA receptors, and their ligand-affinity, is greater in neonates than in older animals [13]. NK-1 receptor density is also maximal in late fetal and early post-natal life, however substance P levels are lower than adult levels at birth [9].

Regarding stress responses, the functional neuroendocrine pathways between hypothalamus and pituitary are present at 21 weeks gestation. Corticotrophin- releasing factor (CRF) may stimulate fetal ACTH and beta-endorphin as early as the second trimester, and cortisol and beta-endorphin increases have been assayed following intrauterine sampling for exchange transfusion. Norepinephrine is present in paravertebral ganglia and adrenal chromaffin cells at 10 weeks gestation and is released with intrauterine stress (asphyxia). Epinephrine is present, in smaller amount, after 23 weeks gestation [14].

The amygdala and midbrain periaqueductal gray (PAG) are regions of interest regarding stress and pain responses in adults [15-17]. In a murine model of stress activation, exposure to a potentially infanticidal adult male rat suppresses pain–related behaviors in pre-weanling but not adult rats [18]. This analgesia is mediated by opioid receptors in the PAG that are innervated by projections from the amygdala. Preproenkaphalin mRNA, measured in the amygdala, increased after the exposure induced heat analgesia in pre-weanling but not adult rats, suggesting a change in stress-induced analgesia during early ontogeny. In 1987, a seminal report regarding analgesia for procedures in the neonatal ICU changed clinical practice [19]. Researchers showed that newborns undergoing thoracotomy for ductus arteriosus closure without adequate anesthesia (e.g., using a high dose of sufentanil) had significant metabolic stress and clinical morbidity, reflected as increased catecholamine, endorphin, glucagon, glucose, and lactate release, increased substrate utilization, and increased post-operative complications, including mortality [20-22]. Recent clinical studies have continued to measure surrogate measures and " biologic markers " of pain reactivity in neonates [23, 24] to assess the efficacy of various analgesic interventions. Such measures include cytokines, cortisol, beta-endorphins, growth hormones, catecholamines, and quantified cardiac autonomic activity.

In is not entirely clear if the neonate, apparently neurologically "primed" for nociception, is also *consciously* hyperalgesic. A debate among pediatric pain specialists currently suggests that, based upon new neurobiologic data concerning neonatal pain, the definition of pain should be modified for the perinatal period. At present, pain is defined as "an unpleasant sensory and emotional *experience*, associated with actual or potential tissue damage or described in terms of such damage." Prior experience with pain is not a prerequisite for neonatal pain. Therefore, an alternative definition is that "pain is an inherent quality of life that appears early in development and serves as a signal for tissue damage " [25]. Ethical discussions now sparked by this debate have medical and legal ramifications. Current data supports that the neonate does have intact mechanisms for acute nociception and potentially deleterious stress responses, but that conscious suffering is a yet to be defined state requiring interaction among several cortical areas serving sensation and emotion, not fully developed or connected in the neonate [26, 27].

The long -term consequences of untreated pain in the developing organism are not yet defined, but some studies suggest that early pain responses influence later pain behaviors [28]. In one murine model, skin wounds on rat pups caused increased innervation and lowered pain thresholds in the area of injury for 3 months post-injury. In the rats that had recurrent painful stimuli from birth, the changes in the receptive fields of the dorsal horn neurons were persistent [29]. Another study exposed rat pups to repeated hind-paw injections over several days. When compared to control pups and at adult age, the rats that experience repeated noxious stimuli showed increased responses to painful and non-painful stimuli relative to their controls. Pathologically, the experimental group showed a loss of nociceptive primary afferents [30]. A third study found that the pain-conditioned behaviors of rats differed according to the timing of the stimulus. Rat pups exposed to early, repetitive noxious stimulation had a decrease in pain threshold compared to control rats. Adult rats given repetitive painful stimuli showed greater stress responses, such as freezing and digging, than controls [31].

Regarding medication trials, infant animal studies are particularly useful, proving initial data which avoids the ethical and practical issues involved with exposing human neonates to potentially toxic agents. As well, infant animal trials may suggest allow direct access to the study of physiologic mechanisms, provide genetic clues through the use of inbred strains, and show potential long-term effects of agents seen in a species with a shorter life span than the human neonate [32]. Some essential single dose or short-term safety and efficacy studies of opioids and local anesthetics in the human have thankfully been obtained and show important physiologic differences between the infant and the adult, providing the following important pharmacologic guidelines [33]:

- Neonates have an immature cytochrome P450 hepatic enzyme system and, therefore, conjugate opioids and local anesthetics slowly. Delayed toxicity with prolonged infusions is possible.
- Renal function, including glomerular filtration and renal tubular secretion, is decreased in the first few weeks of life (longer for premature infants ) compared with adults. The half-life of opioids and, more significantly, their metabolites (MSO4-6-glucuronide), may be increased. Delayed sedation and respiratory depression are limited by increased dosing intervals and decreased doses.

- Neonatal total body water is increased compared to adults. Fat is minimal. Analgesics with high water solubility have a large volume of distribution.
- Neonates have decreased plasma protein binding, albumen and α1 acid glycoprotein, resulting in increased free-drug and greater first-pass toxicity.
- Ventilatory reflexes are immature in the neonate. Infants have a low threshold for hypoventilation secondary to opioids.

In humans, few empiric studies also show late effects of painful stimuli. One report describes that neonatal males who received a eutetic mixture of topical local anesthetics (Emla Cream) prior to circumcision had 12-25% less facial grimacing and tachycardia than randomized control infants without treatment [34]. An earlier study observed that males circumcised within two days of age had longer periods of crying and higher pain ratings than uncircumcised males [35]. Another report compared 18 preterm infants, subject to repeated painful procedures in the NICU, with matched full term infants regarding their somatic complaints at 18 months. Twenty-five percent of mothers of preterm infants with prolonged NICU stays noted a significantly increased number of somatic complaints in their toddlers as compared to mothers of fullterm infants briefly managed in the normal nursery [36]. Alternatively, a recent study of 24 preterm infants compared with matched full-term infants had similar behavioral pain scores when exposed to a finger prick at 4 months of age [24]. Former preterm infants shown illustrations of painful events at ages 8-10 years reported higher ratings of pain than age-matched controls. Longer neonatal intensive care unit (NICU) stays were directly correlated with higher ratings [37]. Immediate effects of adequate analgesia in the NICU may also be seen. The NOPAIN trial [38], a study of preterm neonatal responses to analgesia and sedation, has provided provocative findings on the reduction of physiologic instability and intraventricular hemorrhage (IVH ). The incidence of IVH in the preterm infant during the first few eventful post-natal days in the NICU was minimized by decreased handling and procedures in conjunction with continuous intravenous morphine.

Therefore, in brief, the treatment and evaluation of neonatal pain is scientifically defensible and clinically essential. The neonatal pain transmission system is adequately developed, centrally hyperexcitable, with the necessary components of central sensitization, but still remains generally non-specific in its response to stimuli. Age does influence the organism's response to painful stimuli. Neonates and infants feel pain, but assessment of this phenomenon is an ongoing challenge [26,39]. Long-term effects of neonatal pain are documented and worthy of future investigation.

## Neuropathic Pain

Many current reports suggest that children with "adult "neuropathic disorders have less measurable or reported pain. Such pain problems include brachial plexus injury, peripheral nerve injuries/complex regional pain syndrome (CRPS), and post-amputation syndromes. This general observation seems at odds with the previously described neonatal hyperalgesic state. Infant animal studies may provide some explanation. In the rat spared nerve injury (SNI) and the chronic constriction nerve injury (CCI), mechanical allodynia was measured in adult animals but was absent in animals aged 3, 10, and 21 days at the time of surgery [40]. This finding is in contrast to inflammatory models of infant pain. Another study of early neuropathic injury in animals describes the development of self-mutilation (autotomy) after dorsal rhizotomy of the brachial plexus in infant and adult rats [41]. Self-mutilation behavior was seen only in adult rats, suggesting that a mature neurosensory system is required for autotomy, or, possibly, that neuroplasticity is a robust phenomenon in early development. Such evidence is consistent with human neonatal responses to brachial plexus birth injury. In a study of self-mutilation in young children following neonatal brachial plexus injury, the abnormal behavior was present infrequently and most notably in patients who subsequently underwent brachial plexus microsurgery, possibly related to the surgery, the severity of initial injury, or both factors [42]. In pediatric amputees, one Canadian review of 60 children and adolescents showed that surgical amputation was much more likely to be followed by phantom pain (48.5% patients with pain ) than associated with congenital amputation (3.7%) [43].

Prolonged peripheral neuropathic pain, such as associated with herpes zoster, trigeminal neuralgia, or diabetic neuropathy (IDDM), is also uncommon in pediatric practice. Few epidemiological reviews in children are available [44, 45]. One Icelandic report following Herpes Zoster infection found an incidence of 1.6/1000/year, with no patients reporting pain after 1 month and no post-herpetic neuralgia syndrome [46]. In patients with immunodeficiency and with malignancy, post-herpetic neuralgia is reported but uncommonly persists after 6 months. Treatment-related neuropathic pain is very common and possibly under-recognized in children with cancer and may be one etiology of high dose opioid escalation seen in patients with advanced cancer [47]. In complex regional pain syndrome (CRPS), patients with small fiber neuralgia with associated inflammatory and autonomic changes, children frequently recover following structured physical therapy whereas adults frequently develop a chronic pain syndrome despite extensive pharmacologic and regional anesthetic intervention. [48]. What is the pathophysiologic mechanism underlying these variable clinical presentations? Is there a critical period for restorative neuroplasticity? Is the region of interest peripheral or central nervous system? Are more rostral centers dominant? Specific peripheral mechanisms are shown in a recent study of age-dependent responses to thermal hyperalgesia and mechanical allodynia in a rat model of acute postoperative pain [49]. Younger animals, age 2 weeks, recovered more quickly than older animals, ages 4 and 16 weeks, from mechanical allodynia but not thermal hypersensitivity. This study suggests developmental differences in the modulation of A-fiber sensitization after surgery. C-fiber recovery was not age-specific in this model. These findings may add to the understanding of infant and neonatal responses to post-operative analgesia.

Cortical mechanisms are essential to the *human* experience of pain and suffering. In an ongoing study of functional brain MRI (fMRI) changes in children and adolescents with acute and resolving clinical signs of CRPS, the BOLD signal in previously defined regions of interest for pain is different. Similar provocative adult studies of CRPS show fMRI changes indicating cortical reorganization of somatosensory areas as well as both ipsilateral and contralateral activation of a neural network which includes emotional, attentional, and motoric regions [50-55]. In these investigations, a non-human animal subject would not likely express the human cortical complexity of pain. However, animal data has shown localized and stimulus – dependent BOLD signal changes in the animal nociceptive system at the levels of the somatosensory cortex, thalamus, and brainstem, encouraging the use of this non-invasive technology in the awake human subject [37].

Animal experimentation is an accessible but focused way to acquire data, sometimes producing controvery in the field. In the expanding field of infant animal studies [56], two reports argue against the use of two neuropathic agents for neonatal analgesia, ketamine and nitrous oxide [57]. One report describes increased programmed cell death or apoptosis diffusely in the rat cortex when administered before 7 days of life. Another study shows no analgesic effect of nitrous oxide in rats younger than 21 days (approximately analogous to a school-aged child) [58]. However, both these agents have wide standardized use in pediatric anesthesia [59, 60]. With such discordant information, additional human studies are clearly indicated, taking into account the physiologic issues raised through animal experimentation.

In summary, neuropathic pain mechanisms, described in molecular detail in animal studies at the brainstem, spinal, and peripheral levels, are slowly lending themselves to scrutiny in the pediatric population. Expansion to the more rostral and critical centers of pain modualtion is now possible, following initial animal work in localization, with non-invasive radiologic tools.

# Opioids

In the earlier section on neonatal pain, the early development of endogenous opioids and opioid receptors in the pain transmission system is presented. Studies of opioid effect in the developing organism highlight additional ontologic factors. However, pharmacokinetics in full term infants (older than 3 months) generally reflects adult data for these medications.

In one study of post-natal rats (PND 3-21), the effect of age on analgesic potency was investigated for mu-receptor agonists, morphine, fentanyl, and meperidine. At all ages, these three opioids were analgesic per a tail-flick paradigm but had *different potencies* with equivalent brain and plasma levels. However, meperidine was less effective in the younger rat (PND 3-9) and epileptogenic in the older animal (PND 21 ). This animal data suggests that pharmacokinetics, development of the blood-brain barrier, and the ontogeny of opioid receptor function may have important roles in the sensitivity of post-natal rats to mu receptor agonists [61].

The main three opioid receptor subtypes of the central and peripheral nervous system are expressed at different periods during pre- and post-natal development in the rat. Mu and kappa-opioid receptor mRNA appear early per an in situ hybridization study (G13) with relatively late development of delta mRNA (G 21). As well, a developmental pattern was found in the mesostriatal system. Kappa-opioid receptor mRNA appears first (G15) in the striatum, followed by mu mRNA (G21) and then delta mRNA (P8), suggesting possible modulation of cholinergic and dopaminergic neurons by opioids [62]. Endogenous opioids are also shown to modulate perinatal behavior, such as suckling, maternal-infant interaction, and early learning at the nipple [63, 64]. As well, native opioid peptide [Met5]enkephalin is tonically active influencing cell proliferation and tissue organization, thus serving as a regulator of fetal growth [65]. In human infants, evaluation of the effects of prenatal exposure to opioids is often confounded by the complexity of the prenatal environment, with possible maternal polydrug use, nutritional deprivation, and intrauterine stress. However, clear evidence of abnormalities in coordination of sucking, swallowing, and respiration is seen in infants born to mothers with a history of opioid abuse [66, 67]. Other reports describe prolonged brainstem evoked responses [68], autonomic nervous system instability [69], mild psychomotor delay [70], and higher mean birth weight [71]. Of course, as noted earlier, the absence of opioids to adequately treat pain in the *post-natal* period may also be associated with later childhood developmental difficulties [53, 72].

Opioid tolerance is possibly age-dependent and related to the ontogeny of the NMDA receptor and trans- membrane functions of protein kinases. In one animal study, there is age-dependent morphine tolerance in the neonatal rat [56]. As well, there is a reported transition age, approximately at 21 days, when NMDA antagonists attenuate morphine tolerance, showing no effect at ages 7 and 14 days [56]. Another report indicates that NMDA receptor antagonists are not at all effective in blocking morphine tolerance in the neonatal rat [73]. Nitric oxide synthase (NOS) inhibitors may be more important [74]. A meta analysis of 2 studies evaluating neonatal abstinence syndrome (NAS) in the human found a significant reduction in treatment failure with alternative opioid use rather than diazepam [75]. Clinical reviews also add alpha-adrenergic agents to the armamentarium [76]. A recent chart review of 10,000 pain clinic patients finds that the tendency for opioid tolerance is more prominent in the young than in elderly groups [77], and that young patients with chronic pain escalate opioids more rapidly [78]. It is most likely that a number of factors influence the development of opioid tolerance in patient populations, but individual animal data involving developing organisms does direct attention primarily to the ontogeny of the opioid receptor. Ultimately, endogenous and exogenous analgesia is genetically determined and modified, raising the topic of the pharmacogenetics of analgesia.

## Pharmacogenetics

The study of genetically determined variations in drug response is an area of intense development, catalyzed by increased cataloging of single nucleotide polymorphisms (SNPs) and the linkage of these variant alleles to susceptibility to pain disorders and responses to pharmacotherapeutics [79]. There is an ontogeny of cytochrome P-450 enzymes, including the CYP2C9 and CYP3A substrates, active in the metabolism of multiple analgesics and sedatives. However, not all polymorphisms have been found, as yet, to be clinically significant. Codeine, often administered to infants and children, is one of the notable examples linked to a genetically determined hypoanalgesic effect. Codeine analgesia is dependent upon morphine formation via CYP2D6, which may be rendered ineffective by a genetic polymorphism or pharmacologically inhibited by other competitive medications, such as serotonin-reuptake inhibitors and neuroleptics. Genetic differences in human responsiveness to codeine is documented and supported by animal data. Two rat strains with a marked difference in CYP2C9 enzyme activity, Sprague-Dawley (high metabolizer) and Dark Agouti (low metabolizer), demonstrate age-related differences for codeine metabolism. Both strains show substantially lower codeine efficacy for 3 day old animals but not for rats at 10 days, 21 days, and adulthood [69, 80]. The mu-opioid receptor and its genetic variants may offer clues to human vulnerability to opioid dependence [81] and eventually allow for specific targeting of effective opioids with minimal adverse effects in specific individuals, especially important in vulnerable patients such as ill neonates.

## Conclusion

The promises and challenges of rationally using effective therapeutics due to increased knowledge of pharmacogenetics are just being elucidated. This approach offers a genetically based approach to pain management. The translation of data from pediatric animal models to the human child will likely provide the foundation for this promising future research.

## References

[1] Caldwell PH, Murphy SB, Butow PN, Craig JC: Clinical trials in children. *The Lancet.* 2004; 364: 803-811.

[2] Berde C, Cairns B: Developmental Pharmacology Across Species: Promise and Problems. *Anesth. Analg.* 2000; 91: 1-5.

[3] Roberts R, Rodriguez W, Murphy D, Crescenzi T: Pediatric drug labeling: improving the safety and efficacy of pediatric therapies. *JAMA* 2003; 290: 950-1.

[4] Yakovlev PI, Lecours AR: *The myelogenetic cycles of regional maturation of the brain.* Philadelphia, FA Davis, 1967.

[5] Michael J. Rivkin: Developmental neuroimaging of children using magnetic resonance techniques. *Mental Retardation and Developmental Disabilities Research Reviews* 2000; 6: 68-80.

[6] Gilles FH, Leviton A, Dooling EC: *The developing human brain: growth and epidemiologic neuropathy.* Boston, John Wright, 1983.

[7] Kinney HC, Brody BA, Kloman AS, Gilles FH: Sequence of central nervous system myelination in human infancy. I. An autopsy study of myelination. *Journal of Neuropathology and Experimental Neurology* 1987; 46: 283-301.

[8] Kinney HC, Brody BA, Kloman AS, Gilles FH: Sequence of central nervous system myelination in human infancy. II. Patterns of myelination in autopsied infants. *Journal of Neuropathology and Experimental Neurology* 1988; 47: 217-234.

[9] Fitzgerald M, Anand KJ: *Developmental neuroanatomy and neurophysiology of pain, Pain in infants and children.* Edited by Schecter NL, Berde CB, Yaster M. Baltimore, Williams and Wilkins, 1993, pp 11-31

[10] Woodbury CJ, Ritter AM, Koerber HR: Central anatomy of individual rapidly adapting low-threshold mechanoreceptors innervating the "hairy" skin of newborn mice: early maturation of hair follicle afferents. *The Journal of Comparative Neurology* 2001; 436: 304-23.

[11] Mogil JS, Wilson SG, Bon K, Lee SE, Chung K, Raber P, Pieper JO, Hain HS, Belknap JK, Hubert L, Elmer GI, Chung JM, Devor M: Heritability of nociception II. 'Types' of nociception revealed by genetic correlation analysis. *Pain.* 1999; 80: 67-82.

[12] Fitzgerald M, Koltzenburg M: The functional development of descending inhibitory pathways in the dorsolateral funiculus of the newborn rat spinal cord. *Brain Research.* 1986; 24: 261-70.

[13] Zhu H, Barr GA: Ontogeny of NMDA receptor-mediated morphine tolerance in the postnatal rat. *Pain.* 2003; 104: 437-447.

[14] Fitzgerald M: Neurobiology of fetal and neonatal pain, *Textbook of Pain.* Edited by Wall PD, Melzack R. London, Churchill-Livingstone, 1994, pp 46-52.

[15] Zambreanu L, Wise RG, Brooks JCW, Iannetti GD, Tracey I: A role for the brainstem in central sensitisation in humans. Evidence from functional magnetic resonance imaging. *Pain.* 2005; 114: 397-407.

[16] Borsook D, Burstein R, Becerra L: Functional imaging of the human trigeminal system: Opportunities for new insights into pain processing in health and disease. *Journal of Neurobiology.* 2004; 61: 107-125.

[17] Kwong K, Belliveau J, Chesler D, Goldberg I, Weisskoff R, Poncelet B, Kennedy D, Hoppel B, Cohen M, Turner R, Cheng H, Brady T, Rosen B: Dynamic Magnetic Resonance Imaging of Human Brain Activity During Primary Sensory Stimulation. *PNAS.* 1992; 89: 5675-5679.

[18] Wiedenmayer CP, Goodwin GA, Barr GA: The effect of periaqueductal gray lesions on responses to age-specific threats in infant rats. *Developmental Brain Research.* 2000; 120: 191-198.

[19] Anand KJ, Hickey PR: Pain and its effect in the human neonate and fetus. New England *Journal of Medicine.* 1987; 317: 1321-1329.

[20] Anand KJ, W.G. S, Aynsley-Green A: Randomised trial of fentanyl anaesthesia in preterm babies undergoing surgery: effects on the stress response. *Lancet.* 1987; 1: 62-66.

[21] Friesen RH, Henry DB: Cardiovascular changes in preterm neonates receiving isoflurane, halothane, fentanyl, and ketamine. *Anesth. Analg.* 1986; 90: 6-10.

[22] Crean P, Koren G, Goresky G, Klein J, Macleod S: Fentanyl-oxygen versus fentanyl-N2O/oxygen anaesthesia in children undergoing cardiac surgery. *Can. Anaesth. Soc. J.* 1986; 33: 36-40.

[23] Goldman RD, Koren G: Biological markers of pain in the vulnerable infant. *Clinics in Perinatology.* 2002; 29: 415-25.

[24] Oberlander TF, Grunau RE, Whitfield MF, Fitzgerald C, Pitfield S, Saul JP: Biobehavioral Pain Responses in Former Extremely Low Birth Weight Infants at Four Months' Corrected Age. *Pediatrics.* 2000; 105: e6-

[25] Anand KJ, Craig KD: New perspectives on the definition of pain. *Pain.* 1996; 67: 3-6.

[26] Anand KJ: Consensus statement for the prevention and management of pain in the newborn. *Archives of Pediatric and Adolescent Medicine.* 2001; 155: 173-180.

[27] Ortinski P, Kimford J, Meador MD: Neuronal mechanisms of conscious awareness. *Archives of Neurology.* 2004; 61: 1017-1020.

[28] Goubet N, Clifton RK, Shah B: Learning about pain in preterm newborns. *Journal of Developmental and Behavioural Pediatric.* 2001; 22: 418.

[29] Reynolds ML, Fitzgerald M: Long-term sensory hyperinnervation following neonatal skin wounds. *Journal of Comparative Neurology.* 1995; 358: 487-98.

[30] Reynolds M, Alvares D, Middleton J, Fitzgerald M: Neonatally wounded skin induces NGF-independent sensory neurite outgrowth in vitro. *Developmental Brain Research.* 1997; 102: 275-283.

[31] Anand KJS, Coskun V, Thrivikraman KV, Nemeroff CB, Plotsky PM: Long-Term Behavioral Effects of Repetitive Pain in Neonatal Rat Pups. *Physiology and Behavior.* 1999; 66: 627-637.

[32] Soriano SG, Anand KS, Rovnaghi CR, Hickey PR: Of mice and men: Should we extrapolate Rodent Experimental Data to the care of Human Neonates? *Anesthesiology.* 2005; 102: 866-868.

[33] Berde CB, Masek B: Pain in children, *Textbook of Pain.* Edited by Wall PD, Melzack R. Edinburgh, Scotland, Churchhill Livingstone, 1999, pp 1463-1478.

[34] Taddio A, Goldbach M, Ipp M, Stevens B, Koren G: Effect of neonatal circumcision on pain responses during vaccination in boys. *Lancet.* 1995; 345: 291-2.

[35] Taddio A, Katz J, Ilersich AL, Koren G: Effect of neonatal circumcision on pain response during subsequent routine vaccination. *The Lancet.* 1997; 349: 599-603.

[36] Grunau RV, Whitfield MF, Petrie JH: Pain sensitivity and temperament in extremely low-birth-weight premature toddlers and preterm and full-term controls. *Pain.* 1994; 58: 341-6.

[37] Weisman SJ, Bernstein B, Schechter NL: Consequences of inadequate analgesia during painful procedures in children. *Archives of Pediatric and Adolescent Medicine.* 1998; 152: 147-149.

[38] Anand KJ, Barton BA: Analgesia and sedation in preterm neonates who require ventilatory support: results from the NOPAIN trial. Neonatal Outcome and Prolonged Analgesia in Neonates. *Archives of Pediatric and Adolescent Medicine.* 1999; 153: 331-338.

[39] Taddio A, Ohlsson A, Einarson TR, Stevens B, Koren G: A Systematic Review of Lidocaine-Prilocaine Cream (EMLA) in the Treatment of Acute Pain in Neonates. *Pediatrics.* 1998; 101: e1-

[40] Howard RF, Walker SM, Michael Mota P, Fitzgerald M: The ontogeny of neuropathic pain: Postnatal onset of mechanical allodynia in rat spared nerve injury (SNI) and chronic constriction injury (CCI) models. *Pain.* 2005; 115: 382-389.

[41] Vaculin S, Franek M, Andrey L, Rokyta R: Self-mutilation in young rats after dorsal rhizotomy. *Neuro Endocrinology Letters.* 2005; 26: 25-8.

[42] McCann ME, Waters P, Goumnerova LC, Berde C: Self-mutilation in young children following brachial plexus birth injury. *Pain.* 2004; 110: 123-129.

[43] Wilkins KL, McGrath PJ, Finley GA, Katz J: Phantom limb sensations and phantom limb pain in child and adolescent amputees. *Pain.* 1998; 78: 7-12.

[44] Resnick DK, Levy EI, Jannetta PJ: Microvascular decompression for pediatric onset trigeminal neuralgia. *Neurosurgery.* 1998; 43: 807-8.

[45] Solders G, Thalme B, Aguirre-Aquino M, Brandt L, Berg U, Persson A: Nerve conduction and autonomic nerve function in diabetic children. A 10-year follow-up study. *Acta Paediatrica.* 1997; 86: 361-6.

[46] Petursson G, Helguson S, Gudmundsson S, Sigurdsson JA: Herpes zoster in children and adolscents. *Pediatric Infectious Disease Journal.* 1998; 17: 905-908.

[47] Collins JJ, Grier HE, Kinney HC, Berde CB: Control of severe pain in children with terminal malignancy. *Journal of Pediatrics.* 1995; 128: 864-5.

[48] Lee BH, Scharff L, Sethna NF, McCarthy CF, Scott-Sutherland J, Shea AM, Sullivan P, Meier P, Zurakowski D, Masek BJ, Berde CB: Physical therapy and cognitive-behavioral treatment for complex regional pain syndromes. *The Journal of Pediatrics.* 2002; 141: 135-140.

[49] Ririe DG, Vernon TL, Tobin JR, Eisenach JC: Age-dependent Responses to Thermal Hyperalgesia and Mechanical Allodynia in a Rat Model of Acute Postoperative Pain. *Anesthesiology.* 2003; 99: 443-8.

[50] Maihofner C, Forster C, Birklein F, Neundorfer B, Handwerker HO: Brain processing during mechanical hyperalgesia in complex regional pain syndrome: a functional MRI study. *Pain.* 2005; 114: 93-103.

[51] Pierpaoli C, Jezzard P, Basser PJ, Barnett A, Di Chiro G: Diffusion tensor MR imaging of the human brain. *Radiology.* 1996; 201: 637-48.

[52] Wimberger DM, Roberts TP, Barkovich AJ, Prayer LM, Moseley ME, Kucharczyk J: Identification of "premyelination" by diffusion-weighted MRI. *Journal of Computer Assisted Tomography.* 1995; 19: 28-33.

[53] Inder TE, Huppi PS: In vivo studies of brain development by magnetic resonance techniques. *Mental Retardation and Developmental Disabilities Research Reviews* 2000; 6: 59-67.

[54] Takeda K, Nomura Y, Sakuma H, Tagami T, Okuda Y, Nakagawa T: MR assessment of normal brain development in neonates and infants: comparative study of T1- and diffusion-weighted images. *Journal of Computer Assisted Tomography.* 1997; 21: 1-7.

[55] Neil J, Shiran SI, McKinstry RC, Schefft GL, AZ S, Almli CR, Akbudak E, Aronovitz JA, Miller JP, Lee BC, T.E. C: Normal brain in human newborns: apparent diffusion coefficient and diffusion anisotropy measured by using diffusion tensor MR imaging. *Radiology.* 1998; 209.

[56] Wang Y, Mitchell J, Moriyama K, Kim K-j, Sharma M, Xie G-x, Palmer PP: Age-Dependent Morphine Tolerance Development in the *Rat. Anesth. Analg.* 2005; 100: 1733-1739.

[57] Ikonomidou C, Bosch F, Miksa M, Bittigau P, Vandouml;ckler J, Dikranian K, Tenkova TI, Stefovska V, Turski L, Olney JW: Blockade of NMDA Receptors and Apoptotic Neurodegeneration in the Developing *Brain. Science.* 1999; 283: 70-74.

[58] Fujinaga M, Doone R, Davies MF, Maze M: Nitrous Oxide Lacks the Antinociceptive Effect on the Tail Flick Test in Newborn Rats. *Anesth. Analg.* 2000; 91: 6-10.

[59] Murray DJ, Mehta MP, Forbes RB: The additive contribution of nitrous oxide to isoflurane MAC in infants and children. *Anesthesiology.* 1991; 75: 186-90.

[60] Hickey PR, Hansen DD, Cramolini GM, Vincent RN, Lang P: Pulmonary and systemic hemodynamic responses to ketamine in infants with normal and elevated pulmonary vascular resistance. *Anesthesiology.* 1985; 62: 287-93.

[61] Thornton SR, Compton DR, Smith FL: Ontogeny of mu opioid agonist anti-nociception in postnatal rats. *Developmental Brain Research.* 1998; 105: 269-276.

[62] De Vries TJ, Hogenboom F, Mulder AH, Schoffelmeer AN: Ontogeny of mu-, delta- and kappa-opioid receptors mediating inhibition of neurotransmitter release and adenylate cyclase activity in rat brain. *Brain Research. Developmental brain research.* 1990; 54: 63-9.

[63] Robinson SR, Hoeltzel TC, Cooke KM, Umphress SM, Smotherman WP, Murrish DE: Oral capture and grasping of an artificial nipple by rat fetuses. *Brain Research. Developmental brain research.* 1998; 109: 187-99.

[64] Smotherman WP, Simonik DK, Andersen SL, Robinson SR: Mu and kappa opioid systems modulate responses to cutaneous perioral stimulation in the fetal rat. *Phsiology and Behaviour.* 1993; 53: 751-6.

[65] Zagon IS, Wu Y, McLaughlin PJ: Opioid growth factor and organ development in rat and human embryos. *Brain Research.* 1999; 839: 313-322.

[66] Gewolb IH, Fishman D, Qureshi MA, Vice FL: Coordination of suck-swallow-respiration in infants born to mothers with drug-abuse problems. *Developmental Medicine and Child Neurology.* 2004; 46: 700-5.

[67] LaGasse LL, Messinger D, Lester BM, Seifer R, Tronick EZ, Bauer CR, Shankaran S, Bada HS, Wright LL, Smeriglio VL, Finnegan LP, Maza PL, Liu J: Prenatal drug exposure and maternal and infant feeding behaviour. *Archives of Disease in Childhood. Fetal and Neonatal Edition.* 2003; 88: 391-9.

[68] Lester BM, LaGasse L, Seifer R, Tronick EZ, Bauer CR, Shankaran S, Bada HS, Wright LL, Smeriglio VL, Liu J: The Maternal Lifestyle Study (MLS): Effects of prenatal cocaine and/or opiate exposure on auditory brain response at one month. *The Journal of Pediatrics.* 2003; 142: 279-285.

[69] Bada HS, Bauer CR, Shankaran S, Lester B, Wright LL, Das A, Poole K, Smeriglio VL, Finnegan LP, Maza PL: Central and autonomic system signs with in utero drug exposure. *Archives of Disease in Childhood. Fetal and Neonatal Edition.* 2002; 87: 106-12.

[70] Bunikowski R, Grimmer I, Heiser A, Metze B, Schafer A, Obladen M: Neurodevelopmental outcome after prenatal exposure to opiates. *European Journal of Pediatrics.* 1998; 157: 724-730.

[71] McLaughlin PJ, Tobias SW, Lang CM, Zagon IS: Chronic Exposure to the Opioid Antagonist Naltrexone During Pregnancy: Maternal and Offspring Effects. *Physiology and Behavior.* 1997; 62: 501-508.

[72] Brattberg G: Do pain problems in young school children persist into early adulthood? A 13-year follow-up. *European Journal of Pain.* 2004; 8: 187-199.

[73] Zhu H, Barr GA: Opiate withdrawal during development: are NMDA receptors indispensable? *Trends in Pharmacological Sciences.* 2001; 22: 404-408.

[74] Zhu H, Barr GA: Naltrexone-precipitated morphine withdrawal in infant rat is attenuated by acute administration of NOS inhibitors but not NMDA receptor antagonists. *Psychopharmacology.* 2000; 150: 325-336.

[75] Johnson K, Gerada C, Greenough A: Treatment of neonatal abstinence syndrome. *Archives of Disease in Childhood.* 2003; 88: F2-5.

[76] Taddio A, Katz J: Pain, opioid tolerance and sensitisation to nociception in the neonate. Best Practice and Research. *Clinical Anesthesiology.* 2004; 18: 291-302.

[77] Agin CW, Glass PSA: Tolerance and Aging: Optimizing Analgesia in Pain Management. *Anesth. Analg.* 2005; 100: 1731-1732.

[78] Buntin-Mushock C, Phillip L, Moriyama K, Palmer PP: Age-Dependent Opioid Escalation in Chronic Pain Patients. *Anesth. Analg.* 2005; 100: 1740-1745.

[79] Fishbain DA, Fishbain D, Lewis J, Cutler RB, Cole B, Rosomoff HL, Rosomoff RS: Genetic Testing for Enzymes of Drug Metabolism: Does It Have Clinical Utility for Pain Medicine at the Present Time? A Structured Review. *Pain Medicine.* 2004; 5: 81-93.

[80] Caraco Y, Sheller J, Wood AJ: Pharmacogenetic determination of the effects of codeine and prediction of drug interactions. *The Journal of Pharmacology and Experimental Therapeutics.* 1996; 278: 1165-74.

[81] Hoehe MR, Kopke K, Wendel B, Rohde K, Flachmeier C, Kidd KK, Berrettini WH, Church GM: Sequence variability and candidate gene analysis in complex disease: association of {micro} opioid receptor gene variation with substance dependence. *Hum. Mol. Genet.* 2000; 9: 2895-2908.

In: Translational Pain Research, Volume 2
Editor: Jianren Mao, pp. 253-276
ISBN: 1-60021-205-0
© 2006 Nova Science Publishers, Inc.

*Chapter XIV*

# Selective Serotonin Agonists for the Acute Management of Migraine

*David M. Biondi*[*]

Director, Headache Management Program
Spaulding Rehabilitation Hospital, 125 Nashua Street, Boston, MA 02114, USA
Consultant, Headache Management, Department of Neurology,
Massachusetts General Hospital, 15 Parkman Street, Boston,
MA 02114, USA

## Abstract

Translational research approaches have become widely used in biomedical research. In the field of headache studies, especially related to migraine, translational research has vastly improved knowledge of migraine pathophysiology and clinical management strategies. The triptans, a class of medications that are specifically indicated for the acute management of migraine, were developed based on clinical and laboratory observations. Originally developed for their vasoconstrictive effect, these selective serotonin agonists were later found to have other pharmacological effects on neuronal tissue that are much more likely to be the primary mechanism of action for achieving migraine relief. Recent translational research studies have discovered treatment strategies that improve the clinical efficacy of the triptans based on specific receptor targets and functional neuronal changes occurring with the central processing of pain. In turn, the triptans have played an important role in revealing and further delineating the pathophysiological basis of migraine. As knowledge of migraine mechanisms improves, so shall the opportunity to discover novel therapeutic targets and develop more effective mechanism-based treatment strategies. This chapter will review the clinical presentation of migraine, contemporary pathophysiological model of migraine, pharmaceutical development of selective 5-HT$_1$ (serotonin) agonists as a "migraine specific" treatment, and use of

---

[*] Address correspondence: David M Biondi, DO. Spaulding Rehabilitation Hospital, 125 Nashua Street, Boston, MA 02114. Phone: 617-573-2106. Email: dbiondi@partners.org

triptans in clinical practice. The chapter will also explore novel pharmacological targets and future directions for the developing an ideal medication for the acute management of migraine.

# Introduction

The clinical management of migraine has flourished over the last 15 years as knowledge of migraine pathophysiology has improved. Translating clinical observations into laboratory models and preclinical scientific data into clinical medicine has been an effective strategy for the discovery of novel therapeutic targets, development of new pharmacological agents, and improvement of treatment efficacy for migraine. No longer considered a primary vascular disorder, migraine is now believed to be an intricate cascade of events that is primarily neurogenic in origin but has the consequence of secondary changes in cerebral cortical perfusion [1]. Astute clinical observations, quantitative neurosensory testing [2], and heightened cortical sensitivity to transcranial magnetic stimulation [3] have suggested the presence of cerebral cortical hyperexcitability in subjects who have migraine. The pain of migraine is a consequence of the activation and sensitization of peripheral and central trigeminal pathways. The early phase of migraine pain appears to be an inflammatory or nociceptive pain resulting from the development of neurogenic inflammation around cranial blood vessels and sensitization of peripheral trigeminal nerve terminals [1]. There is modest evidence that this early inflammatory phase of the migraine process might be similar to the underlying mechanism of tension-type headache [4]. However the clinical observation that allodynia, hyperalgesia, and expansion of nociceptive fields occur during the majority of well-established migraine attacks not only provides a clinical means of differentiation from tension-type headache but also indicates sensitization of central pain pathways [5]. These clinical features of an established migraine attack are evocative of those associated with neuropathic pain [6].

The hypothesis that cortical hyperexcitability, trigeminal mediated neurogenic inflammation, sensitization of perivascular trigeminal nerve terminals, and sensitization of central pain pathways are stages in the development of migraine pain and its associated symptoms permits the advancement of mechanism-based treatment strategies that can improve both the abortive and preventive management of migraine. For example, serotonin (5-HT) is recognized to be an important neurotransmitter in the descending nociceptive inhibitory control of pain transmission and for a number of decades has been implicated as an important mediator of migraine activity [7,8]. The identification of specific changes in serotonergic activity occurring during migraine attacks led to the development of serotonin receptor agonists that specifically target the $5\text{-HT}_{1B}$ and $5\text{-HT}_{1D}$ receptors [9], the pharmacological class of medications commonly called the triptans. Discovery of the triptans has revolutionized acute migraine management strategies and vastly improved the efficacy of acute migraine treatment for the majority of migraineurs but improvements in the efficacy outcomes and tolerability of migraine abortive treatments are still needed [10].

# Clinical Presentation of Migraine

Migraine is a highly prevalent medical disorder having a wide range of activation triggers, clinical manifestations, and treatment options. Migraine is a paroxysmal neurological disorder that is generally characterized by recurrent attacks of moderate to severe head pain that is accompanied by physical and cognitive impairment as well as a number of symptoms including nausea, vomiting, photophobia, and phonophobia [11]. Migraine affects approximately 13% of the general population and is about 3 times more prevalent in adult females [12]. A family history of migraine or similar headaches can be identified in over 90% of cases [13]. The revised International Classification of Headache Disorders (ICHD II) provides diagnostic criteria for the many different varieties of headache including migraine. [Table 1] [11] The well-known clinical features of migraine include unilateral head pain, throbbing or pulsating head pain quality, moderate to severe pain intensity, and several associated symptoms such as nausea, vomiting, photophobia, and phonophobia. Patients with migraine are often hypersensitive to sensory stimuli other than light and sound, such as olfactory scents and tactile stimuli [15]. Other symptoms experienced by the migraineur during and between attacks include chronic nausea, diminished appetite, poor sleep quality, dizziness, disequilibrium, fatigue, cognitive inefficiency, mood alterations, and behavioral changes. Migraine pain often exhibits side-shift or alternation of pain unilaterality within or between attacks.

Over-emphasis placed on a diagnostic requirement to exhibit any one of the well-known clinical features might contribute to the misdirected diagnosis of a headache condition other than migraine (i.e. tension-type or "sinus" headache). Notwithstanding the classic features of a migraine attack, migraine related head pain could be bilateral in 40% of cases [14] and non-throbbing in about 30% [16]. The well recognized visual auras of migraine, photopsia (flashing lights) or fortification spectra (angular prismatic visual hallucinations also called teichopsia), are experienced by only 15-20% of migraineurs and even then it is only associated with some of their migraine attacks [17]. Migraine auras are focal neurological symptoms that are most often visual but can also be sensory and occur before or early in the course of a migraine attack. Aura symptoms gradually develop over 5-20 minutes and resolve within 60 minutes [11]. Although nausea and vomiting are features that often contribute to migraine disability, they need not be present to establish a diagnosis of migraine in accordance with the ICHD II. Other clinical symptoms and signs that can misdirect the diagnosis away from a correct diagnosis of migraine are sinus pressure, nasal congestion, rhinorrhea and lacrimation, which are common features of migraine that are wrongly ascribed to "sinus headache" [18]. Neck pain is likewise a common accompaniment of migraine and can sometimes mislead a clinician to establish a diagnosis of tension-type headache [19]. Sinus and tension-type headaches are rarely disabling, therefore patients with recurrent, disabling headache regardless of associated symptoms require further evaluation and consideration for alternative headache disorders such as migraine.

The pain associated with typical migraine attacks has a duration ranging between 4 and 72 hours and usually results in temporary impairment or disability. Many intrinsic and extrinsic circumstances such as hormonal cycles especially estrogen, stress, hunger, physical exertion, illness, exposure to bright light or loud noise, strong odors, dramatic ambient temperature variations, or weather changes can exacerbate migraine-related pain and other associated symptoms. Despite a much greater prevalence in the general population, tension-type headache is rarely a primary complaint of patients in medical clinics. [20] It is the intense pain and disability associated with most migraine attacks that prompt migraineurs to seek medical attention.

**Table 1. Migraine Diagnostic Features (modified from the ICHD II) [11]**

| Migraine without aura |
|---|
| *Diagnostic criteria:*<br>  A. At least five attacks fulfilling criteria B-D.<br>  B. Headache attacks lasting 4 to 72 hours (untreated or unsuccessfully treated).<br>  C. Headache has at least two of the following characteristics:<br>    1. Unilateral location.<br>    2. Pulsating quality.<br>    3. Moderate or severe pain intensity.<br>    4. Aggravation by or causing avoidance of routine physicalactivity (e.g., walking or climbing stairs).<br>  D. During headache there is at least one of the following:<br>    1. Nausea and/or vomiting.<br>    2. Photophobia and phonophobia.<br>  E. Headache is not attributed to another disorder. |
| **Typical aura with migraine headache** |
| *Diagnostic criteria:*<br>  A. At least two attacks fulfilling criteria B-D.<br>  B. Aura consisting of at least one of the following but no motor weakness:<br>    1. Fully reversible visual symptoms including positive features (i.e. flickering lights, spots, or lines) and/or negative features (i.e., loss of vision).<br>    2. Fully reversible sensory symptoms including positive features (i.e., pins and needles) and/or negative features (i.e., numbness).<br>    3. Fully reversible dysphasic speech disturbances.<br>  C. At least two of the following:<br>    1. Homonymous visual symptoms and/or unilateral sensory symptoms.<br>    2. At least one aura symptom develops gradually over >5 minutes and/or different aura symptoms occur in succession over >5 minutes.<br>    3. Each symptom lasts >5 minutes and <60 minutes.<br>  D. Headache fulfilling criteria B-D for "1.1. Migraine without aura" begins during the aura or follows aura within 60 minutes.<br>  E. Not attributed to another disorder. |

# A Contemporary Pathophysiological Model of Migraine

Migraine was once believed to be a primary disorder of cranial circulation or blood vessels thereby fostering its association with the moniker, "vascular headache", which is now considered a misnomer by a majority of scientists and clinicians who work in the field of headache studies. The vascular theory of migraine arose from the astute clinical observations and work of Harold G Wolff, John R Graham, and colleagues in the late 1930s [21]. Wolff hypothesized that the visual aura and other neurological manifestations of migraine resulted from intracranial vasoconstriction and cerebral ischemia while the pain of migraine resulted from subsequent extracranial vasodilatation. Despite the popularity of this model, clinical observations such as unilateral head pain and the side shifting nature of migraine-related head pain remained difficult to explain based on vascular mechanisms. Other clinicians and scientists began to promote the neurogenic theory of migraine, which was based on the hypothesis that the clinical features associated with migraine were solely the consequence of abnormal brain or neuronal activity.

The contemporary model of migraine pathophysiology has evolved from the predominantly vascular theories promoted over several decades to that of a complex neurovascular process involving cerebrocortical hypersensitivity, altered neurotransmitter activity, changes in pain modulation and nociceptor function, neurogenic inflammation in the dura and around cranial blood vessels, sensitization of peripheral and central trigeminal pain pathways, activation of various components of the autonomic nervous system, and altered brain perfusion [22, 23,24]. Migraine can be best described as an episodic neurological and neurovascular disorder. Clinical research supports the conclusion that migraine is genetically determined in a large majority of cases. Genetic studies have suggested the presence of a heterogeneous genotype which gives rise to different phenotypic expressions [25]. The cerebral cortex of migraineurs is generally believed to exhibit lower activation thresholds for depolarization than non-migraineurs. The consequence of this neurophysiological alteration is believed to initiate the complex cascade of neurological events that result in the clinical features of a migraine attack. The trigeminal nerve is the primary sensory pathway for most headaches, although other nerves, such as the upper cervical sensory afferents, may be primarily involved in some types of headache. The pain of migraine is initiated by inflammation in or around pain sensitive structures of the head such as the meninges, dural vascular structures, and cranial blood vessels. Although the presence of scalp sensitivity during a migraine attack has long been observed in clinical practice [26], the recognition that this clinical feature of migraine is a form of allodynia [5], a clinical marker for central sensitization and hallmark of neuropathic pain, changed the way that many scientists and clinicians conceptually understand migraine.

The earliest clinical feature of a migraine attack in up to 70% of migraineurs is a "prodrome", which is a constellation of premonitory symptoms occurring up to 48 hours prior to the onset of a migraine aura or headache [27]. Prodromal symptoms can include feelings of fatigue, mood changes, food cravings, excessive yawning, vertigo, difficulty concentrating and cognitive inefficiency. It is not known what physiological events underlie these symptoms but it is possibly related to early alterations in specific neurotransmitters (i.e. dopamine) [28] or neurotransmitter receptor activity. In the aura phase of migraine, a "wave" of spreading cortical activation (depolarization) is believed to result in the clinical symptoms of aura experienced by some migraineurs [29]. Typical migraine auras are "positive", transient, and migratory neurological phenomena such as photopsia, spreading visual hallucinations, and migrating paresthesiae. In the wake of the depolarizing wave there is suppression of spontaneous and evocable cortical activity a phenomenon known as "cortical spreading depression". The suppression of cortical excitability likely contributes to the "negative" clinical symptoms of migraine such as visual blind spots (scotoma), numbness, weakness, word finding difficulties, and cognitive inefficiency. Cortical recovery time or repolarization appears to be delayed in migraineurs, which might explain the persistence of neurological migraine attack symptoms for several minutes to hours. If the migraine attack fails to progress to the next stage, the patient may experience migraine visual aura or other neurological symptoms without associated headache, conditions also referred to as "ophthalmic migraine", "acephalgic migraine", or "migraine equivalent" [11]. If the attack progresses to the next stage, the trigeminal nerve is activated through an as yet unknown mechanism but believed to be either directly by the spreading cortical depolarization or through a brainstem "reflex" [30]. Trigeminal activation is believed to incite the release of vasoactive, proinflammatory, and algogenic substances from its terminals in the dura and around cranial blood vessels thereby resulting in neurogenic inflammation manifested by mast cell degranulation, vasodilation, and plasma protein extravasation [1]. If the process fails to proceed beyond this stage or if its progression is arrested by an appropriate treatment, the head pain might have qualities similar to those experienced with tension-type headache. It is not unusual for migraineurs to experience both tension-type and migraine headaches [31]. In migraine, the majority of attacks are associated with throbbing pain, which likely occurs as the perivascular trigeminal nerve terminals become sensitized thereby resulting in painful responses to previously innocuous stimuli such as blood vessel stretching and pulsations [5]. Ensuing activation of structures within central pain pathways such as the trigeminal nucleus caudalis and thalamus is believed to result in referred pain patterns and expansion of nociceptive sensory fields to regions of the neck and upper torso. Activation of parasympathetic fibers in the superior salivatory nucleus results in symptoms of nasal congestion, rhinorrhea, and tearing. In the next stage of migraine, the effects of protracted perivascular inflammation and peripheral trigeminal sensitization are hypothesized to incite sensitization of central pain pathways in the brainstem, upper spinal cord, thalamus and cortex [1,5]. Central sensitization, recruitment and activation of brainstem structures, as well as activation of autonomic pathways result in several well-known clinical features of migraine including photophobia, phonophobia, nausea, nasal congestion, and rhinorrhea. Another potential feature of this late migraine stage is allodynia affecting the face, scalp, and contiguous regions of the neck and torso [31]. Allodynia is not only a clinical marker for sensitization of central pain pathways but appears to be an important marker for treatment efficacy [32], which will be discussed later in this chapter. During the resolution stage of a severe or prolonged migraine attack, many migraineurs will experience a "postdrome" that can last several hours to a day in duration. Common postdromal symptoms include fatigue, lassitude, irritability, myalgia, and cognitive inefficiency.

## Neurotransmitter Involvement in Migraine

Experimentally induced activation of trigeminal sensory neurons in animal models elicits the release of substance P (SP), calcitonin gene-related peptide (CGRP), and neurokinin A

(NKA) from nociceptive trigeminal terminals thereby inciting the initiation of neurogenic inflammation in the dura and around dural blood vessels [33]. During migraine attacks, CGRP concentration is elevated in external jugular venous blood of human subjects [34]. The central processing of pain is believed to be a complex balance between the facilitation and inhibition of pain signaling. Glutamate (Glu), protein kinase C (PKC), and nitric oxide (NO) have important roles in the prolongation and amplification of the pain response, development of clinical neuropathic pain characteristics, and initiation of neural plasticity [34, 35, 36]. In the current model of migraine pathophysiology, sensitized trigeminal nociceptors are believed to activate second-order neurons in the primary sensory nucleus and nucleus caudalis of the trigeminal nerve. As in other pain states, the transmission of pain signaling is modulated or inhibited partly by descending monoaminergic (i.e. serotonergic) pathways from the rostral ventromedial nucleus (RVM) and endogenous opioid systems in the periaqueductal gray (PAG) of the brainstem. Early observations of changes in circulating serotonin (5-HT) stimulated interest in understanding the role of this neurotransmitter in the migraine process. It was demonstrated that intravenously administered serotonin could trigger migraine attacks in some migraineurs. [37] Other work demonstrated reduced concentrations of circulating (platelet) serotonin and elevated levels of urinary serotonin metabolites during migraine attacks [38, 39]. These findings suggested that serotonin was released during a migraine attack. Still other observations suggested that serotonin had a complex mechanism of action in migraine pathophysiology, for example the observed exacerbation of migraine by medications that deplete endogenous monoamines such as reserpine and the observed migraine preventive effects of serotonin antagonists such as the ergot derivative, methysergide [40]. Contrary to the studies demonstrating that parenteral serotonin triggered migraine attacks, other studies found that intravenous serotonin and norepinephrine provided relief of migraine attacks already in progress [41].

Multiple 5-HT receptor subtypes and autoregulatory processes that are intended to maintain a state of homeostasis in the nervous system might explain the complex and seemingly paradoxical effects of serotonin observed in migraine research. To date, seven 5-HT receptor families ($5-HT_1$-$5-HT_7$) and several different receptor subtypes have been identified [42]. Enhancing serotonin concentrations in the central nervous system is generally believed to have antinociceptive effects [43]. Consequently several types of antidepressants that enhance the concentrations of serotonin and norepinephrine in the CNS through various mechanisms of action (i.e. tricyclics-TCA, monoamine oxide inhibitors-MAOI, serotonin-norepinephrine reuptake inhibitors-SNRI) are clinically useful as migraine preventives. [44] Agonists of $5HT_2$ receptors are generally believed to facilitate central pain transmission; therefore $5HT_{2B/2C}$ receptor antagonists such as propranolol, methysergide, and cyproheptadine are found useful for migraine prevention presumably through inhibition of certain pain transmissions [44]. The tricyclic antidepressants (TCAs), in addition to their pharmacological effect of enhancing monoaminergic activity in the CNS, are believed to act in part through the down-regulation of postsynaptic $5-HT_2$ receptors. [45] Finally, at least five $5-HT_1$ receptor subtypes have been identified in human subjects ($5-HT_{1A}$, $5-HT_{1B}$, $5-HT_{1D}$, $5-HT_{1E}$, and $5-HT_{1F}$). [46] Selective agonists that have parallel pharmacological effects at the $5-HT_{1B}$, $5-HT_{1D}$, and $5-HT_{1F}$ receptors have demonstrated potent efficacy for the abortive and symptomatic management of migraine attacks [47].

# Development of 5-HT₁ Receptor Agonists for Migraine Attack Management

As introduced previously, an important role for serotonin (5-HT) in the pathogenesis of migraine was suggested by the reduction of circulating 5-HT levels and simultaneous increase in urinary levels of the 5-HT metabolite, 5-hydroxyindoleacetic acid (5-HIAA), during migraine attacks. Clinical observations demonstrated extracranial vasodilation during migraine attacks [21] and resolution of migraine after intravenous serotonin was administered [41]. These findings combined with the belief that migraine pain resulted from cranial vasodilation motivated the search for a serotonin receptor agonist with vasoconstrictive activity. In 1972, Patrick Humphrey and colleagues set out to identify novel therapeutic agents for the acute management of migraine based on these criteria. In 1984 they identified and studied a compound that was chemically related to serotonin but with selective affinity for what had been known as a 5-HT₁-like receptor subtype, which was found primarily expressed on cranial vasculature [9, 48, 49]. Although the compound, eventually named sumatriptan, was originally developed for its vasoconstrictive effect, it was later found to have another and potentially more important pharmacological action on similar 5-HT receptors that populate nerve terminals in the brain and sympathetic nerve terminals innervating some peripheral vessels. Sumatriptan was eventually found to have selective affinity for 5-HT$_{1B}$ and 5-HT$_{1D}$ receptors that are primarily expressed on cerebral vasculature and trigeminal nerve terminals respectively [50].

Table 2. Triptans Available in the United States [56]

| 5-HT$_{1A/B}$ Agonists (Triptans) |
|---|
| 1. Sumatriptan |
|     a. Subcutaneous injection |
|     b. Oral tablet |
|     c. Nasal spray |
| 2. Zolmitriptan |
|     a. Oral tablet |
|         i. Conventional |
|         ii. Oral disintegrating |
|     b. Nasal spray |
| 3. Rizatriptan |
|     a. Oral tablet |
|         i. Conventional |
|         ii. Oral disintegrating |
| 4. Naratriptan |
|     a. Oral tablet |
| 5. Almotriptan |
|     a. Oral tablet |
| 6. Frovatriptan |
|     a. Oral tablet |
| 7. Eletriptan |
|     a. Oral tablet |

The efficacy of sumatriptan and other triptans in the acute management of migraine is believed to result from one or more pharmacological mechanisms including the normalization of dilated intracranial arteries through vasoconstriction [51], neuronal inhibition in the peripheral trigeminal system [52], and inhibition of second-order neuronal sensitization in the trigeminocervical complex [53]. Later studies demonstrated that triptan administration reduced the elevated CGRP levels in cranial venous blood [54] and attenuated but did not reverse the increase in rostral brainstem activity as demonstrated by positron emission tomography (PET) [55] during migraine attacks.

Since its release for clinical use in 1991, the success of subcutaneous sumatriptan for the acute management of migraine has inspired the development and release of 7 different triptans in oral tablet formulations [56]. Two of these triptans were later developed as nasal spray formulations. Sumatriptan remains as the only triptan available as an injection and, in Europe, as a rectal suppository (Table 2).

## Triptans in Clinical Practice

Migraine abortive treatments are used to provide acute pain relief, symptom relief (i.e. antinausea), and reduction of disability associated with migraine attacks. Some migraineurs will find efficacy from using nonspecific analgesic medications such as simple analgesics (i.e. acetaminophen), nonsteroidal anti-inflammatory drugs (NSAIDs), or combination analgesics (i.e. acetaminophen, aspirin, caffeine combination products) if they are administered very early at the onset of a migraine attack and while pain intensity is mild [57]. The clinical features of an individual patient's migraine attack might help to determine the most appropriate medication and its route of administration. Migraine attacks that are associated with early onset or severe nausea, vomiting, severe headache upon awakening, or the rapid escalation of migraine pain intensity might respond best to a non-oral route of administration such as parenteral injection, rectal suppository, or nasal spray. Sometimes a combination of medications (rational multiple drug treatment) is needed to achieve the best results [58]. For example, the concomitant administration of a NSAID and triptan might have better efficacy than either medication used alone.

The triptan class of medications has demonstrated unquestionable efficacy for the abortive management of migraine attacks in adults (18 years or older). Clinical research has demonstrated that triptans generally deliver better efficacy and have greater tolerability when compared with the nonspecific analgesic medications [59, 60], and these data are supported by patient preference [61]. An evidence-based literature review conducted by the US Headache Consortium and published in 2000 found that triptans had demonstrated a pronounced statistical and clinical benefit for the acute management of migraine attacks in adults. A Practice Parameter published by the American Academy of Neurology following the evidence-based review established the following guideline: triptans are effective and relatively safe for the acute treatment of migraine headaches and are an appropriate initial treatment choice for patients with moderate to severe migraine who have no contraindication for their use [44]. In 2001, the results of a large meta-analysis that included 53 high-quality clinical trials (published and unpublished) of oral triptan safety, efficacy, and tolerability encompassing over 24,000 adult subjects were reported [62]. It was determined that all oral triptans had better treatment efficacy than placebo. Overall the differences in treatment outcomes among the oral triptans were small. The absolute 2-hour headache response rate (moderate or severe pain intensity reduced to pain-free or mild pain intensity at 2 hours after treatment) generally ranged between 50% and 70 %. The absolute 2-hour pain free (moderate or severe pain intensity reduced to pain-free at 2 hours after treatment) generally ranged between 20% and 40 %. Placebo subtracted outcomes were less robust. The authors concluded that all oral triptans were effective and well tolerated. There were statistical differences in some outcome measures when comparing various triptans but the clinical significance of these differences remains uncertain. Another evidence-based review published in 2003 by the Cochrane Collaboration concluded that sumatriptan was effective for the acute treatment of migraine attacks [63]. The review determined that sumatriptan was well tolerated although minor adverse events were not uncommon. Other oral triptans were found to be similar in efficacy and tolerability to sumatriptan while the combination of ergotamine tartrate and caffeine was found to be significantly less effective. It was also determined that drugs used for the acute management of migraine other than triptans and ergot derivatives were not sufficiently studied to draw firm conclusions regarding treatment efficacy and tolerability. It is important to recognize that the early clinical trials of triptans and all Federal Drug Administration (FDA) mandated regulatory trials of triptans required that study subjects delay treatment until their pain was subjectively rated at the moderate to severe intensity level. Post hoc analyses of some clinical trials suggested that subjects who violated study protocol and treated at mild pain intensity experienced greater treatment efficacy [64]. Efficacy outcomes demonstrated a greater likelihood to achieve a pain-free outcome and greater likelihood to achieve a sustained pain-free outcome (pain free at 2 hours without pain recurrence in the 24 hour period following treatment) when the triptan was administered at mild pain intensity. In experimental models, triptans have not demonstrated efficacy in reversing central sensitization possibly related to the finding that central (2$^{nd}$ order) trigeminal neurons do not express a high density of 5-HT$_{1D}$ receptors. Correspondingly, in clinical use, triptan efficacy is diminished when allodynia is present during a migraine attack [65]. Recent prospective trials have demonstrated substantial improvement of efficacy outcomes when the patient was instructed to treat at a mild level of pain intensity [66, 67, 68, 69, 70]. Cumulative outcome results have generally demonstrated a doubling of the pain-free efficacy outcomes for oral triptans when they are administered during a mild level of pain intensity.

## Brief Reviews of Individual Tripans

Table 3 summarizes the triptans that are available in the United States (US), commonly used dosages in clinical practice, and selected pharmacokinetic data [56]. A brief synopsis of each triptan will be found in the paragraphs to follow. This information is not intended to be a comprehensive summary of the triptans, therefore readers are directed to review the scientific literature and FDA-approved product package labeling specific to each triptan.

## Table 3. Triptans available in the US, selected dosages and pharmacokinetic data [56]

| Triptan | Dosage (mg) | Bioavailability (%) | Tmax (hr) | T1/2 (hr) | Metabolism |
|---|---|---|---|---|---|
| Sumatriptan | 6mg sc | 96 | 0.17 | 2 | MAO-A, hepatic |
| | 100mg po | 14 | 1.5 | 2-3 | |
| | 20mg in | 15.8 | 1.5 | 1.8 | 60% renal unchanged |
| | (also available in 25mg and 50mg tablet strengths) | | | | |
| Zolmitriptan | 5mg po | 46 | 1.5 | 2.3 | MAO-A, hepatic, P450 |
| | 5mg in | 47 | 1.5-2 | 2-3 | |
| | (also available in 2.5mg tablet strength) | | | | |
| Rizatriptan | 10mg po | 45 | 1.0 | 2-3 | MAO-A, hepatic, 30% renal unchanged |
| Naratriptan | 2.5mg po | 74 | 2.0 | 5.5 | hepatic P450 isoenzymes |
| | (also available in 1mg tablet strength) | | | | not MAO-A 50% renal unchanged |
| Almotriptan | 12.5mg po | 70 | 2.1 | 3.1 | Hepatic CYP3A4 and 2D6, MAO-A, 40% renal unchanged |
| | (also available in 6.25mg tablet strength) | | | | |
| Frovatriptan | 2.5mg po | 21(m); 30(f) | 2.3 | 27 | Hepatic CYP1A2 not MAO-A, 32% renal unchanged |
| Eletriptan | 40mg po | 50 | 18 | 4 | Hepatic CYP3A4 |
| | (also available in 20mg tablet strength) | | | | Not MAO-A |

sc: subcutaneous injection
mg: milligram
f: female
in: intranasal spray
hr: hour
MAO-A: monoamine oxidase type A inhibitor
po: oral tablet
m: male

## Sumatriptan

Sumatriptan was the first 5-HT$_1$ receptor agonist available for clinical use. It was initially released in Europe in 1991 and subsequently released in the United States in 1993 as a subcutaneous injection. Sumatriptan binds with high affinity to 5-HT$_{1D}$ and 5-HT$_{1B}$ receptors [56]. Sumatriptan is indicated for the acute treatment of migraine attacks with or without aura in adults. Sumatriptan subcutaneous injection is also indicated for the acute treatment of cluster headache episodes in adults. Sumatriptan is available in 6mg subcutaneous injection; 25 mg, 50 mg, and 100 mg tablets; and 5 mg and 20 mg nasal spray formulations. Clinical studies and clinical experience has shown sumatriptan to be rapidly effective in providing relief from migraine pain, migraine-associated symptoms (i.e. nausea and photophobia), and migraine-associated disability. The 6 mg subcutaneous injection, which can be self-administered, has demonstrated the highest efficacy of all triptans with 0.5, 1, and 2-hour headache responses of 63, 73, and 70% respectively when taken at moderate to severe pain intensity. Comparable placebo responses are 15, 24, and 21% respectively. The 1 and 2 hour pain-free outcomes after a 6mg subcutaneous dose were 48% and 64% respectively compared to placebo responses of 5 and 11%. The usual dose for a sumatriptan subcutaneous injection is 6 mg. A second dose can be given in 1 hour but studies have failed to show clear benefit if the initial dose is not effective. The maximum daily dosage of the injectable sumatriptan is 12 mg. The adverse event profile of the subcutaneous injection is greater than that observed after tablet administration. The sumatriptan oral tablet has demonstrated efficacy after single doses of 25 mg, 50 mg, and 100 mg. The 50 mg and 100 mg dosages are generally more effective than the 25 mg dose in clinical practice. A second dose can be taken 2 hours after the initial dose if needed up to a daily maximum dosage of 200 mg. Sumatriptan nasal spray was found to have a faster onset of therapeutic effect than the tablet form but the 2 hour headache response was not substantially better than that achieved with the tablet [71]. The initial dose of sumatriptan nasal spray commonly used in clinical practice is 20 mg. A second dose can be administered in 2 hours if needed up to a maximum daily dosage of 40 mg. The probability of achieving a headache response at 2 hours is approximately 60% with the sumatriptan 50 mg or 100 mg tablet and approximately 65% with the sumatriptan 20 mg nasal spray when taken at the moderate to severe level of pain intensity. The comparable placebo responses were approximately 20% for the tablet and 30% for the nasal spray formulations. Clinical trials and experience suggest that the nasal spray formulation tends to have an inconsistent response from attack to attack. Its overall clinical usefulness has been limited by the medication's undesirable taste. The injectable is a good choice for patient's who develop nausea and vomiting during their attack or when a rapid therapeutic effect is desirable. The nasal spray might be a good choice when nausea occurs early in the migraine attack. The headache recurrence rates for sumatriptan generally ranged between 30 and 40% but administering the medication when migraine pain is mild has resulted in a substantial reduction of migraine recurrence [66].

## Zolmitriptan

Zolmitriptan binds with high affinity to human recombinant $5\text{-}HT_{1D}$ and $5\text{-}HT_{1B}$ receptors [56]. It has a modest affinity for $5\text{-}HT_{1A}$ receptors. The active N-desmethyl metabolite of zolmitriptan has identical receptor affinity relative to the active compound. Zolmitriptan is indicated for the acute treatment of migraine attacks with or without aura in adults. Zolmitriptan is available in 2.5 mg and 5 mg oral tablets and 5 mg nasal spray formulations. The tablet is available as a conventional tablet or an orally disintegrating preparation. The disintegrating tablet might be a good choice for patients who are not able to take conventional tablets or have nausea early in the course of their attacks. Contrary to what might be implied by the delivery formulation, zolmitriptan from the orally disintegrating tablet is not absorbed through the oral mucosa but is swallowed in the saliva and absorbed from the gastrointestinal tract. The zolmitriptan nasal spray formulation is partially absorbed through the nasopharyngeal mucosa and has demonstrated early detectable serum drug levels. Accordingly the zolmitriptan nasal spray has a rapid onset of therapeutic effects. It is generally better tolerated than the sumatriptan nasal spray owing to the overall improved taste and demonstrated of a more consistent response in multiple attack studies. The probability of achieving a headache response at 2 hours is approximately 67% with the zolmitriptan 2.5mg or 5mg tablets and 72% with the zolmitriptan 5mg nasal spray when administered at moderate to severe head pain intensity. The comparable placebo response was approximately 36% for all formulations.

As mentioned previously the nasal spray route of drug delivery may be desirable for patients with nausea or who need a more rapid response than that experienced with a tablet. The typical dosages used in clinical practice are the 2.5 mg tablet and 5 mg nasal spray. The 2.5 mg and 5 mg tablet strengths were similar in treatment efficacy outcomes in clinical trials although some patients do respond better to the larger dosage. The 2.5 mg dose is generally associated with a lower adverse event profile. The maximum daily dosage of zolmitriptan is 10mg. Headache recurrence rates ranged between 22 and 37% and, as is common to all triptans, treating at mild pain intensity reduces the probability of recurrence [67]. There have been no substantial increases in therapeutic gain when comparing efficacy of zolmitriptan with that of sumatriptan but clinical experience has suggested that sumatriptan non-responders might respond to zolmitriptan.

## Naratriptan

Naratriptan binds with high affinity to $5\text{-HT}_{1D}$ and $5\text{-HT}_{1B}$ receptors [56]. Naratriptan is indicated for the acute treatment of migraine attacks with or without aura in adults. Naratriptan is available in 1 mg and 2.5 mg tablet strengths. The 2.5mg dose is most commonly used in clinical practice and is generally more effective than the 1mg dose. A second naratriptan dose can be taken 4 hours after the initial dosage for a daily maximum of 5 mg. Pharmacokinetic studies of Naratriptan demonstrate a longer time to maximum serum concentration (Tmax) and 50% clearance of serum concentration (T1/2) after a single dose when compared to sumatriptan. Placebo controlled studies of naratriptan have demonstrated that it has less efficacy for headache response at a 2-hour outcome endpoint. The 4-hour headache responses after administration of naratriptan are generally comparable to the 2-hour response of all other oral triptans except frovatriptan, which has a treatment efficacy profile that is comparable to naratriptan. The probability of achieving a headache response at 4 hours is approximately 67% when naratriptan 2.5 mg is taken at the moderate to severe level of pain intensity. The comparable placebo response at 4 hours was approximately 40%. Headache recurrence was relatively low and ranged between 17 and 28% when evaluated after a 4-hour headache response. In clinical trials, naratriptan generally has a favorable side effect profile, which is comparable to the profile associated with placebo. Headache responses can be expected to improve when the medication is taken at mild pain but specific studies to evaluate this clinical observation have not be completed. Naratriptan might be a good triptan choice for patients who experience a slow progression of individual migraine attacks or experience adverse side effects with other triptans.

## Rizatriptan

Rizatriptan binds with high affinity to human cloned 5-$HT_{1D}$ and 5-$HT_{1B}$ receptors [56]. It has a weak affinity for 5-$HT_{1A}$, 5-$HT_{1E}$, 5-$HT_{1F}$, and 5-$HT_7$ receptors. Rizatriptan is indicated for the acute treatment of migraine attacks with or without aura in adults. Rizatriptan is available in 5 mg and 10 mg tablet strengths. The tablet is available as a conventional tablet or an orally disintegrating preparation. The disintegrating tablet might be a good choice for patients who are not able to take conventional tablets or have nausea early in their attack. As with the zolmitriptan orally disintegrating tablet, rizatriptan from the orally disintegrating tablet is not absorbed through the oral mucosa but is absorbed from the gastrointestinal tract. The 10 mg tablet is the dosage strength most commonly used in clinical practice and has demonstrated greater efficacy than the 5 mg dose. Clinical efficacy is generally greatest when the medication is taken at mild head pain intensity [68]. A second or third rizatriptan dose can be taken 2 hours after the previous dose up to a daily maximum of 30 mg if necessary. Due to a pharmacokinetic interaction, the 5 mg tablet is recommended for patients taking propranolol and this dose can be repeated 3 times as outlined above up to a maximum daily dosage of 15 mg. Rizatriptan has demonstrated fast action and high efficacy at 2 hours after dosing. The probability of achieving a headache response at 2 hours is approximately 70% when rizatriptan 10 mg (conventional or oral disintegrating tablet) is taken at the moderate to severe level of head pain intensity. The comparable placebo response was approximately 35%. There appears to be a greater likelihood of achieving a pain-free outcome when directly compared with sumatriptan, zolmitriptan, and naratriptan [72]. Rizatriptan's fast onset of action, high efficacy (headache response and pain-free), as well as its sustained pain freedom was also demonstrated in the meta-analysis reported by Ferrari and colleagues [62]. Headache recurrence rates ranged between 30% and 47%.

## Almotriptan

Almotriptan binds with high affinity to the 5-$HT_{1D}$, 5-$HT_{1B}$, and 5-$HT_{1F}$ receptors [56]. It has a weak affinity for the 5-$HT_{1A}$ and 5-$HT_7$ receptors. Almotriptan is indicated for the acute treatment of migraine attacks with or without aura in adults. Almotriptan is available in 6.25 mg and 12.5 mg tablet strengths. The 12.5 mg tablet is most commonly used in clinical practice and has demonstrated greater efficacy than the 6.25 mg dose. Clinical efficacy is generally greatest if the medication is taken at the mild stage of pain [69]. A second dose of almotriptan can be taken 2 hours after the first if necessary and the maximum daily dosage is 25 mg for a healthy adult. The medication has demonstrated a fast onset of action and a high likelihood of achieving a pain-free response at 2 hours after dosing. The probability of achieving a headache response at 2 hours is approximately 60% when almotriptan 12.5mg is taken at the moderate to severe level of pain intensity. The comparable placebo response was approximately 38%. Almotriptan has generally demonstrated better overall tolerability than other triptans with similar pharmacokinetics [62]. Drug related adverse events associated with almotriptan 12.5 mg dose compared favorably with those reported after taking placebo specifically a 16% adverse event rate was associated with almotriptan compared to 15% for placebo. Headache recurrence rates ranged between 18% and 29%.

## Frovatriptan

Frovatriptan exhibits high affinity to $5\text{-}HT_{1D}$ and $5\text{-}HT_{1B}$ receptors [56]. An active metabolite, desmethyl frovatriptan, has weaker affinity for the $5\text{-}HT_{1B}$ and $5\text{-}HT_{1D}$ receptors than the parent compound. Frovatriptan is indicated for the acute treatment of migraine attacks with or without aura in adults. Frovatriptan is available in 2.5 mg tablets. The initial dose is a 2.5 mg tablet. Second and third dosages can be taken at least 2 hours after the previous dose up to a daily maximum of 7.5 mg in healthy adults. Frovatriptan has the longest elimination half-life of all oral triptans at approximately 26 hours. The probability of achieving a headache response at 2 hours has ranged between 37 and 46% when frovatriptan 2.5mg is taken at the moderate to severe level of pain intensity. The comparable placebo responses ranged between 21 and 27%. Frovatriptan has generally demonstrated a low headache recurrence rate ranging between 7 and 25% when compared to placebo. Frovatriptan has demonstrated good tolerability [73].

## Eletriptan

Eletriptan binds with high affinity to the $5\text{-}HT_{1D}$, $5\text{-}HT_{1B}$, and $5\text{-}HT_{1F}$ receptors [56]. It has a modest affinity for the $5\text{-}HT_{1A}$, $5\text{-}HT_{1E}$, $5\text{-}HT_{2B}$, and $5\text{-}HT_7$ receptors. Eletriptan is indicated for the acute treatment of migraine attacks with or without aura in adults. Eletriptan is available in 20 mg and 40 mg tablet strengths. The 40 mg tablet is most commonly used in clinical practice and has demonstrated greater efficacy than the 20 mg dose. Clinical efficacy is generally greatest if the medication is taken at the mild stage of head pain [70]. A second eletriptan dose can be taken 2 hours after the first if necessary up to a maximum daily dosage of 80mg for a healthy adult. Because eletriptan is metabolized by hepatic CYP3A4, it is recommended that it not be given within 72 hours of potent CYP3A4 inhibitors such as ketoconazole, itraconazole, nefazodone, troleandomycin, clarithromycin, ritonavir, and nelfinavir because of the potential for a greater than expect eletriptan serum concentration. The clinical significance of this potential interaction is uncertain. Eletriptan has demonstrated a fast onset of action and high likelihood of achieving a pain-free response at 2 hours after dosing. The probability of achieving a headache response at 2 hours is approximately 60% when eletriptan 40mg is taken at the moderate to severe level of pain intensity. The comparable placebo response was approximately 25%. Eletriptan has demonstrated efficacy superior to sumatriptan in head-to-head comparison trials [74]. The migraine recurrence rate for eletriptan is approximately 30%.

## Safety Concerns Associated with the 5-HT Agonists

Isolated reports of serious cardiovascular adverse events and the occurrence of chest symptoms mimicking angina pectoris have raised clinicians' concern about the safety of triptans. Results from clinical trials and post-marketing surveillance analyses have demonstrated that the risk of serious cardiovascular adverse events is extremely low when patients are appropriately selected [75]. Coronary blood vessels express 5-HT$_{1B}$ receptors and the triptans can cause vasoconstriction when interacting with these receptors [76]. It is for this reason that triptans, as a medication class, are contraindicated for use in patients who have a history of ischemic heart disease (i.e. angina pectoris, history of myocardial infarction, or documented silent ischemia), or otherwise have symptoms or findings consistent with ischemic heart disease, coronary artery vasospasm, Prinzmetal's variant angina, or other significant underlying heart disease [56]. Despite careful selection, there have been a few extremely rare occurrences of adverse cardiovascular events in patients without a previously known history of cardiac disease [75]. The underlying cause of these unpredictable cardiac events is not known but it might be related to previously unrecognized cardiovascular or vasospastic disease. No triptan has been determined safer than another with respect to cardiovascular adverse events. Chest pain or other chest symptoms are recognized side effects of the triptans and have been reported in 1% to 7% of patients taking therapeutic doses of oral triptans [75]. Although the etiologies of these symptoms are not known, there is evidence to suggest that these "chest symptoms" are not related to myocardial ischemia [77, 78, 79, 80]. In vitro studies have demonstrated that triptans cause very little arterial constriction in solution concentrations that are similar to serum concentrations resulting from the administration of recommended dosages for clinical practice [81, 82]. A study of myocardial perfusion using positron emission tomography and electrocardiography found no changes in myocardial perfusion or electrocardiographic patterns after patients with no cardiovascular symptoms were administered a sumatriptan 6mg subcutaneous injection [83]. The triptans are also contraindicated for use in patients with a history of basilar and hemiplegic migraine [56]. Despite this warning, clinical investigators have published reports of using triptans in cases of basilar migraine, migraine associated with prolonged aura, and hemiplegic migraine with no occurrence of serious adverse events [84]. The use of triptans is also contraindicated within 24 hours of taking another chemically distinct triptan (5-HT1 agonist) and any ergotamine containing compound or derivative (i.e. dihydroergotamine, ergotamine tartrate, methysergide) [56].

In 2002, the American Headache Society convened a panel of neurologists, cardiologists, primary care physicians, pharmacologists, and epidemiologists to formulate a consensus statement regarding the concern of cardiovascular safety and triptan use [85]. The expert panel's consensus was that the safety profile of triptans appeared well defined and the risk of adverse cardiovascular events was extremely low when patients were selected according to the recommendations outlined in the FDA-approved product package labeling. Triptan class labeling in the United States includes the contraindication for use in patients with history, symptoms, or signs of ischemic cardiac, cerebrovascular, or peripheral vascular syndromes. It is also strongly recommended that triptans not be given to patients in whom unrecognized coronary artery disease is predicted by the presence of risk factors such as hypertension, hypercholesterolemia, obesity, strong family history of coronary artery disease, tobacco use, men over 40 years of age, and menopausal women unless a cardiovascular evaluation provides satisfactory clinical evidence that cardiovascular disease is absent. The panel was not able to find compelling evidence to implicate a greater risk of triptan associated serious cardiovascular adverse events in patients with coronary artery disease when compared to other subjects. The panel acknowledged that the vast majority of reviewed data was obtained from populations of patients without known cardiovascular disease and there were isolated cases of serious cardiovascular adverse events in patients without previously recognized coronary artery disease, In clinical practice, good medical judgment is required before prescribing any triptan but uncertainty and concern of cardiovascular risks shared by some clinicians has limited triptan availability to many migraine patients who could otherwise benefit from them.

## Satisfaction with Migraine Treatments: Clues to an Ideal Migraine Abortive Medication

Triptans have generally demonstrated treatment superiority over analgesics or other "non-specific" migraine treatments used for the abortive or symptomatic management of migraine attacks [59, 60]. Despite the high degree of efficacy and patient satisfaction offered by the triptans, there remains opportunity for improvement. Studies have suggested that the most important determinants of patient satisfaction are fast action and complete migraine relief [10]. Complete migraine relief includes freedom from pain as well as total relief from all migraine related symptoms such as nausea, vomiting, photophobia, and phonophobia. Patients ideally desire to achieve a sustained response from acute treatment without recurrence of migraine pain or other symptoms and consistency of treatment response from attack to attack. [86] When specifically evaluating the triptan class of medications, patients and physicians generally agree upon the desirable attributes of an ideal triptan [87]. In triptan naïve patients, treatment efficacy was given highest priority followed by treatment tolerability and treatment consistency respectively. Triptan experienced patients also prioritized efficacy first but reported treatment consistency to be a higher priority attribute than tolerability. This intergroup difference might have been influenced by good triptan-related tolerability already experienced by the triptan-experienced group. Regarding specific efficacy measures such as 1-hour pain freedom, 2-hour pain freedom, and sustained pain freedom defined as pain freedom at 2 hours with no recurrence or need for rescue medication for 24 hours after initial treatment, patients preferred fast relief (pain freedom at 1 hour) whereas physicians generally preferred that their patients achieve a sustained pain free outcome.

Clinical research has attempted to improve treatment efficacy and therefore patient satisfaction by matching the pharmacokinetic and pharmacological attributes of a specific triptan to patients' concepts of the ideal migraine abortive medication [88, 89]. Despite these efforts, an individual patient's response to a specific triptan is difficult to predict based on the triptan's pharmacokinetic variables or statistical differences in clinical outcomes from comparative drug trials or meta-analyses. Currently, the most reliable strategy for improving treatment efficacy with triptans has been achieved by educating patients to take triptans early in a migraine attack while the pain is mild and prior to the development of clinical markers for sensitization of central trigeminal pain pathways (i.e. cutaneous allodynia of the face or scalp). Another effective treatment strategy in clinical practice has been the rational combination of therapeutic agents that have different but complementary pharmacological effects (i.e. a triptan and nonsteroidal anti-inflammatory drug) [58].

## Future Directions in Developing Migraine Abortive Medications

As knowledge of migraine mechanisms improves so shall the opportunity to discover and develop mechanism-based treatment strategies by exploiting translational research tactics. These treatments will specifically target one or more steps in the cascade of events that compose the migraine attack. Candidate pharmacological targets continue to expand but there is enthusiasm for agents that act as $5\text{-HT}_{1F}$ agonists [90], CGRP antagonists [91], NOS inhibitors [92], AMPA-kainate receptor antagonists [93], NMDA receptor antagonists [94], centrally acting cyclooxygenase-2 antagonists [95], adenosine A1 receptor agonists [96], and cannabinoid receptor agonists [97].

The new candidate medication for the acute management of migraine will ideally have fast, reliable, and pain-free treatment outcomes without migraine symptom recurrence. It will also provide complete relief from all migraine-associated symptoms other than pain such as nausea, vomiting, and sensitivities to various physical stimuli. The candidate medication will be easy to administer, have excellent tolerability, and exceptional safety thereby allowing unrestricted use and return to normal functioning after treatment administration. The medication will be effective when taken at any point in the migraine attack regardless of pain intensity or presence of cutaneous allodynia.

## Conclusion

Although the abortive management of migraine has been greatly improved by the discovery of sumatriptan and all of the other triptans that followed, the search for a new class of migraine abortive medications possessing better treatment efficacy outcomes, tolerability, and safety is motivated by the actuality that triptans are not effective or tolerated by all migraineurs while others have contraindications for their use. But until a novel therapeutic target and effective pharmacological agent is identified, the selective $5\text{-HT}_{1B/1D}$ receptor agonists, a group of medications commonly known as triptans, will continue to be preferred treatment for the abortive management of episodic migraine attacks.

# References

[1] Goadsby PJ: Migraine Pathophysiology. *Headache.* 2005; 45 (Suppl 1): S14-24.
[2] Burstein R, Cutrer FM, Yarnitsky D: The development of cutaneous allodynia during a migraine attack: clinical evidence for sequential recruitment of spinal and supraspinal nociceptive neurons in migraine. *Brain.* 2000, 123:1703–1709.
[3] Aurora SK, Welch KM, Al-Sayed F. The threshold for phosphenes is lower in migraine. *Cephalalgia.* 2003; 23(4): 258-263.
[4] Ashina S, Bendtsen L, Ashina M. Pathophysiology of tension-type headache. *Curr. Pain Headache Rep.* 2005;9(6):415-22.
[5] Burstein R, Yarnitsky D, Goor-Aryeh I, et al.: An association between migraine and cutaneous allodynia. *Ann. Neurol.* 2000, 47:614–624.
[6] Mersky H and Bogduk N (Eds), *IASP Pain Terminology In Classification of Chronic Pain,* Second Ed. Seattle, WA, USA. IASP Press 1994. 209-214.
[7] Ostfeld AM, Chapman LF, Goodell H, Wolff HG. Studies in Headache: Summary of evidence concerning a noxious agent active locally during migraine headache. *Psychosom. Med.* 1957; 19: 199.
[8] Humphrey PP. 5-hydroxytryptamine and the pathophysiology of migraine. *J. Neurol.* 1991; 238 (Suppl 1): S38-34.
[9] Humphrey PP. Preclinical studies on the anti-migraine drug, sumatriptan. *Eur. Neurol.* 1991; 31 (5): 282-290.
[10] Davies GM, Santanello N, Lipton R. Determinants of patient satisfaction with migraine therapy. *Cephalalgia.* 2000;20: 554-560.
[11] Headache Classification of the International Headache Society: The International Classification of Headache Disorders, 2nd Edition. *Cephalalgia.* 2004; 24 (Suppl 1): 1-160.
[12] Lipton RB, Stewart WF. Prevalence and impact of migraine. *Neurol. Clin.* 1997;15:1-13.
[13] Peroutka SJ. Genetic basis of migraine. *Clin. Neurosci.* 1998;5(1):34-37.
[14] Vingen JV, Sand T, Stover LJ: Sensitivity to various stimuli in primary headaches: a questionnaire study. *Headache.* 1999, 39:552–558.
[15] Selby G, Lance JW. Observation on 500 cases of migraine and allied vascular headaches. *J. Neurol. Neurosurg. Psychiatry* 1960; 23: 23-32.
[16] Stewart WF, Schechter A, Lipton RB. Migraine heterogeneity: disability, pain intensity, attack frequency, and duration. *Neurology.* 1994; 44: S24-S39.
[17] Rasmussen BK, Olesen J. Migraine with aura and migraine without aura: an epidemiological study. *Cephalalgia.* 1992; 12: 221-228.
[18] Cady R, Dodick DW, Levine HL, Schreiber CP, et al. Sinus headache: a neurology, otolaryngology, allergy, and primary care consensus on diagnosis and treatment. *Mayo. Clin. Proc.* 2005 Jul;80(7):908-16.

[19] Kaniecki RG. Migraine and tension-type headache: an assessment of challenges in diagnosis. *Neurology.* 2002; 58 (9Supp16): S15-S20.

[20] Tepper SJ, Dahlof CG, Dowson A, Newman L, et al. Prevalence and diagnosis of migraine in patients consulting their physician with a complaint of headache: data from the Landmark Study. *Headache.* 2004 Oct;44(9):856-64.

[21] Graham JR,Wolff HG. Mechanisms of migraine headache and action of ergotamine tartrate. *Arch. Neurol. Psychiatry.* 1938; 39: 737-763.

[22] Moskowitz MA: The neurobiology of vascular head pain. *Ann. Neurol.* 1984, 15:157–168.

[23] Goadsby PJ, Zagami AS, Lambert GA. Neural processing of craniovascular pain: a synthesis of the central structures involved in migraine. *Headache.* 1991; 31: 365-371.

[24] Pietrobon D, Streissnig J. Neurobiology of migraine. *Nat. Rev. Neurosci.* 2003; 4(5): 386-398.

[25] Ferrari MD. Migraine. *Lancet.* 1998; 351: 1043-1051.

[26] Drummond PD. Scalp tenderness and sensitivity to pain in migraine and tension headache. *Headache.* 1987; 27(1):45-50.

[27] Kelman L. The premonitory symptoms (prodrome): a tertiary care study of 893 migraineurs. *Headache.* 2004;44(9):865-72.

[28] Peroutka SJ. Dopamine and migraine. *Neurology.* 1997;49(3):650-656.

[29] Hadjikhani N, Sanchez del Rio M, Schwartz D, Bakker D, et al. Mechanisms of migraine aura revealed by functional MRI in human visual cortex. *Proc. Natl. Acad. Sci. U S A.* 2001;98(8):4687-92.

[30] Bolay H, Reuter U, Dunn AK, et al. Intrinsic brain activity triggers trigeminal meningeal afferents in a migraine model. *Nat. Med.* 2002; 8: 136-142.

[31] Burstein R, Cutrer FM, Yarnitsky D: The development of cutaneous allodynia during a migraine attack: clinical evidence for sequential recruitment of spinal and supraspinal nociceptive neurons in migraine. *Brain.* 2000. 123:1703-1709.

[32] 32. Burstein R, Collins B, Jakubowski M.Defeating migraine pain with triptans: A race against the development of cutaneous allodynia. *Ann. Neurol.* 2004;55: 19-26.

[33] Goadsby PJ, Edvinsson L. The trigeminovascular system and migraine: studies characterizing cerebrovascular and neuropeptide changes seen in humans and cats. *Ann. Neurol.* 1993; 33: 48-56.

[34] Goadsby PJ, Edvinsson L, Ekman R. Vasoactive peptide release in the extracerebral circulation of humans during migraine headache. *Ann. Neurol.* 1990; 28: 183-187.

[35] Sarchielli P, Alberti A, Codini M, et al. Nitric oxide metabolites, prostaglandins and trigeminal vasoactive peptides in internal jugular vein blood during spontaneous migraine attacks. *Cephalalgia.* 2000; 20: 907-918.

[36] Ramadan NM. The link between migraine and glutamate. *CNS Spectrum.* 2003; 8: 446-449.

[37] Ostfeld AM. Some aspects of cardiovascular regulation in man. *Angiology.* 1959; 10: 34-42.

[38] Ferrari MD, Odink J, Tapparelli C, et al. Serotonin metabolism in migraine. *Neurology.* 1989; 39: 1239-1242.

[39] Sicuteri T, Testi A, Anselmi B. Biochemical investigations in headache: increase in hydroxyindoleacetic acid excretion during migraine attacks. *Int. Arch. Allergy. Appl. Immunol.* 1961; 19: 55-58.

[40] Curzon G, Barrie M, Wilkerson MI. Relationships between headache and amine changes after administration of reserpine to migrainous patients. *J. Neurol. Neurosurg. Psychiatry.* 1969;32(6):555-61.

[41] Kimball RW, Friedman AP, Vallejo E. Effects of serotonin in migraine patients. *Neurology.* 1960; 10: 107-111.

[42] Hoyer D, Clarke DE, Fozard JR, et al. International Union of Pharmacology classification of receptors for 5-hydroxytryptamine (serotonin). *Pharmacol. Rev.* 1994; 46: 157-203.

[43] Furst S. Transmitters involved in antinociception in the spinal cord. *Brain. Res. Bull.* 1999;48(2):129-41.

[44] Silberstein SD. Practice parameter: evidence-based guidelines for migraine headache (an evidence-based review). Report of the Quality Standards Subcommittee of the American *Academy of Neurology. Neurology.* 2000;55:754-762.

[45] Chaput Y, de Montigny C, Blier P. Presynaptic and postsynaptic modifications of the serotonin system by long-term administration of antidepressant treatments. An in vivo electrophysiologic study in the rat. *Neuropsychopharmacology.* 1991; 5: 219-229.

[46] Peroutka SJ. 5-Hydroxytryptamine receptor subtypes and the pharmacology of migraine. *Neurology.* 1993;43(6 Suppl 3):S34-38.

[47] Peroutka SJ. Developments in 5-hydroxytriptamine receptor pharmacology in migraine. *Neurol Clinics* 1990; 8: 829-839.

[48] Humphrey PP, Feniuk W, Perren MJ, et al. Serotonin and migraine. *Ann. NY. Acad. Sci.* 1990; 600: 587-598.

[49] Feniuk W, Humphrey PP, Perren MJ, et al. Rationale for the use of 5-HT1-like agonists in the treatment of migraine. *J. Neurol.* 1991; 238 (Suppl 1): S57-S61

[50] Hoskin KL, Kaube H, Goadsby PJ. Sumatriptan can inhibit trigeminal afferents by an exclusively neural mechanism. *Brain.* 1996;119:1419-28

[51] Humphrey PP, Goadsby PJ. The mode of action of sumatriptan is vascular? A debate. *Cephalalgia.* 1994;14(6):401-10.

[52] Moskowitz MA, Cutrer FM. Sumatriptan: a receptor-targeted treatment for migraine. *Annu. Rev. Med.* 1993;44:145-154.

[53] Goadsby PJ. The pharmacology of headache. *Prog. Neurobiol.* 2000;62(5):509-525.

[54] Buzzi MG, Carter WB, Schimizu T. Dihydroergotamine and sumatriptan attenuate levels of CGRP in plasma in rat superior sagittal sinus during electrical stimulation of the trigeminal ganglion. *Neuropharmacology.* 1991;30(11):1193-1200.

[55] Diener HC. Positron emission tomography studies in headache. *Headache.* 1997;37(10):622-625.

[56] *Physicians Desk Reference.* 60th edition. Thomson PDR, Montvale NJ 2006.

[57] Goldstein J, Silberstein SD, Saper JR, et al. Acetaminophen, aspirin, and caffeine versus sumatriptan succinate in the early treatment of migraine: results from the ASSET trial. *Headache.* 2005;45(8):973-82.

[58] Smith TR, Sunshine A, Stark SR, et al. Sumatriptan and naproxen sodium for the acute treatment of migraine. *Headache.* 2005; 45(8): 983-991.

[59] Lipton RB, Bigal ME, Goadsby PJ. Double-blind clinical trials of oral triptans vs other classes of acute migraine medication-a review. *Cephalalgia.* 2004; 24: 321-332

[60] Pini LA, Fabbri L, Cavazzuti L. Efficacy and safety of sumatriptan 50 mg in patients not responding to standard care, in the treatment of mild to moderate migraine. The Sumatriptan 50 mg Italian Study Group. *Int. J. Clin. Pharmacol. Res.* 1999;19(2):57-64.

[61] Ceballos Hernansanz MA, Sanchez RR, Cano Org, Lopez-Gil A. Migraine treatment patterns and patient satisfaction with prior therapy: a substudy of a multicenter trial of rizatriptan effectiveness. *Clin. Ther.* 2003;25(7):2053-2069.

[62] Ferrari MD, Roon KI, Lipton RB, Goadsby PJ. Oral triptans (serotonin 5-HT1B/1D agonists) in acute migraine treatment: a meta-analysis of 53 trials. *Lancet.* 2001; 358: 1668-1675.

[63] McCrory DC, Gray RN. Oral sumatriptan for acute migraine. *Cochrane Database Syst. Rev.* 2003; 3:CD002915.

[64] Cady RK, Sheftell F, Lipton RB, et al. Effect of early intervention with sumatriptan on migraine pain: retrospective analyses of data from three clinical trials. *Clin. Ther.* 2000 Sep;22(9):1035-48.

[65] Lainez MJA. Clinical benefits of early triptan therapy for migraine. *Cephalalgia.* 2004; 24 (Suppl 2): 24-30

[66] Scholpp J, Schellenberg R, Moeckesch B, Banik N. Early treatment of a migraine attack while pain is still mild increases the efficacy of sumatriptan. *Cephalalgia.* 2004;24(11):925-33.

[67] Klapper J, Lucas C, Rosjo O. Benefits of treating highly disabled migraine patients with zolmitriptan while pain is mild. *Cephalalgia.* 2004;24(11):918-24.

[68] Mathew NT, Kailasam J, Meadors L. Early treatment of migraine with rizatriptan: a placebo-controlled study. *Headache.* 2004;44(7):669-73.

[69] Mathew NT. Early intervention with almotriptan improves sustained pain-free response in acute migraine. *Headache.* 2003;43(10):1075-9.

[70] Brandes JL, Kudrow D, Cady R, et al. Eletriptan in the early treatment of acute migraine: influence of pain intensity and time of dosing. *Cephalalgia.* 2005;25(9):735-42.

[71] Ryan R, Elkind A, Baker CC, et al. Sumatriptan nasal spray for the acute treatment of migraine: results of two clinical studies. *Neurology.* 1997; 49: 1225-1230.

[72] Adelman JU, Lipton RB, Ferrari MD, et al. Comparison of rizatriptan and other triptans on stringent measures of efficacy. *Neurology.* 2001; 57: 1377-1383.

[73] Buchan P, Keywood C, Ward C. The pharmacokinetics of frovatriptan (VML 251/SB209509) in male and female subjects. *Func. Neurol.* 1998; 13: 177.

[74] Sandrini G, Farkkila M, Burgess G, et al. Eletriptan vs sumatriptan: a double-blind, placebo-controlled, multiple migraine attack study. *Neurology.* 2002;59(8):1210-7.

[75] Dodick DW, Martin VT, Smith T, Silberstein S. Cardiovascular tolerability and safety of triptans: a review of clinical data. *Headache.* 2004; 44 (Suppl 1): S20-S30.

[76] Maassen VanDenBrink A, Reekers M, Bax WA, et al. Coronary side-effect potential of current and prospective antimigraine drugs. *Circulation.* 1998; 98: 25-30.

[77] Muir DF, McCann GP, Swan L, et al. Hemodynamic and coronary effects of intravenous eletriptan, a 5-HT1B/1D receptor agonist. *Clin. Pharmacol. Ther.* 1999;66: 85-90.

[78] MacIntyre PD, Bhargava B, Hogg KJ, et al. The effect of i.v. sumatriptan, a selective 5-HT1 receptor agonist, on central haemodynamics and the coronary circulation. *Br. J. Clin. Pharmacol.* 1992;34: 541-546.

[79] MacIntyre PD, Bhargava B, Hogg KJ, et al. Effect of subcutaneous sumatriptan, a selective 5-HT1 agonist, on the systemic, pulmonary, and coronary circulation. *Circulation.* 1993;87: 401-405.

[80] Hood S, Birnie D, Swan L, et al. Effects of subcutaneous naratriptan on systemic and pulmonary haemodynamics and coronary artery diameter in humans. *J. Cardiovasc. Pharmacol.* 1999;34: 89-94.

[81] van den Broek RW, Maasseb VanDenBrink A, de Vries R, et al. Pharmacological analysis of of contractile effects of eletriptan and sumatriptan on human isolated blood vessels. *Eur. J. Pharmacol.* 2000; 407: 165-173.

[82] Longmore J, Hargreaves RJ, Boulanger CM, et al. Comparison of the vasoconstrictor properties of the 5-HT$_{1B/1D}$ receptors agonists rizatriptan and sumatriptan in human isoloated coronary artery: outcome of two independent studies using different experimental protocols. *Func. Neurol.* 1997; 12:3-9.

[83] Lewis PJ, Barrington SF, Mardsen PK, et al. A study of the effects of sumatriptan on myocardial perfusion in healthy female migraineurs using 13NH3 positron emission tomography. *Neurology.* 1997; 48: 1542-1550.

[84] Klapper J, Mathew N, Nett R. Triptans in the treatment of basilar migraine and migraine with prolonged aura. *Headache.* 2001;41(10):981-4.

[85] Dodick D, Lipton RB, Martin V, et al. Consensus statement: Cardiovascular safety profile of triptans (5-HT1B/1D agonists) in the acute treatment of migraine. *Headache.* 2004; 44: 414-425.

[86] Lanteri-Minet M. What do patients want from their acute migraine therapy? Eur Neurol 2005; 53 (Suppl 1):3-9.

[87] Lipton RB, Stewart WF. Acute migraine Therapy: Do doctors understand what patients with migraine want from therapy? *Headache.* 1999; 39 (Suppl 2):S20-S26.

[88] Goadsby PJ, Dodick DW, Ferrari MD, et al. TRIPSTAR: prioritizing oral triptan treatment attributes in migraine management. *Acta Neurol. Scand.* 2004; 110: 137-143.

[89] Farrari MD, Goadsby PJ, Lipton RB, et al. The use of multiattribute decision models in evaluating triptan treatment options in migraine. *J. Neurol.* 2005;252(9):1026-32.

[90] Ramadan NM, Skljarevski V, Phebus LA, Johnson KW. 5-HT1F receptor agonists in acute migraine treatment: a hypothesis. *Cephalalgia.* 2003;23(8):776-85.

[91] Edvinsson L. Clinical data on the CGRP antagonist BIBN4096BS for treatment of migraine attacks. *CNS Drug. Rev.* 2005;11(1):69-76.

[92] Lassen LH, Christiansen I, Iversen HK, et al. The effect of nitric oxide synthase inhibition on histamine induced headache and arterial dilatation in migraineurs. *Cephalalgia.* 2003;23(9):877-86.

[93] Sang CN, Ramadan NM, Willihan RG, et al. LY293558, a novel AMPA/GluR5 antagonist, is efficacious and well-tolerated in acute migraine. *Cephalalgia.* 2004; 24: 596-602.

[94] Classey JD, Knight YE, Goadsby PJ. The NMDA receptor antagonist MK-801 reduces Fos-like immunoreactivity within the trigeminocervical complex following superior sagittal sinus stimulation in the cat. *Brain Res.* 2001; 907:117-124.

[95] Rassmussen MK, Binzer M. Non-steroidal anti-inflammatory drugs in the treatment of migraine. *Curr. Med. Res. Opin.* 2001;17 (Suppl 1):S26-S29.

[96] Goadsby PJ, Hoskin KL, Storer RJ, et al. Adenosine A1 receptor agonists inhibit trigeminovascular nociceptive transmission. *Brain.* 2002; 125: 1392-1401.

[97] Akerman S, Kaube H, Goadsby PJ. Anandamine is able to inhibit trigeminal neurons using an in vivo model of trigeminovascular-mediated nociception. *J. Pharmacol. Exp. Ther.* 2004; 309:56-63.

*Chapter XV*

# Gender Differences in Clinical Pain Management

*Anita Holdcroft*[*]
Reader in Anaesthesia and Honorary Consultant Anaesthetist,
Imperial College London, Magill Department of Anaesthesia,
369 Fulham Road, London SW10 9NH

## Abstract

Sex and gender differences have been distinguished by biological and behavioural properties respectively, but it is becoming increasingly recognised that they interact at any one time and across the lifespan of an individual. In humans, biological differences are becoming identified through genetic studies. Molecular biology is revealing that receptors in the pain pathway may exert recognisable physical effects in humans and that gonadal hormones can modify genomic activity at different levels in the nervous system. Mechanisms for gender-related differences in clinical pain may not only originate through cellular activity that creates a spectrum of silent to hypersensitive 'pain memory' but also through networks of neural and other cells to integrate a response that is unique to an individual. Gender differences in autonomic and cognitive responses to pain stimuli have been technologically visualised through brain imaging studies that have pieced together complex activity with outputs in motor and affective as well as sensory systems. Chronic pain management has now progressed to recognise gender differences in risk factors, epidemiology, neurobiology, symptoms, behaviour and psychosocial interactions. Multidisciplinary therapies are being utilised that have varied effects between males and females. Study design to measure gender differences has only recently been formalised and this will have a major impact on future research.

---

[*]Reader in Anaesthesia and Honorary Consultant Anaesthetist, Imperial College London, Magill Department of Anaesthesia, 369 Fulham Road, London SW10 9NH. Tel: 020 8746 8816. Fax: 020 8237 5109

# Introduction

The start of the present interest in sex and gender differences in medicine was derived from the recognition of the lack of gender research in clinical trials coupled with a growing scientific and public lobby for initiatives in women's health. Pain then became one of the areas of gender-related medicine through pioneering work of a small group of clinicians such as Professor Maria Adele Giamberardino and basic scientists such as Professor Karen Berkley that culminated in 1999 in the formation of the International Association for the Study of Pain (IASP) Special Interest Group on Sex, Gender and Pain. Professor Roger Fillingim and Professor Anna Maria Aloisi were elected joint chairs and in 2000 the first textbook on 'Sex, Gender, and Pain' was published by the IASP [1]. Of the 32 scientific contributors less than a third were health care professionals. This relationship between basic science and clinical activity still holds for numbers of publications. Nevertheless at the beginning of 2005 a landmark consensus document was produced that clearly outlined methodological designs for laboratory and clinical research [2]. If the recommendations of this publication are used as standards by grant awarding bodies and reviewers then this will strengthen the ability of researchers to provide comparative results for measuring sex and gender differences.

# Sex and Gender

One of the fundamental distinctions between basic science and clinical research in pain has been in the terminology. Molecular and cellular biologists do not distinguish the genetic differences between male and females cells; animal research is reported according to sex and human studies vary between using the words 'sex' and 'gender' interchangeably or separately. The first question to consider here is: what are the differences, if any, between sex and gender and do they have relevance particularly in a clinical setting?

Following an initiative by the Institute of Medicine in the United States, a book on broad aspects of sex differences was produced that sought to characterize these words [3]. Sex was defined as the classification of living things generally as male or female according to reproductive organs and functions assigned by chromosomal complement. Gender was defined as a person's self representation as male or female, or how that person is responded to by social institutions on the basis of the individual's gender presentation. One interpretation of this identification of sex with biological constructs such as genetics and physiology, and gender with more qualitative features such as psychology, sociology, culture and the environment, leads to dichotomisation of mechanisms for sex/gender differences. Thus in basic science literature the results of experiments to determine sex differences do not refer to gender because the characteristics of gender as defined above are related to human behaviour. Likewise in humans, since sex is not determined in many experiments, the word gender appears to be more appropriate. However, these distinctions are not real because throughout life sex-and gender-related factors interact, they influence one another and change as biology ages. Such recognition is important in the interpretation of laboratory studies since the housing conditions of animals may have behavioural effects on experimental results that are not recognised unless a broader view of 'sex' differences is applied. For example, exposure of female rodents to males may alter their behaviour. In humans the complex relation between sex and gender can be illustrated by the chronic pain condition, irritable bowel syndrome (IBS). IBS is characterised by the combination of bowel habit disturbance and sensory symptoms. Women, compared with men, in many studies report longer episodes of pain, more constipation, bloating, and other gastrointestinal symptoms [4, 5, 6, 7]. Although there are physiological sex differences in gut transit times and in hormonal effects on gastrointestinal function that may account for menstrual fluctuations in symptoms, these do not explain all the findings in IBS [4, 8]. In considering additional causes for the different symptoms between males and females, gender issues are relevant. For example, there may be differences in pain expression or reporting style or factors that exacerbate symptoms. Of significance is the greater female than male usage of over the counter analgesics [9]. Many of these drugs have side effects on the gastrointestinal tract e.g. constipation from codeine (opioid) use, that have the potential to modify symptoms. Thus in IBS it is probable that it is the combination of the sex and gender-related effects that contribute to the clinical differences.

The application of gender-related research is to identify those factors relevant to individual symptoms that may be generated not only by biological but also by behavioural contributions so that a pain history and subsequent therapies can be focussed more appropriately. In a comprehensive review of therapies for IBS it was concluded that the majority of studies did not factor outcomes dependent on gender [10]. What the authors found did emerge from research into specific medications for use in women with IBS is serotonin receptor-based pharmacological treatments. The rationale for this therapeutic approach is that serotonin neurones contain both oestrogen beta and progestin receptors; these receptors are targets for gonadal sex steroids which can modify gene expression and hence alter pain transmission. For non-constipated patients the recommended drug is a $5-HT_3$ antagonist, Alosetron and for diarrhoea-predominant IBS a partial $5-HT_4$ receptor agonist Tegaserod, both drugs having shown efficacy in clinical trials in females with IBS [11, 12]. However the design of the clinical trials on which these recommendations are based have been criticized because the higher frequency of IBS in females has skewed the sex distribution such that only a small number of men were included. Studies with larger numbers of males are now required to eliminate gender bias. Furthermore, research into the mechanisms by which these drugs produce their effects is needed in order to explain why serotonin receptor pharmacology is specifically relevant to IBS, and also the significant influence of oestrogen on this system [13].

## Genetics

One of the most publicly acclaimed results from gender research in pain is that of the sensitivity of red haired women to analgesic drugs. This research can be traced from humans into animals. First in male and female humans, various types of stressors occur in different frequencies and influence nociception and pain responses [14]. These stressors are trauma, abuse and major life events such as childbearing in women. When applied to animals, stress induced analgesia can recruit neurochemically distinct mechanisms. The two that predominate are the opioid and N-methyl-D-aspartate (NMDA) systems [15]. A sex difference in stress induced opioid analgesia depends on the pain stimulus and the genotype of the rodent tested [16]. In rodents in contrast with the opioid system, the NMDA system functions such that an NMDA antagonist only blocks stress induced analgesia in males and not females yet the stress stimulus produces the same amount of analgesia in males and females despite there being similar NMDA neuronal circuitry. The key to this difference was found to be in the activation of the system; it was stimulated by oestrogen, the sex steroid hormone associated with female characteristics [17]. These findings then led to genetic studies to determine the underlying mechanisms. The candidate gene that was postulated was the melanocortin-1 receptor. Not only is this receptor expressed in brain glial cells, the locus coeruleus and in the midbrain periaqueductal gray, all of which are known functional brain areas in pain modulation, but it is homozygous in 60% of red-haired females making population screening relatively easy. Thus human experiments followed and in women homozygous for the gene, greater analgesia to the kappa opioid analgesic pentazocine was demonstrated [18]. Further translation of the linkage with the NMDA system would be difficult to determine in humans for ethical reasons. However, this important outcome has started people to question whether analgesics should be given to humans based on their genetics, gender or other physical characteristics.

# Pain Responses from Viscera

## A. Brain-Gut Interactions

The main anatomical differences between females and males are their reproductive structures that are chiefly visceral organs in the pelvis, but reproduction also has a dichotomized central nervous system control. Thus although this organization is functionally for procreation, neuroendocrinological activity may have more generalised effects one of which is the response to visceral stimulation. For example, results from applying a rectal stimulus to activate the cortex using functional magnetic resonance imaging demonstrated no sensory scoring differences between males and females but interesting regional activations in the brain that may have relevance to clinical pain syndromes [19]. Males showed activity in the sensory and parieto-occipital regions in contrast to females whose activity was in the anterior cingulate and insular regions. In a recent Positron Emission Tomographic study [20] with IBS patients during rectal inflation or an expected painful visceral distension, i.e. a psychological stimulus, the same differences were shown for both tests. The men showed activation of their cognitive (dorsolateral prefrontal cortex) and central autonomic regions (insula, periaqueductal gray) and inhibition of limbic (e.g. amygdala) regions compared with females who showed greater activation of affective (mid and posterior cingulate) and autonomic regions. It is possible that these results may explain some of the affective, autonomic and antinociceptive responses to visceral stimulation. Altered autonomic responses in IBS to a visceral stress have recently been demonstrated with an increased sympathetic and decreased parasympathetic response in males compared with females [21].

This result compliments the laboratory studies of colorectal distension that measured different neuroendocrine function in male and female rats in relation to visceral stress [22]. Such findings across species would indicate that multiple levels of the central nervous system are activated during visceral stimulation whether in normal or pathological conditions and that these activities may vary with the sex of the species.

A mechanistic hypervigilance model for gender-related IBS symptoms proposed by Meyer [23] describes the relationship of these subcortical integrative networks of cognitive, autonomic and antinociceptive responses to their outputs, as the 'emotive motor system'. In this biobehavioural perspective, the model incorporates outputs from cortical networks such as attitudes, beliefs and coping with pain memories, autonomic responses and inhibition of nociception. Another model integrating somatovisceral sensory pathways with cortical activity and effector responses is based on cross-system convergence responses to pelvic afferent stimulation [24]. Both these dynamic models bring to human experience of chronic pain a concept of individual pain memories (possibly with sensitisation of multiple brain regions) as well as the biopsychosocial constructs (that include gender-relevant 'significant others' and health care personnel/interactions) of gender-related pain mechanisms [25]. In clinical medicine these pointers have to be viewed with the seriousness of epidemic precautions. The reasons for this caution are that once central nervous system sensitisation has occurred it is much harder to manage than if it is prevented and, because it is unique to an individual, management may require multiple approaches at different levels and systems in the central nervous system. Thus processes for blocking or inhibiting noxious impulses may differ in each sex and be altered by gender-related factors. One of the fundamental questions of pain management is why chronic pain develops in some people and not in others. It is possible that part of the answer lies in sex/gender-related mechanisms. This process has implications for access to medical services (e.g. fast onset of pain relief), diagnosis and investigations (e.g. treat infections) such that men and women in pain are treated equitably. It is important to remember lessons from gender differences in cardiac pain management where women over a decade ago were excluded from adequate diagnostic and treatment facilities before gender differences were recognised and acknowledged [26, 27]. These results may have to be re-learned in other specialties.

## B. Viscero-Visceral and Viscero-Somatic Hyperalgesia

### i) Hyperalgesia

Acute, recurrent and chronic pains from reproductive organs appear to be more frequent in women than men and include dysmenorrhoea, labour and postpartum pain and pelvic inflammatory disease [28]. Following research into the hypothesis that this higher frequency in females may be the result of sensitisation in the nervous system, it has been demonstrated in both animals and humans that there is a greater co-occurrence in females of other painful conditions, so-called viscero-visceral and viscero-somatic hyperalgesia [29, 30]. The term hyperalgesia describes the perception of a painful stimulus as more painful than usual and results from sensitisation in the nervous system. Sensitisation can occur peripherally e.g. in response to inflammation, or centrally in the spinal cord or higher centres. It is manifest by increased neuronal activity to a noxious stimulus (with a shift to the left of the stimulus response curve) that can continue long after the pathology has resolved, an expanded receptive field size and spread of hyperexcitability to the spinal cord, relaying in the thalamus and onto the cerebral cortex. The normal response to an afferent stimulus from skin, muscle or viscera is a convergence onto spinal cord segments. If sensitization has occurred as a result of pathophysiology in a visceral organ, there is widespread divergence of neural information. Thus the interactions between somatic and/or visceral afferents e.g. from inflamed reproductive organs, may influence functions in segments remote from the original site. For example, in women during menstruation muscle hyperalgesia may occur cyclically in sites distant from the reproductive tract; in animals this is exemplified in rats with endometriosis that demonstrate referred muscle hyperalgesia [31].

One of the interesting facets of clinical pain from viscera such as the commonly occurring IBS is that it has co-morbidities with other pain syndromes. In a systematic review of the literature IBS had common features associated with fibromyalgia, chronic fatigue syndrome, temporomandibular joint disorder and chronic pelvic pain [32]. Since these conditions have a female prevalence, investigations into cerebral function in women with co-morbidities of IBS and fibromyalgia have been conducted. Central pain processing differs in these women in the presence of IBS and fibromyalgia and this is considered by different groups of researchers to be one explanation for these co-morbidities [33, 34]. The cortical response is likened to a hyperalgesic state such that an abnormal sensory response occurs to normal homeostatic and urge-related reflex activities [33].

## ii) Diagnosis of Visceral Pathophysiology

Pain was described as the fifth vital sign in 2001 by the Joint Commission of Health Care Organisations to bring it into prominence with the pulse rate, respiratory rate, blood pressure and temperature so that adequate pain relief is provided by health care establishments. Pathophysiology in a viscus may produce vague dull or cramp-like pain, or pain referred to skin or muscle, or tenderness in skin and muscle. Unfortunately for health care administrators seeking to deliver targets, it may also be silent with no pain/sensation at any site. A close comparison to this concept in terms of pathophysiology is an unsuspected abnormally high blood pressure that can lead to complications before diagnosis. One example that threatens women more than men is silent myocardial ischaemia [35]. Generally, complications of silent dysfunction in one organ appear to result in hidden or exaggerated dysfunction in another [31].

A common clinical presentation of visceral pathophysiology is referred hyperalgesia. It may occur intermittently or continuously in conditions even where visceral stimulation is only intermittent e.g. dysmenorrhoea or ureteric colic (see Table 1 for visceral pain phenomena [36, 37, 38, 39, 40, 41, 42, 43, 44, 45, 46, 47, 48]). Its effects may be prolonged because the hyperalgesia persists long after the original stimulus has finished [48]. A typical complaint is muscle or subcutaneous tenderness in the referral segment. Accompanying symptoms may include autonomic responses such as nausea and vomiting. It was the poor pain localisation, widespread muscle pains and nausea typical of a visceral origin of pain that confused the diagnosis of coronary heart disease in women compared with men before gender differences were clarified. One of the confounding factors was that the differential diagnosis of such symptoms also related to the gastrointestinal tract (and interestingly to basic scientists, pathophysiologically to the same spinal segments) and so for women their pains were more frequently diagnosed as indigestion rather than coronary artery disease.

**Table 1. Gender-related abdominal visceral pain phenomena**

| Pathology | Pain phenomena | References Human | References Animal |
|---|---|---|---|
| Interstitial cystitis | Females > Males | [36] | |
| Irritable bowel syndrome | Females > Males | [37] | |
| + *fibromyalgia* | ↑ pain | [38] | |
| | Comorbidity | [39, 32, 33] | |
| (convergence colon/uterus) | ↑ pain | | [40] |
| Bile stones | Females > Males | [41] | |
| | Pancreatitis Males>females | [42, 43] | |
| | ↑ angina frequency | [44, 45] | |
| Ureteric stones | *Viscero-visceral, viscero-somatic hyperalgesia* | | |
| | Muscle hyperalgesia (cyclical reproductive changes in females) | | [46, 47] |
| + *endometriosis* | ↑ pain | [48] | [31] |

In the long term visceral symptoms may become better localised, that is lateralised and sharper. They may have a clear relationship with hormonal menstrual changes; this relationship may be tested while keeping a joint pain/menstrual diary. Such relationships have been described for interstitial cystitis and they point the direction of therapies towards hormonal modulation [49]. Other visceral symptoms to consider include tropic changes with a reduction in muscle volume and an increase in subcutaneous tissue thickness [44].

The diagnostic profile of painful symptoms for a diagnostic entity requires further research and precisely documented findings. For women the tendency for viscero-visceral interactions contributes to greater symptom diversity. Also for men there have been issues of misdiagnosis and lack of accurate data. For example in interstitial cystitis where there is a purportedly higher frequency in women there has been a reluctance to diagnose the condition in men leading to misdiagnosis as chronic prostatitis [36, 50].

### iii) Viscero-Visceral and Viscero-Somatic Hyperalgesia

In humans an acute noxious stimulus of a visceral organ e.g. by balloon distension, can replicate pain sensations felt during chronic pain conditions. Normally low threshold sensory receptors from the viscera do not respond with pain but as the stimulus intensity increases e.g. to empty the bowel, the sensation becomes more dominant and urges the subject to take notice of the stimulus [51]. These low threshold mechanoreceptors have been extensively investigated in the laboratory and are involved in normal physiological function of the gut e.g. peristalsis and secretion. High-threshold mechanoreceptors activate in the noxious range of distending pressures but if sensitized also fire at low pressures [52]. In patients with bowel disorders such as IBS, a decrease in threshold to stimulation with a balloon can be measured [53]. This is primary hyperalgesia. The areas of secondary hyperalgesia will include undamaged tissues either in the same viscus or in another viscus, so-called viscero-visceral hyperalgesia, or on the body wall in the area of referral (viscero-somatic hyperalgesia). These mechanisms for IBS symptoms can be considered to originate in abnormal peripheral nociceptive processing. The question then arises, how do these results fit with the theories on brain function expounded above?

### iv) Visceral Protection – Interpreting Disparate Results

Clinically the viscera are the most protected of our tissues except for the male sexual organs, but even they move inward in a cold threatening environment. In contrast, the limbs are exposed regularly to trauma. For flight and fight responses the viscera are almost all deprived of blood in order for the sympathetic nervous system to switch on energy supply to skeletal and cardiac muscles. For species protection reproductive function is likewise dominant with nervous system control of sexual function and parturition. In laboratory studies such a coordinated methodological approach that includes whole body responses is rare. Even clinical medical specialties have become system targeted (e.g. urology, gastroenterology, gynaecology) so that a broad diagnostic approach to capture viscero-visceral interactions is unusual. Hence the pain clinician may have to make therapeutic choices for patients that are cross-specialties and cross-systems. One of the key points that we make in our analysis of gender-related treatments is highly applicable to this conundrum [54]. It is that a multimodal approach is likely to be more effective than a single mode. The challenge is to select the best combinations for an individual patient based on hypothesis-driven research, on patient's choice (influenced by cognition, gender, sociocultural and other factors) and response to therapies. The greatest threat for chronic pain patients and especially women is for their pain to be considered normal (i.e. 'reproductive' in origin) and symptomatic treatment offered rather than mechanism-based therapies.

## Back Pain

Back pain is one of the commonest pain conditions both within communities and across hospital referral networks. Apart from gender, other risk factors are also strong predictors of back pain e.g. economic and occupational. In the transition from acute to chronic back pain gender-related causes predominate such as cognition (e.g. beliefs), behaviour (coping, alcohol abuse) and emotion (anxiety, stress). For example, a person who is highly anxious often focuses on a stimulus and amplifies their response to it, so-called hypervigilance as described above for IBS. Thus fear of potential injury may lead to inactivity that in turn leads to stiffness, muscle weakness and imbalance. In women back pain commonly occurs during pregnancy when significant hormonally induced changes occur in the musculoskeletal system. The addition of muscle hyperalgesia of visceral origin (see Table 1) adds to these female-related factors. When pain becomes chronic many patients are referred to pain clinics. In multidisciplinary clinics there has been a shift of emphasis from providing pharmacological pain relief with strong analgesics to improving cognitive, behavioural and emotional functions. In a descriptive study of 240 chronic pain patients with back pain, pain severity, disability and opioid use was compared between males and females [55]. Opioid use was related to disability and not pain severity, but of those who used opioids, the affective distress of men was significantly higher than women.

One of the puzzles of laboratory animal research has been why some animals develop neuropathic pain behaviours after nerve lesions and others do not. However, when back pain has a pathological origin in nerve root damage a gender perspective may not be anticipated because an intervention to prevent further damage is indicated. Nevertheless, the role of sex and genetic factors has recently been investigated in a rodent lumbar radiculopathy model [56]. Interestingly it was not the nature of the injury that determined the pain response but the strain of rodent and its sex, such that female Sprague Dawley and Long Evans rats demonstrated increased hypersensitivity compared with males of the same strain. Thus the pathological causes of back pain may have to be re-examined in humans and where nerve damage may be present, genetic factors including sex may be a key elements in diagnosis. Hence painful or non-painful presentations of somatic (or visceral) dysfunction may be relevant to gender-based investigations.

# Therapies

Laboratory research fails to recognise system failures and health care professional behaviours that may have a significant gender bias even when evidence on gender differences in pain mechanisms is substantial. Some of the possible barriers to adequate pain relief are listed in Table 2. They have been relatively under-researched and exist outside the research framework for drug discovery yet they may offer substantial gender-related effects on patient therapies. Some of these cognitive and behavioural issues have become well recognised through population studies as described below.

**Table 2. Barriers to adequate pain relief**

|   | Description | Gender issues |
|---|---|---|
| Physician | - Lack of communication<br>- Lack of knowledge about opioids<br>- 'Opiophobia' -negative attitude to prescribing opioids<br>- Inadequate pain assessment skills | - Male patients may not acknowledge cognitive dysfunction<br>- Prescribing habits may differ with gender<br>- Gender-related attitudes and beliefs may influence choice of analgesic<br>- Pain variation with hormonal changes may not be recognised |
| Patient | - Lack of communication<br>- Fears of addiction | - Males do not present so frequently as females with pain<br>- Possible effect on use of patient controlled analgesia (females>males) |
| Health Care | - Regulatory scrutiny | - Male physicians have more commonly than females been subject to regulatory scrutiny in the UK |

## A. Pharmacoepidemiology

Patterns of prescription medications for the top 15 used drugs in the US indicate that it is at adolescence when gender differences appear and the number of prescriptions for analgesics become higher for females than males [57]. This result is not unexpected given the alterations in endogenous gonadal hormones at puberty and the beginning of menstrual-related pains in women. In a cross sectional Scottish survey of over 1500 patients, non-prescription analgesics (mainly drug combinations) accounted for a quarter of over the counter sales and 59% of self-medicated drugs were analgesics [58]. Female sex was a significant predictor of drug use in this study. The conclusions highlighted (1) the use of multiple analgesics that could lead to potential interactions between analgesics and also with other drugs; (2) over the counter drugs were being used to supplement those used by health care practitioners to treat pain; and (3) improved pharmacovigilance was needed in pain management. In a larger cross sectional population survey from Sweden, almost twice as many women as men had used analgesics in the two weeks previous to the survey; this increased use was related to pain severity but not to an overall increase in pain complaints [59]. Again the contribution of these results to the risks of adverse effects of analgesics in women was highlighted.

There are few studies of pain management that combine drugs or compare combinations of pharmacological and behavioural therapies yet population studies indicate that in the community patients take more than one type of drug. A laboratory based trial of an anticholinergic medication (hyoscine-N-butylbromide) with a non-steroidal anti-inflammatory agent (ketoprofen) to treat muscle hyperalgesia of ureteric origin reduced pain behaviours with the combined therapy compared when the two drugs were used alone [60]. A popular combination for mild to moderate pain management is that of codeine (an opioid because of its metabolism to morphine) and acetaminophen (paracetamol) yet there are few clinical trials in chronic pain and none specifically focussed on identifying gender differences.

Even in hospitals pain may be largely untreated despite access to many types of analgesics. In a large in-patient study, 91% of hospitalised patients had pain complaints yet only 29% received analgesic medication and of these there were more women than men (Odds Ratio 1.33) [61]. Opioid drugs are a group of analgesic drugs that are more often prescribed in hospitals than in the community. Gender-related studies of their use in the clinical setting have been based on postoperative rather than chronic pain. However, for spinal injury patients where the pain intensity is similar in males and females, there is an increased use of opioids in female patients [62]. One difficulty in studying gender effects in a spinal injury group is that the ages of the patients are not comparable since young men and older women have spinal cord injuries from different pathologies. A study of osteoarthritis in older male and female patients (n = 11298) may be more relevant to assessing prescribing habits [63]. Although both males and females were prescribed non-steroidal anti-inflammatory drugs, female patients were prescribed a significant amount more and had a greater total supply than males even when confounding risk factors were controlled for. Questions on gender-based prescribing were raised by the researchers such as what are the reasons for the gender variations and what impact does this type of behaviour have on outcome and quality of pain management. Until this research is completed a clinician should not only consider the gender-based evidence from clinical trials but also have cognisance for their own behaviour towards male and female pain patients.

## B) Analgesics

Extensive reviews of sex differences and analgesics have identified gonadal hormone and other effects on mu and kappa opioid responsiveness [64, 65, 66]. One of the key species differences that has an important translational interpretation is that male rodents have greater analgesic responses to morphine whereas male humans show less than females. Although rodent strain differences, a bias in pain measures and stimuli type may be responsible for part of the preclinical results, the combined evidence from multiple laboratories is this one-way sex difference. Another species difference is that the active glucuronide metabolites of morphine, morphine-3-glucuronide (M3G) and morphine-6-glucuronide (M6G) are both formed in humans but only M6G in rodents [67]. M3G in humans may have no analgesic action and may even antagonise morphine analgesia; this is in contrast with M6G, which has a potency similar to or greater than that of morphine. Hence if morphine is administered systemically to animals the active opioid profile may differ considerably from that in humans. Accordingly, results from opioid analgesia in animals should be cautiously translated into human research. Human volunteer studies have attempted to clarify some of these issues. One pharmacokinetic study observed gender differences in the contribution of M6G to morphine analgesia [68]. Another study of morphine on experimental pain found no sex differences with heat, pressure and ischaemic noxious stimuli but females reported more side effects than males [69]. A further volunteer study of M6G alone has not identified sex differences in pharmacodynamics [70]. The possible pharmacodynamic mechanisms for morphine gender-related differences in analgesia and adverse reactions not only include metabolic products but also receptor availability, type and site. The growing clinical use of opioids for a long-term use may generate hypothesis-driven studies to test which of these mechanisms predominate in disease populations as well as volunteers. It appears from epidemiological studies that in long term pain conditions, women require more analgesia than men. It is possible that the long term use of analgesic drugs in chronic pain may contrast with short term administration and produce different pharmacokinetic and pharmacodynamic gender-related effects.

In humans there are temporal effects of opioids, some of which can be repeatedly demonstrated in postoperative pain management. Following a review of the overall results from 18 studies it was concluded that females consumed less opioids than males on the days after surgery [64]. A missing variable was the amount of pain experienced. Thus a prospective study was initiated to measure both pain intensity and opioid consumption. The result confirmed the original observation and also that pain intensity was comparable between the gender groups [71]. These studies however are in contrast with those conducted immediately after surgery in the recovery period from anaesthesia where females wake earlier than males. At this time women experience more pain and require more morphine than men to achieve the same degree of analgesia [72, 73]. In a younger population of 12-18 year old adolescents, gender differences in pain and its relief were measured after surgery such that the amount of opioid use was the same, but it was the preoperative anticipation of pain that was associated with more postoperative pain in women and not in men [74]. These results may be used to design strategies to reduce postoperative pain through coping mechanisms.

## C) Multidisciplinary Care

Evidence for gender-related effects on the outcome of multidisciplinary care is now accumulating. One of the earlier studies was randomised and observer blind and compared intensive exercises with conventional physiotherapy or control measures for the treatment of low back pain [75]. The women improved best with the intensive exercises and the men with conventional physiotherapy. One of the observations on the differences in the groups, apart from gender, was that the men had more physically demanding jobs. After work-related injury, exercise combined with psychological behaviour therapy was administered to 1827 patients. The sites of the injuries were different; women had more neck and men more lower back injuries. After one year's follow up the men had better outcomes for disability, physical fitness and psychosocial effects [76]. In another prospective cohort study of a mixed group of chronic pain clinic patients, measures taken after an intensive in-patient course recorded differences in pain and distress scores between men and women at three month's follow up [77]. The men had maintained their improvement whereas women reported the same pain and distress as prior to the course. In a specific group of patients with chronic spinal pain a randomised placebo controlled multi-centre trial of cognitive behavioural therapy compared with control or physical therapy found that women had a better outcome as measured with the SF36 and quality of life questionnaires than men [78]. The same group more recently reported a similarly designed study with three year follow up of outcomes for back and neck pain which also included a fourth full time therapy group with combined cognitive behavioural therapy and physical therapy [79]. This latter group was most effective in women not only for psychological assessments but also for cost-effectiveness.

Laboratory research as outlined above in the sections on brain imaging would indicate that the cognitive and behavioural aspects of pain management are rapidly gaining recognition. It is only recently that the results of randomised controlled studies of gender differences in multidisciplinary care have been available. Major confounding factors in chronic pain studies are the difficulties in controlling for similar patient groups and the stability of populations for an adequate length of follow up for outcome measures. Important outcomes for the patient include pain, mood and disability but others relating to cost-effectiveness are applicable for both the patient and health care systems. Multidisciplinary health care may only be funded if the outcome is positive. Hence employment issues are a recurring theme in most of these studies and the observed gender differences often reflect social inequality. Thus studies at some stage will have to reconcile these confounding factors in order to achieve definitive benefits.

# Conclusion

Gender-related factors contribute to chronic pain management in many ways. The numbers of women seeking health care are higher than men and although this demand is often for drug-based therapies, analgesics are disproportionately available to women. This effect may be systems based rather than patient led and more research is needed into prescribing habits. The behaviours and beliefs of professionals are also relevant to the development and application of diagnostic criteria for chronic pain conditions that have multiple symptoms.

Laboratory research has identified mechanisms for pain that may apply to human pain states although more appropriate models would be welcomed. Many mechanisms may be categorised as sex- and gender-related but these terms overlap in clinical practice. The mechanisms include gonadal hormone modulation, neuroendocrine and autonomic nervous system functions, affective, psychosocial, familial, cognitive and behavioural activity, anatomical, physiological and genomic effects that interact not only in the nervous system but also in other body systems. A clinical approach has to be multidisciplinary in order to define and select the relevant therapies.

# References

[1] Fillingim, R. *Sex, Gender, and Pain*. Seattle: International Association for the Study of Pain Press; 2000.

[2] Becker, JB; Arnold, AP; Berkley, KJ. et al. Strategies and methods for research on sex differences in brain and behaviour. *Endocrinology.* 2005, 146, 1650-1673.

[3] Wizemann, TM: Pardue, M-L. Eds. *Exploring the Biological Contributions to Human Health.* Does sex matter? Washington: National Academy Press; 2001, page 13.

[4] Heitkemper, M; Jarrett, M; Bond, EF; et al. Impact of sex and gender on irritable bowel syndrome, *Biological Research for Nursing* 2003, 5, 56-65.

[5] Talley, NJ. Diagnosing an irritable bowel: does sex matter? *Gastroenterology.* 1991, 100, 834-837.

[6] Corney, RH: Stanton, R. Physical symptom severity, psychological and social dysfunction in a series of outpatients with irritable bowel syndrome. *J. Psychosom. Res.* 1990, 34, 483-491.

[7] Taub, E; Cuevas, JL; Cook, EW; Crowell, M; Whitehead, WE. Irritable bowel syndrome defined by factor analysis. Gender and race comparisons. *Dig. Dis. Sci.* 1995, 40, 2647-2655.

[8] Heitkemper, MM; Cain, KC; Jarrett, ME: et al. Symptoms across the menstrual cycle in women with irritable bowel syndrome. *American Journal of Gastroenterology.* 2003, 98, 420-430.

[9] Isacson, D; Bingefors K. Epidemiology of analgesic use: a gender perspective. *European Journal of Anaesthesiology.* Supplement 2002, 26, 5 –15.

[10] Nabiloff, BD; Heitkemper, MM; Chang, L; Mayer, EA. Sex and Gender in Irritable Bowel Syndrome. Chapter 16 in *Sex, Gender, and Pain*. Fillingim, R., Ed.: Seattle, IASP Press, Seattle, 2000, 327-353.

[11] Camilleri, M; Mayer, EA; Drossman, DA, Heath, A; Dukes, GE; McSorley et al. Improvement in pain and bowel function in female irritable bowel patients with alosetron, a 5-HT3 receptor antagonist. *Alimentary Pharmacology and Therapeutics* 1999, 13, 1149-1159.

[12] Baker, DE. Tegaserod for the treatment of constipation-predominant irritable bowel syndrome. *Rev. Gastroenterol. Disord.* 2001,1, 187-198.

[13] Bethea, CL; Lu, ZN; Gundlah, C; Streicher, JM. Diverse actions of ovarian steroids in the serotonin neural system. *Frontiers in Neuroendocrinology.* 2002, 23, 41-100.

[14] Holdcroft, A; Snidvongs, S; Cason, A. et al. Pain and uterine contractions during breast feeding in the immediate post-partum period increases with parity. *Pain.* 2003, 104, 589-596.

[15] Craft, RM. Sex differences in drugs and non-drug induced analgesia. *Life Sciences.* 2003, 72, 2675-2688.

[16] Mogil, J.S.: Chesler, E.J.: Wilson, S.G. et al. Sex differences in thermal nociception and morphine antinociception in rodents depend on genotype. *Neurosci. Biobehav. Rev.* 2000, *24*, 375-325.

[17] Sternberg, W.F.: Mogil, J.S.: Kest, B.et al. Neonatal testosterone exposure influences neurochemistry of swim-induced analgesia in adult mice. *Pain.* 1996, 63, 321-326.

[18] Mogil, J.S.: Wilson, S.G.: Chesler, E.J. et al. The melanocortin-1 receptor gene mediates female-specific mechanisms of analgesia in mice and humans. *Proc. Natl. Acad. Sci.* USA 2003, 100, 4867-4872.

[19] Kern, MK; Jaradeh S, Arndorfer, RC, Jesmanowicz, A; Hyde, J; Shaker, R. Gender differences in cortical representation of rectal distension in healthy humans. *Am. J. Physiol. Gastrointest. Liver. Physiol.* 2001, 281, G1512-1523.

[20] Nabiloff, BD; Berman, S; Chang, L; Derbyshire, SWG; Suyenobu, B; Vogt, BA. et al. Sex-related differences in IBS patients: central processing of visceral stimuli. *Gastroenterology.* 2003, 124, 1738-1747.

[21] Tillisch, K; Mayer, EA; Labus, JS; Stains, J; Chang, L; Naliboff, BD. IBS have altered autonomic responsiveness to visceral stressor. *Gut.* 2005, 54, 1396-1401.

[22] Holdcroft, A; Sapsed-Byrne, S; Ma, D; Hammal, D; Forsling, M.L. Sex and oestrous cycle differences in visceromotor responses and vasopressin release in response to colonic distension in male and female rats anaesthetised with halothane. *British Journal of Anaesthesia.* 2000, 85, 907-910.

[23] Mayer, EA. The neurobiology of stress and gastrointestinal disease. *Gut.* 2000, 47, 861-869.

[24] Berkley, KJ. A life of pelvic pain. *Physiology and Behavior.* 2005, 86, 272-280.

[25] Fillingim, RB; Maixner, W. Gender differences in the responses to noxious stimuli. *Pain Forum.* 1995, 4, 209-221.

[26] Kuhn, FE; Rackley, CE. Coronary artery disease in women. Risk factor evaluation, treatment and prevention. *Archives of Internal Medicine.* 1993, 36, 2626-2636.

[27] Herlitz,J; Bang,A; Karlson,BW. Is there a gender difference in aetiology of chest pain and symptoms associated with acute myocardial infarction? *European Journal of Emergency Medicine.* 1999, 6, 311-315.

[28] Giamberardino, M.A. Sex differences in visceral pain. In *Sex, gender and pain.* Fillingim, R., Ed.: IASP Press, Seattle, 2000; 135-163.

[29] Berkley, KJ. Multiple mechanism of pelvic pain: lessons from basic research. In: MacLean, AB; Stones, RW. Thornton, S. Eds. *Pain in obstetrics and gynecology.* RCOG Press, London, 2001, 26-39.

[30] Giamberardino, M.A. Referred muscle pain/hyperalgesia and central sensitization. *J. Rehab. Med.* 2003, 41 suppl., 85-88.

[31] Giamberardino, MA; Berkley, KB; Affaitati, G; Lerza, R; Centurione, L; Lapenna, D. et al. Influence of endometriosis on pain behaviors and muscle hyperalgesia induced by ureteral calculosis in female rats. *Pain.* 2002, 95, 247-257.

[32] Whitehead, WE; Palsson, O; Jones, KR. Systematic review of the comorbidity of irritable bowel syndrome with other disorders: what are the causes and implications? *Gastroenterology.* 2002, 122, 1140-1156.

[33] Chang, L; Berman, S; Mayer, EA; Suyenobu, B; Derbyshire, S; Naliboff, B; Vogt, B; Fitzgerald, L; Mandelkern, MA. Brain responses to visceral and somatic stimuli in patients with irritable bowel syndrome with and without fibromyalgia. *American Journal of Gastroenterology.* 2003, 98, 1354-1361.

[34] Kwan, CL; Diamant, NE; Pope, G; Mikula, K; Mikulis, DJ; Davis, KD. Abnormal forebrain activity in functional bowel disorder patients with chronic pain. *Neurology.* 2005, 65, 1268-1277.

[35] Forslund, L; Hjemdahl, P; Held, C; Bjorkander, I; Eriksson, SV; Rehnqvist, N. Ischaemia during exercise and ambulatory monitoring in patients with stable angina pectoris and healthy controls. Gender differences and relationships to catecholamines. *European Heart Journal.* 1998, 19, 535-537.

[36] Clemens, JQ; Meenan, RT; O'Keeffe Rosetti, MC; Brown, SO; Gao, SY; Calhoun, EA. Prevalence of interstitial cystitis symptoms in a managed care population. *Journal of Urology.* 2005, 174, 576-580.

[37] Mayer, EA; Bernam, S; Chang, L; Naliboff, BD. Sex-based differences in gastrointestinal pain. *European Journal of Pain.* 2004, 8, 451-463.

[38] Lubrano, E; Iovino, P; Tremolattera, F; Parsons, WJ; Ciacci, C; Mazzacca, G. Fibromyalgia in patients with irritable bowel syndrome. An association with the severity of the intestinal disorder. *International Journal of Colorectal Disease.* 2001, 16, 211-215.

[39] Frissora, CL; Koch, KI. Symptom overlap and comorbidity of irritable bowel syndrome with other conditions. *Current Gastroenterology Reports.* 2005, 7, 264-271.

[40] Berkley, KJ; Hubscher, CH; Wall, PD. Neuronal responses to stimulation of the cervix, uterus, colon and skin in the rat spinal cord. *Journal of Neurophysiology.* 1993, 69, 533-544.

[41] Enochsson, L; Lindberg, B; Swahnm F; Arnelo, U. Intraoperative endoscopic retrograde cholangiopancreatography (ERCP) to remove common bile duct stones

during routine laparoscopic cholecystectomy does not prolong hospitalisation: a 2-year experience. *Surgical Endoscopy.* 2004, 18, 367-371.
[42] Berkley, KJ. Sex differences in pain. *Behavioral Brain Research.* 1997, 20, 371-380.
[43] Taylor, TV; Rimmer, S; Holt, S; Jeacock, J; Lucas, S. Sex differences in gallstone pancreatitis. *Annals of Surgery.* 1991, 214, 667-670.
[44] Giamberardino, MA. Recent and forgotten aspects of visceral pain. *European Journal of Pain.* 1999, 3, 77-92.
[45] Foreman, RD. Mechanisms of cardiac pain. *Ann. Rev. Physiol.* 1999, 61, 143-147.
[46] Roza, C; Laird, JM; Cervero, F. Spinal mechanisms underlying persistent pain and referred hyperalgesia in rats with an experimental ureteric stone. *Neurophysiology.* 1998, 79, 1603-1612.
[47] Giamberardino, MA; Affaitati, G; Valente, R; et al. Changes in visceral pain reactivity as a function of estrous cycle in female rats with artificial ureteral calculosis. *Brain Research.* 1997, 74, 234-238.
[48] Giamberardino, MA; Laurentis, S; Affaitati, G; Lerza, R; Lapenna, D, Vecchiet, L. Modulation of pain and hyperalgesia from the urinary tract by alogenic conditions of the reproductive organs in women. *Neuroscience Letters.* 2001, 304, 61-64.
[49] Powell-Boone, T; Ness, TJ; Cannon, R; Lloyd, LK; Weigent, DA; Fillingim, RB. Menstrual cycle affects bladder pain sensation in subjects with interstitial cystitis. *Journal of Urology.* 2005, 174, 1832-1836.
[50] Kusek, JW; Nyberg, LM. The epidemiology of interstitial cystitis: is it time to expand our definition? *Urology.* 2001, 57, 95-99.
[51] Cevero, F. Sensory innervation of the viscera: peripheral basis of visceral pain. *Physiological Reviews.* 1994, 74, 95-138.
[52] Cevero, F; Laird, JMA. Visceral pain. *Lancet.* 1999, 353, 2145-2148.
[53] Mayer, EA; Naliboff, BD; Chang, L. Basic pathophysiologic mechanisms in irritable bowel syndrome. *Digestive Diseases.* 2001, 19, 212-218.
[54] Holdcroft, A; Berkley, KJ. *"Sex and Gender Differences in Pain and its Relief"* for the 5th Edition of the 'Wall and Melzack's Textbook of Pain' Chapter 75, Eds S. McMahon and M. Koltzenburg (Elsevier Churchill Livingstone, Edinburgh) 2006 pages 1181-1197.
[55] Fillingim, RB; Doleys, DM; Edwards, RR; Lowery, D. Clinical characteristics of chronic back pain as a function of gender and oral opioid use. *Spine.* 2003, 28, 143-150.
[56] LaCroix-Fralish, ML; Rutkowski, MD; Weinstein JN; Mogil, JS; Deleo, JA. The magnitude of mechanical allodynia in a rodent model of lumber radiculopathy is dependent on strain and sex. *Spine.* 2005, 30, 1821-1827.
[57] Roe, CM; McNamara, AM, Motheral, BR. Gender- and age-related prescription drug use patterns. *Annals Pharmacotherpautics.* 2002, 36, 30-39.
[58] Porteus, T; Bond, C; Hannford, P; Sinclair, H. How and why are non-prescription analgesics used in Scotland? *Family Practitioner.* 2005, 22, 78-85.
[59] Isacson, D; Bingefors, K. Epidemiology of analgesic use: a gender perspective. *European Journal of Anaesthesiology.* Supplement 2002, 26, 5 – 15.

[60] Giamberardino, MA; Valente, R; DeBigontina, P; Iezzi, S; Vecchiet, L. Effects of spasmolytic and/or non-steroidal anti-inflammatory drugs on muscle hyperalgesia of ureteral origin in rats. *European Journal of Pharmacology.* 1995, 278, 97-101.

[61] Visentin, M; Zanolin, E; Trentin, L; Sartori, S; deMarco, R. Prevalence and treatment of pain in adults admitted to Italian hospitals. *European Journal of Pain.* 2005, 9, 61-67.

[62] Noorbrink Budh, C; Lund, I; Hultling, C; Levi, R; Werhagen, L; Ertzgaard, P; Lundeberg, T. Gender related differences in pain in spinal cord injured individuals. *Spinal Cord.* 2003, 41, 122-128.

[63] Dominick, KL; Ahern, FM; Gold, CH; Heller, DA. Gender differences in NSAID use among older adults with osteoarthritis. *Annals of Pharmacotherapeutics.* 2003, 37, 1566-1571.

[64] Miaskowski, C; Gear, RW; Levine, JD. Sex-related differences in analgesic responses. In *Sex, Gender, and Pain. Progress in Pain Research and Management.* Vol 17 Fillingim, RB, Ed. Seattle, IASP Press 2000, 209-230.

[65] Craft, RM; Mogil, JS; Aloisi, AM. Sex differences in pain and analgesia: the role of gonadal hormones. *European Journal of Pain.* 2004, 8, 397-411.

[66] Fillingim, RB; Gear, RW. Sex differences in opioid analgesia: clinical and experimental findings. *European Journal of Pain.* 2004, 8, 413-425.

[67] Milne, RW; Nation, RL; Somogyi, AA. The disposition of morphine and its 3- and 6-glucuronide metabolites in humans and animals and the importance of the metabolites to the pharmacological effects of morphine. *Drug Metabolism Review.* 1996, 28, 345-472.

[68] Murthy, BR; Pollack, GM; Brouwer, KL. Contribution of morphine-6-glucuronide to antinociception following intravenous administration of morphine to healthy volunteers. *Journal of Clinical Pharmacology.* 2002;42, 569-576.

[69] Fillingim, RB; Ness, TJ; Glover, TL; Campbell, CM; Hastie, BA; Price, DD; Staud, R. Morphine responses and experimental pain: sex differences in side effects and cardiovascular responses but not analgesia. *Journal of Pain.* 2005, 6, 116-124.

[70] Romberg, R; Olofsen, E; Sarton, E; den Hartigh, J; Taschner, PE; Dahan, A. Pharmacokinetic-pharmacodynamic modelling of morphine-6-glucuronide-induced analgesia in healthy volunteers: absence of sex differences. *Anesthesiology.* 2004, 100, 120-133.

[71] Chia, YY; Chow, LH; Hung, CC; Liu, K; Ger, LP; Wang, PN. Gender and pain upon movement are associates with the requirements for postoperative patient-controlled iv analgesia: a prospective survey of 2298 Chinese patients. *Canadian Journal of Anaesthesia.* 2002, 49, 249-255.

[72] Capada, MS; Carr, DB. Women experience more pain and require more morphine than men to achieve a similar degree of analgesia. *Anesthesia and Analgesia* 2003, 97, 1464-1468.

[73] Aubrun, F; Salvi, N; Coriat, P; Riou, B. Sex- and age-related differences in morphine requirements for postoperative pain relief. *Anesthesiology.* 2002, 103, 156-160.

[74] Logan, DE; Rose, JB. Gender differences in postoperative pain and patient controlled analgesia use among adolescent surgical patients. *Pain.* 2004, 109, 481-487.

[75] Hansen, FR; Bendix, T; Skov, P; Jensen, CV; Kristensen, JH, Krohn, L; Schioeler, H. Intensive, dynamic back muscle exercises, conventional physiotherapy or placebo control treatment of low-back pain. *Spine.* 1993, 18, 98-108.

[76] McGreary, DD; Mayer, TG; Gatchel, RJ; Anagnostis, C; Proctor, TJ. Gender-related differences in treatment outcomes for patients with musculoskeletal disorders. *Spine.* 2003, 3, 197-302.

[77] Keogh, E; McCraken, LM; Eccleston, C. Do men and women differ in their response to interdisciplinary chronic pain management? *Pain.* 2005, 114, 37-46.

[78] Jensen, IB; Bergstrom, G; Ljungquist, T; Bodin, L; Nygren, AL. A randomised controlled component analysis of a behavioural medicine rehabilitation programme for chronic spinal pain, are the effects dependent on gender? *Pain* .2001, 91, 65-78.

[79] Jensen, IB; Bergstrom, G; Ljungquist, T; Bodin, L. A 3-year follow-up of a multidisciplinary rehabilitation programme for back and neck pain. *Pain.* 2005, 115, 273-283.

*Chapter XVI*

# Clinical Management of Cancer Pain

*Anca Popescu[1] and E. Daniela Hord[2]*
[1]Robert Wood Johnson Medical School, USA
[2]Massachusetts General Hospital and Harvard Medical School, USA

## Abstract

Management of cancer pain has evolved into a separate subspecialty of medicine and requires a thorough understanding of the pathophysiology and prognosis of the tumor. This chapter is a brief overview for pain researcheres of available cancer pain treatment modalities: opioid and non-opioid analgesics, radiopharmaceuticals, radiation therapy and surgery. This chapter will focus less on the doses of each medication and more on the benefits and shortcomings of each treatment modality and on the combination therapy for the cancer pain management.

## Introduction

Treatment of cancer pain has evolved in the last decades from a palliative to a mechanism-based approach while the molecular mechanisms of pain and pain modulation are being deciphered. Advances in knowledge at the level of nociceptive receptors, ion channels, nociceptive pathways and modulators have led to more effective treatment of pain, increases in life expectancy and life quality. Whereas tumor resection is not solely effective in pain relief, a multi-modality approach tailored to the specific type of tumor offers the best chances of a symptom-free survival.

# Pharmacologic Treatment of Cancer Pain

## Non-Opioid Analgesics

Unlike opioids, non-opioid medications do not cause physiologic dependence, but they may have ceiling effects (in contrast to the opioids). They are often used for their synergism with opioids, allowing lower doses of each agent to be administered. This may reduce the potential toxicity of each agent. Those patients who do not respond to one first-line analgesic can be switched to another, or another co-analgesic agent with a different mechanism of action can be added.

*1) Non-steroidal anti-inflammatory drugs (NSAIDs)* are useful additives to the opioids in patients with metastatic bone disease. NSAIDS are widely prescribed and often provide real benefit. However, since it is common for liver or kidney function to be impaired in cancer patients, caution must be used when prescribing these medications.

Ketorolac is the only NSAID that can be given parenterally for analgesia in the USA. This medication is rarely used in a chronic pain, but it is useful for the short-term management of acute pain and is as efficacious as morphine for mild to moderate pain.

There are two classes of NSAIDs on the market at this time, the non-selective COX inhibitors (e.g. aspirin, ibuprofen, naproxen sodium) and the COX 2 selective inhibitors or *coxibs* (currently, from this class, only celecoxib is in use). The non-selective group causes a higher incidence of side effects related to gastric distress and platelet dysfunction. Celecoxib causes fewer gastrointestinal adverse effects. NSAIDs are still being assessed in cancer patients. Recently they have been associated with adverse thrombotic effects such as myocardial infarction and stroke, so their use is under intense scrutiny at present. Their risks are still uncertain, and it remains unclear whether they should be replaced.

*2) Acetaminophen* is a useful analgesic and anti-pyretic, but should be avoided in patients with impaired liver function since it is potentially hepatotoxic. Combinations of NSAIDs, acetaminophen and opioids have an opioid sparing effect [1]. It should be used as single agent in mild pain or added to the opioid regimen (in an attempt to decrease the opioid requirement if their side effects are significant). Various combinations of acetaminophen, opioids and non-opioid agents are commercially available, and when the total daily dose of acetaminophen is calculated, these have to be considered. Acute ingestion by an adult of 7.5-10 grams/day of acetaminophen, chronic ingestion of 4 grams/day or more than 2.5 grams/day (while also consuming 2 ounces of alcohol) may lead to hepatic failure [2].

*3) Tramadol* is a modulator of descending inhibitory pathways, a weak opioid agonist with selective serotonin reuptake inhibitor (SSRI)-like properties. It is used for mild to moderate pain, especially for patients who do not wish to take opioids. It is occasionally useful for severe pain in combination with other non-opioid analgesics and/or adjuncts in patients who cannot tolerate opioids. It is known to lower seizure thresholds so it must be used with caution in patients with seizure disorders or brain pathology. Tramadol competes for protein binding sites and may potentiate the effects of coumadin. It should also be avoided in combination with tricyclics, selective serotonin reuptake inhibitors and dextromethorphan.

*4) Anticonvulsants* are currently used in an effort to manage refractory neuropathic pain. At the present time, gabapentin has the most evidence base in cancer pain [3]. This drug is an anticonvulsant with an obscure primary mechanism of action, possibly interacting with alpha subunit of N-type calcium channels. It has a proven efficacy in different neuropathic pain syndromes associated with cancer [3, 4]. It has a good adverse effect profile, is not metabolized in the liver, and has no known drug-drug interactions. Treatment usually starts at with 100-300 mg per day, and dose titration usually continues until benefit occurs, side effects supervene, or the total daily dose is at least 3600 mg per day. Some patients respond to 600 mg per day in divided doses, whereas others do not reach a maximal response until the dose is increased to 3600 mg per day, or more.

Most of the anticonvulsant drugs other than gabapentin have been used off-label for neuropathic pain: carbamazepine, oxcarbazepine, phenytoin, valproic acid, clonazepam, lamotrigine, topiramate, tiagabine, zonisamide and levetiracetam. All anticonvulsants are administered using the dosing schedules typically employed for treatment of epilepsy. More details about ion channel blockers are discussed in a separate chapter in this volume.

*5) Corticosteroids* have beneficial multifaceted effects in cancer, including analgesic, appetite stimulant, antiemetic, and improve the sense of well being and overall quality of life [5]. They decrease edema around neural tissues, therefore are useful in painful plexopathies associated with cancer invasion, metastatic bone pain and pain associated with stretching of liver capsule [6]. Current data are inadequate to evaluate drug-selective differences, dose-response relationships, predictors of efficacy, or the durability of favorable effects. Because the risk of adverse effects increases with both the dose and duration of use, long-term therapy usually involves the administration of relatively low doses to patients with advanced disease, whose overriding need for symptom control justifies the risk. Typically, prednisone, 5 to 10 mg, or dexamethasone, 1 to 2 mg, is administered once or twice daily. Dose escalation for worsening symptoms is appropriate if benefits decline with progressive disease, particularly at the end of life.

Another approach to corticosteroid therapy is a high dose regimen, which may be suitable for selected patients with severe pain. The usual scenario is the occurrence of rapidly worsening pain related to a nerve injury. This high dose regimen may begin with dexamethasone 24-100 mg intravenously, followed by 6-24 mg daily and can be given once a day due to the long half-life [1]. This dose is gradually tapered over weeks as an alternative analgesic approach is implemented.

*6) Antagonists at the N-Methyl-D-aspartate (NMDA) receptor* are undergoing intensive investigation [7-10]. Four such drugs, the dissociative anesthetic ketamine, the antitussive dextromethorphan, memantine and the antiviral amantadine, already are commercially available in the United States. Memantine is available in many other countries, and is mainly prescribed for dementia although literature supports its effect on neuropathic pain as well. Ketamine has a difficult side effect profile, which includes nightmares and hallucinations, but its efficacy in some challenging patients with neuropathic pain has encouraged its use, either by continuous infusion or by oral administration, in highly selected patients [2]. Similarly, dextromethorphan has been used at relatively high daily doses to treat refractory neuropathic pain. The starting dose, which can be as high as 120 to 240 mg/d in 3 to 4 divided doses, can be increased gradually and doses higher than 1 g have been administered safely; it is likely that the analgesic dose will be at least 350 mg per day. Experience with amantadine as an analgesic is very limited.

*7) Antidepressant drugs* are nonspecific analgesics and are used primarily for neuropathic pain. In cancer pain they are useful for pain associated with surgery, radiation therapy, chemotherapy or pain due to malignant nerve infiltration [2]. The tricyclic antidepressants (TCAs) have been most extensively studied and there is strong evidence that both the tertiary amine TCAs (e.g., amitriptyline, doxepin and imipramine), and the secondary amine TCAs (e.g., desipramine and nortriptyline) can be effective. There are few controlled trials of other subclasses, but the extant data do support the analgesic efficacy of several SSRIs, such as paroxetine, and several drugs with noradrenergic effects or combined serotonin and noradrenergic effects, including maprotiline, venlafaxine, duloxetine and bupropion.

Although amitriptyline is the best studied TCA, it has a relatively high side effect liability and may not be well tolerated by many patients with serious medical comorbidities. A baseline EKG should be obtained prior to initiation of treatment to exclude patients with conduction abnormalities (bundle branch block, AV block, prolonged QT interval) [2]. Patients who are unable to tolerate amitriptyline, or are predisposed to its sedative, anticholinergic, or hypotensive effects, should be considered for a trial with a secondary amine TCA, such as desipramine. Given the relatively better side effect profile, trials of the newer antidepressants, such as one of the SSRIs, is appropriate for those who cannot tolerate a secondary amine TCA or are strongly predisposed to side effects from these drugs.

Antidepressants do not exert their therapeutic effects rapidly. Dose titration from a low starting dose is typically necessary, but the dose effective for pain relief is less than the antidepressant dose. The response to antidepressant drugs varies and sequential trials are warranted if pain remains refractory.

*8) Sympatholytic agents* are also be used in cancer pain. The alpha-2-adrenergic agonists, such as clonidine and tizanidine, have established analgesic efficacy in a variety of pain syndromes [11] and may be considered nonspecific analgesics. Like the antidepressants, they usually are considered as adjuvant analgesics for selected indications in medically ill populations. Clonidine is usually considered for refractory neuropathic pain, and tizanidine often is tried for neuropathic pain or pain due to muscle spasm. Given its better side effect profile, tizanidine is usually administered first. Epidurally-administered clonidine is effective in cancer pain and relatively more effective for neuropathic pain [12].

*9) Topical analgesic therapies* may particularly benefit medically ill patients with chronic pain by providing pain relief that complements a systemic analgesic regimen without the risk of additional side effects. Topical therapies include local anesthetics, NSAIDs, capsaicin, and other drugs [13].

Topical local anesthetics can be administered by patch or cream. A lidocaine 5% impregnated patch is approved for use in patients with postherpetic neuralgia [14]. This formulation is well accepted by patients and should be considered for any patient who is a candidate for topical local anesthetic therapy.

A 1:1 mixture of lidocaine and prilocaine known as EMLA (eutectic mixture of local anesthetics) can produce dense cutaneous anesthesia if applied thickly under an occlusive dressing. Cutaneous anesthesia may not be necessary to yield analgesic effects in patients with neuropathic pains, however, and patients can alternative methods of application, as well as pure lidocaine creams (e.g., lidocaine 5%).

There is evidence that topical NSAIDs can be effective for cancer pain [15-18] and the complications of cancer treatment and these drugs can be even administered via a subcutaneous route [15].

## Opioid Analgesics

Opioids are the mainstay of cancer pain treatment and their use can markedly improve the quality of life of cancer patients with pain. There is a concern among patients, families and practitioners that they can cause addiction, which is sometimes limiting the treatment options for these patients. In an effort to raise awareness of and functional pain management treatment protocols for the treatment of cancer pain, the World Health Organization (WHO) developed a step-wise treatment algorithm, which was widely disseminated around the world.

The "WHO analgesic ladder" is based on three steps which can be outlined as follows: *Step 1*: Start with non-opioid analgesics for mild pain; *Step 2:* Begin using opioids such as hydrocodone or codeine for mild to moderate pain, with or without non-opioid analgesics; and *Step 3:* Use the more potent opioids such as morphine or hydromorphone for moderate to severe pain, with or without non-opioid analgesics. Other adjuvant medications (see below) can be added at any step of the ladder.

Some practitioners worry that the ladder concept may be misconstrued such that all patients are treated with the same protocol despite differences in their pain level and mechanisms of pain. For example, some patients may present with severe pain and need to be treated at a higher step of the ladder rather than at step one. Obviously, the WHO analgesic ladder is meant to act as a guide, not a mandatory treatment schedule.

There is significant variability in the individual response to morphine due to variability in receptor function, which may be due to a single aminoacid substitution [19]. This may lead to variations in pain relief as well as in the side effects (sedation and respiratory depression [20]. In addition, genetic factors influence individual pain perception [21].

The most common side effects of opioids as a class are: constipation, sedation, nausea, vomiting, respiratory depression, myoclonus, hallucinations, confusion, sleep disturbances, pruritus, sexual dysfunction (amenorrhea, infertility in women and inability to attain or maintain an erection in men), and urinary retention [2].

Opioids may be used in combination in situations of opioid partial switches, to potentiate the response to one opioid with the second and to reduce the toxic side effects [22]. Combination opioids may desensitize opioid receptors (due to different receptor activation and endocytosis) and reduce tolerance (via NMDA receptors) [22]. Experimentally, in mice, the combination of morphine and methadone may be synergistic, whereas others (fentanyl, oxycodone, morphine, oxymorphone) are only additive [23].

*1) Morphine* is the first line treatment in cancer pain indicated by the World Health Organization due to multiple routes of administration, clinical experience, low cost and non-inferiority to other potent opioids [24]. However, it has poor oral availability, wide interindividual response variability and neurotoxic metabolites that accumulate especially in renal failure

*2) Hydromorphone* is equivalent to morphine in pain relief [25]. It causes less pruritus and sedation. It is renally excreted and is not superior to morphine in patients with renal failure [26]. It is available in oral and intravenous formulation. It can also be delivered through the subcutaneous infusion pump, intrathecally or rectally.

*3) Transdermal fentanyl* is the only opioid available in this form and allows a direct absorption from the skin into the bloodstream by bypassing the enterohepatic circulation. After absorption through the skin, it is deposited into the subcutaneous tissues and forms a reservoir. Thus, the therapeutic effect is seen between 12-16 hours. A steady state in the serum is achieved in 48 hours. Until this is achieved, the patients should have immediate-release opioids available. Similarly, when a patch is discontinued, the effects may be seen for another 12-16 hours. The conversion ratio between oral morphine and transdermal fentanyl can be 45-90 mg/day to 25 mcg/hour, supplying the medication for 72 hours [27, 28]. The advantages of transdermal fentanyl are: less constipation, daytime drowsiness and interference with daily activities [29] and increased safety in the setting of renal failure [30]. Some of these effects may be related to the bypassing the gastrointestinal tract, but more studies are needed to clarify this issue. Morphine is equally efficacious as transdermal fentanyl [31]

*4) Oral transmucosal fentanyl citrate* is in part rapidly absorbed through the oral mucosal into the bloodstream and in part swallowed and metabolized through the GI tract (and undergoes hepatic first pass). It is used for breakthrough pain in patients who are receiving more than 60 mg/day of morphine or 50 mcg/hr of transdermal fentanyl for seven days and are presumed to be tolerant to the opioid side effects [2]. The onset of analgesia may be as short as 5 minutes.

*5) Methadone* is the least expensive long-acting opioid and produces similar analgesia as morphine [32]. It is the safest opioid in renal failure [26]. It requires less dose escalation [33]. However, it has a long half life, drug interactions and complex pharmacokinetics [34].

Oral opioids are available as capsules, tablets, liquid forms, immediate and controlled-release formulations. Controlled release tablets (e.g. MSContin, OxyContin and Oramorph SR) do not allow crushing because they lose the long-acting effect and become immediate release. Kadian and Avinza (sustained-release morphine) can be opened and sprinkled on food or given through feeding tubes.

Rectal administration is useful in patients with nausea and vomiting or who are not allowed the oral route of administration immediately before or after a surgical procedure. The opioids can be placed in a colostomy bag if the outflow from the stoma is slow enough to allow mucosal absorption of the drug [35].

Spinal opioids (delivered epidurally or intrathecally) may allow better control of pain in patients in whom systemic administration is associated with significant side effects and incomplete pain relief. This method of delivery bypasses the enterohepatic circulation and thus decreases the levels of toxic metabolites. The primary indication is persistent pain refractory to analgesic and co-analgesic use especially in patients with bilateral or midline pain. The mixture between morphine and local anesthetics is useful in incident pain; clonidine added to morphine improves neuropathic pain control [36]. Side effects that are specific to this route are hypogonadotropic hypogonadism, pruritus, lower extremity edema, tolerance, respiratory depression, urinary retention, constipation, pruritus, device failure and infection. Epidural catheters and external pumps should be used in case of expected survival less than 3 months. Intrathecal catheters with implantable pumps should be considered if survival is longer than 3 months [37].

Intraventricular administration of opioids may be considered in patients with painful head and neck cancers or tumors invading the brachial plexus. It requires an intraventricular catheter connected to a subcutaneous reservoir or infusion pump [38].

## Issues Related Opioid Analgesics

Opioid tolerance and opioid-induced hyperalgesia may limit the clinical utility of opioids in controlling chronic as well as pain. Even brief exposures to mu-receptor agonists induce long-lasting hyperalgesic effects for days. After repeat administration, a delayed type of acute tolerance to morphine develops and limits the antinociceptive potency of morphine [39]. Both tolerance and hyperalgesia occur within 1 month of initiating opioid therapy [40]. They are associated with pronociceptive neuroplastic changes in the primary afferent fibers and the spinal cord require sustained opiate administration and specific interactions with opiate receptors [41]. Therefore, opioids can activate both pain inhibitory and pain facilitatory systems. Acute receptor desensitization via uncoupling of the receptor from G proteins, upregulation of the cAMP pathway, activation of the NMDA receptor system and descending facilitation have been proposed as potential mechanisms underlying opioid-induced hyperalgesia [42]. Administration of ketamine, an NMDA-receptor antagonist, in animal models of opioid induced hyperalgesia, delays the decrease in nociceptive threshold caused by opioids [43] and may even restore the opioid effectiveness in opioid-resistant pain models [44]. Other strategies to decrease or prevent opioid-induced hyperalgesia include alpha 2-agonists, NSAIDs, opioid rotation, or combinations of opioids with different receptor selectivity [42].

High doses of morphine administered intrathecally may also cause hyperalgesia and allodynia. These effects are mediated by nociceptive neurotransmitters (substance P, glutamate and dynorphin), neurokinin 1 (NK1) receptors, multiple sites of the NMDA receptor complex in the dorsal spinal cord, leading to Ca2+ influx and production of nitric oxide (NO) by activation of NO synthase. Morphine-3-glucuronide, a morphine metabolite, evokes nociceptive behaviour similar to that of intrathecal high-dose morphine [45].

# Radiation Therapy for Cancer Pain

In patients with widespread bone metastases, relief of pain can be obtained via a multimodality approach, combining analgesics, bisphosphonates, chemotherapy, radiotherapy, hormonal therapy and bone seeking radiopharmaceuticals.

Radioisotopes have a more favorable therapeutic ratio compared with wide-field external-beam radiotherapy for scattered metastatic bone pain and at present seem more clinically and cost-effective than bisphosphonates in this setting. The efficacy of radioisotopes has been assessed in clinical trials with small sample sizes and short-term evaluations of the outcomes. There is some evidence indicating that radioisotopes may give complete reduction in pain over one to six months with no increase in analgesic use, but adverse effects, specifically leukocytopenia and thrombocytopenia, have also been experienced [46].

## Modalities and Issues of Radiation Therapy

Conventional external beam radiotherapy lacks the precision to allow delivery of large single-fraction doses of radiation and simultaneously limit the dose to radiosensitive structures such as the spinal cord.

Beta-emitting, bone-seeking radiopharmaceuticals represent a good alternative or adjuvant to external beam radiotherapy for palliation of painful osteoblastic bone metastases. They are administered systemically and localize to sites of active bone turnover and emit beta particles (electrons, with a long half life) and gamma (photons, which allow external mapping of distribution in the body).

Myelosuppression is the main side effect of radionuclide therapy, with relative contraindications for treatment include osteolytic lesions, pending spinal cord compression or pathologic fracture, preexisting severe myelosuppression, urinary incontinence, inability to follow radiation safety precautions, and severe renal insufficiency. Prior to consideration for radionuclide therapy, recent bone scans should be evaluated in order to determine if the patient has painful osteoblastic lesions likely to respond to therapy.

The most frequently used radiopharmaceutical for this purpose is strontium 89, followed by samarium 153, and infrequently phosphorus 32 orthophosphate. Strontium-89 and samarium-153 are radioisotopes that are approved in the USA and Europe for the palliation of pain from metastatic bone cancer, whereas rhenium-186 and rhenium-188 are investigational. Radioisotopes are effective in providing pain relief with response rates of between 40% and 95%. Pain relief starts 1-4 weeks after the initiation of treatment, continues for up to 18 months, and is associated with a reduction in analgesic use in many patients. Thrombocytopenia and neutropenia are the most common toxic effects, but they are generally mild and reversible. Repeat doses are effective in providing pain relief in many patients. The effectiveness of radioisotopes can be greater when they are combined with chemotherapeutic agents such as cisplatin. Some studies with 89Sr and 153Sm indicate a reduction of hot spots on bone scans in up to 70% of patients, and suggest a possible tumoricidal action [47].

Approximately 70% of patients with prostate and breast cancer will have a reduction in pain in response to radionuclide therapy, beginning within 2 to 4 weeks and lasting between 2 and 6 months [48]. There may be a transient flare in pain after the administration of these compounds. Patients who are expected to live 3 or more months are more likely to benefit than patients with shorter duration life expectancy [48].

Strontium89 is cleared rapidly from the blood with at least 50% localized in the skeleton. The uptake in bone metastasis 10 times higher than in normal bone [49]

The proportion classified as complete responders to 89Sr ranged from 8% to 77%, with a mean value of 32%, and the proportion showing no response ranged from 14% to 52% (mean 25%). Within this range 44% of patients had some degree of response to 89Sr treatment, giving a mean overall response of 76%. Delay in the start of response was between 4 days and 28 days, with response duration of up to 15 months [47].

A reduction in analgesic use was reported in 71-81% of patients [50], [51]. 89Sr combined with chemotherapy may have therapeutic advantage over 89Sr alone [47].

Samarium153 (153Sm) can be compounded with the calcium salt of ethylene-diamine-tetramethylene phosphonic acid (EDTMP) to give 153Sm-EDTMP. After intravenous administration, it is cleared rapidly from the blood and completely excreted in urine in 6 hours. Palliation in pain may be seen in 70-95% of patients and is independent of the dose given [52] but patients who are administered higher doses have more pain reduction and improvement in sleep than those who receive lower doses [53]. Pain relief is typically noted within 5–10 days and can last up to 4 months. Analgesic consumption decreases significantly [54].

Men with primary lung cancer, lesions in the vertebra or pelvis, and concurrent metastases in the legs tend not to respond to 153Sm [55]. Repeat dosing of 153Sm-EDTMP can improve the duration of pain response and survival [56].

Rhenium 186 and 188 are still experimental. 186Re is compounded with 1-1-hydroethylidene diphosphate (186Re-HEDP), which binds to hydroxyapatite crystals by forming hydroxide bridges in a hydrolysis reaction probably mediated by osteoclasts. 186Re-HEDP binds to plasma proteins in a time-dependent interaction, and is cleared from the plasma with a half-life of 41 h. About 70% of the activity is excreted in the urine within 24 hours. It has been used in patients with hormone-refractory prostate cancer with a significant decrease in pain scores [57]. 188Re-HDP has a mean effective biological half-life in bone of about 16 hours, 11 hours for bone marrow and 12 hours for the whole body [58]. About 40% of the activity received is excreted in the urine within 8 h. It has been shown to decrease pain in 64%-81% of patients with prostate cancer and painful bony metastases [59] and in patients with mixed tumor types [60], [61],[62]. Pain relief starts 1–8 weeks after treatment and lasted up to 3 months [58].

Alpha-emitter radium-223 (223Ra) in breast and prostate cancer patients with skeletal metastases is well tolerated at therapeutically relevant dosages. Pain relief was reported by 52%, 60%, and 56% of the patients after 7 days, 4 weeks, and 8 weeks, respectively [63].

Systemic metabolic radiotherapy for pain treatment, using samarium-153 ethylene diamine tetramethylene phosphonic acid (Sm-153-EDTMP) can be offered to patients with painful metastatic osteosarcoma or in case of recurrent bone sites inaccessible to local therapies (surgery, external irradiation) [64].

The combined kyphoplasty and spinal radiosurgery treatment paradigm (Cyberknife) was found to be clinically effective in patients with pathological fractures; there was no significant spinal canal compromise. In this technique two minimally invasive surgical procedures are combined to avoid the morbidity associated with open surgery while providing both immediate fracture fixation and administering a single-fraction tumoricidal radiation dose [64], [65]. Palliative minimally invasive radiofrequency ablation with concurrent osteoplasty can be effective in individual cases giving a better quality of life and mobility [66].

Spinal radiosurgery (single-fraction) was found to be feasible, safe, and clinically effective for the treatment of spinal metastases from breast carcinoma. The results indicate the potential of radiosurgery in the treatment of patients with spinal breast metastases, especially those with solitary sites of spine involvement, to improve long-term palliation. The most common indication for radiosurgery treatment was pain, followed by primary treatment modality, for radiographic tumor progression, as a postsurgical boost, and for a progressive neurologic deficit [65], [67].

Spinal cord epidural metastasis (SEM) is a common complication of systemic cancer with an increasing incidence. Prostate, breast and lung cancer are the most common offenders. Metastasis usually arises in the posterior aspect of vertebral body with later invasion of epidural space. Pathophysiologically, vascular insufficiency is more important than direct spinal cord compression. The most common complaint is pain, and two thirds of patients with SEM have motor signs at initial diagnosis. Radiotherapy has an important role, particularly in treatment of radiosensitive tumors and in patients who are not candidates for surgery [68].

Radiotherapy has multiple roles in the treatment of leptomeningeal cancer. While it is uncommon for patients to experience regression of neurologic deficits due to leptomeningeal cancer, focal radiotherapy often provides significant palliation of pain, increased intracranial pressure and other focal symptoms. Focal radiotherapy may also be used to eliminate blockages of cerebrospinal fluid (CSF) and allow for safe administration of intrathecal chemotherapy. Craniospinal irradiation (CSI) is most often used as prophylaxis for patients at high risk of leptomeningeal tumor dissemination, but may result in symptom palliation and prolonged disease control for patients with active leptomeningeal tumor [69].

Painful skeletal metastases are a common problem in cancer patients. Although external beam radiation therapy is the current standard of care for cancer patients who present with localized bone pain, 20-30% of patients treated with this modality do not experience pain relief, and few further options exist for these patients. For many patients with painful metastatic skeletal disease, analgesics remain the only alternative treatment option. Recently, image-guided percutaneous methods of tumor destruction have proven effective for treatment of this difficult problem. for palliation of painful skeletal metastases For palliation of painful skeletal metastases, some of these techniques involve injection of ethanol, methyl methacrylate, laser-induced interstitial thermotherapy (LITT), cryoablation, and percutaneous radiofrequency ablation (RFA) [70].

Renal cell carcinoma has previously been described as being less responsive to radiotherapy than other tumor types. A prospective study to assess the effect of radiotherapy on symptoms and quality of life (QOL) in patients with metastatic RCC showed that palliative radiotherapy dose of 30 Gy in 10 fractions can result in a significant response rate and the relief of local symptoms in patients with bone metastases. Improvements in global pain and QOL appear to be limited by the effects of progressive systemic disease [71]. CyberKnife radiosurgery improves pain control and maintains QOL in patients treated for spinal tumors [72].

Despite numerous randomized trials investigating radiotherapy (RT) fractionation schedules for painful bone metastases, there are very few data on RT for bone metastases causing pain with a neuropathic component. The Trans-Tasman Radiation Oncology Group undertook a randomized trial comparing the efficacy of a single 8 Gy (8/1) with 20 Gy in 5 fractions (20/5) for this type of pain. 8/1 was not shown to be as effective as 20/5, nor was it statistically significantly worse. Outcomes were generally poorer for 8/1, although the quantitative differences were relatively small [73].

The current pharmaceutical approach is to target bone metastases by developing drugs that specifically target tumor cells in bone in addition to bone stroma since skeletal metastases are more resistant to treatment, present the highest bulk of tumor mass in the body, serve as site for secondary spread of tumor cells, and are associated with significant morbidity. The scope of future advancements is immense and includes innovative therapeutics and delivery systems aimed to improve skeletal affinity, selectivity, and efficacy of drugs [74].

In animal models of tumors with bone invasion, radiotherapy decreases the objective level of pain. The underlying mechanism seems to be related to the $Ca^{2+}$-signaling cascade or control of vesicular trafficking. Protein synthesis in the spinal cord (secretagogin, syntenin, P2X purinoreceptor 6 (P2X6), and $Ca^{2+}$/Calmodulin-dependent protein kinase 1 are initially increased several fold as result of tumor with pain associated behavior. This increase may be reversible after radiation [75].

Guidelines for radiation safety restrict the use of radioisotopes to specialized centers. Gamma rays can pass out of the patient's body, presenting an external risk to bystanders; consequently, patients should be treated in special lead-lined rooms. Beta particles emitted by radioisotopes destroy malignant cells, but they have a short range and are not harmful to nearby persons. Bremsstrahlung X-rays are formed by the deceleration of beta particles as they pass through shielding materials. Therefore lead is not the best shielding material for radioisotopes such as 89Sr [47].

## Other Medical Treatments

### Bisphosphonates

The most common metastatic cancers to the bone are lung, breast, prostate and multiple myeloma. Bone metastases cause pain by bone resorption by osteoclasts, osteoporosis, microfractures or pathologic fractures, and hypercalcemia. Bone has significant amounts of nociceptive A-delta and C fibers and vanilloid (VR1) receptors, which can be activated by bone catabolism (which decreases bone pH and releases proinflammatory cytokines such as transforming growth factor beta) [76-78].

Osteoclasts are derived from monocytes under the catalyst effect of macrophage-stimulating factor and NFkB (a transcription factor activated by tumor necrosis factor alpha). Osteoblasts release the ligand for its receptor-activator (RANK), while osteoprotegerin binds to RANK ligand at the receptor site and prevents the binding of the activator to the receptor. In the setting of cancer, there is an increase in RANK ligand versus release of osteoprotegerin and thus osteoclasts are activated. Bisphosphonates, once absorbed into the bone, have a long half-life in the skeleton. They inhibit the activation of osteoclasts (shortening their life span), stimulate their apoptosis and stimulate the release of osteoprotegerin [76-78]. Randomized, double blind, placebo controlled studies have shown that they reduce pain and opioid/ analgesic use, but also the risk of skeletal complications (by increasing the time until disease progression that requires radiation or surgery). Although the need for palliative radiation is decreased from 45% to 28%, there is no difference in the rate of pathologic vertebral fractures between treated and non-treated groups [2]. The newer bisphosphonates (pamidronate, zoledronate and ibandronate) have a more durable response than clodronate, a first generation drug. Loading doses of ibandronate may relieve opioid refractory bone pain in 7 days [79] and its effect may last up to 2 years [80].

The most common side effects of this category of medications are dyspepsia, nausea and esophagitis. An unusual side effect, which can lead to a paradoxical increase in bony pain, is osteonecrosis/ osteopetrosis, partcularly painful refractory bone exposures in the jaw [81].

## Calcitonin

Calcitonin is a hormone that inhibits osteoclast-induced bone resorption and is recommended for treatment of hypercalcemia of malignancy. It has the potential to relieve pain, and also retain bone density, thus reducing the risk of fractures.

Even though small trails and clinical experience have shown that calcitonin is a useful additive to the armamentarium of cancer pain management, the Cochrane Database however did not find evidence that calcitonin is effective in controlling complications due to bone metastases; for improving quality of life; or patients' survival [82]. This underscores the importance of randomized controlled trials sufficiently powered to show an effect. In cancer pain patients, it is rarely possible to withhold other therapies that could have an effect on pathological fractures and pain, thus calcitonin's contribution may be less evident.

## Interventional Procedures for Cancer Pain

### Local Anesthesia, Nerve Blocks

*1) Trigger point injections, epidural steroids injections or nerve root blocks* may decrease the peritumoral edema and inflammation caused by tumor compression, which may provide analgesia for a few days to a few weeks. If these give pain relief of sufficient magnitude (usually at least 50%), the patient may be a candidate for more defintive destructive procedures as detailed below.

*2) Peripheral neurolysis with radiofrequency, cryoneurolysis or injection of alcohol or phenol* may destroy peripheral nerves and alleviate pain. An injection of local anesthetic should be perfomed prior to the neurolytic blockade to evaluate efficacy and side effects. This type of neurolysis is performed for visceral (sympathetic-mediated) pain. Neurolytic substances may also be administered intrathecally to destroy nerve root function in a localized distribution. Between 50 and 80% of patients who undergo a neurolytic block for cancer pain have prolonged benefit [2]. Their effect is irreversible. Complications include postural hypotension, paralysis, bowel or bladder dysfunction. Therefore, neurolytic blocks should be reserved for patients who have failed surgical, medical and radiation therapy. Non-destructive analgesics can be delivered constantly via a catheter inserted at the sympathetic ganglia.

*3) CT-guided percutaneous cryoablation* of small (< or = 4-cm) renal lesions appears to require less analgesia than percutaneous radiofrequency ablation [83].

*4)* The stellate *or lumbar sympathetic ganglion block* with a neurolytic agent may relieve sympathetic-mediated pain involving the head/face/arm and leg, respectively.

*Celiac and hypogastric plexus blocks* are useful in visceral pain from pancreatic cancer and cancer of the pelvic organs.

*5) Multimodality treatment: a)* combined use of thoracic paravertebral block and general anesthesia may decrease the VAS score and postoperative administration of analgesics in patients having major breast cancer surgery [84]; *b)* Combined palliative treatments including bypass operation, celiac plexus block and radiation therapy prolongs survival of patients with unresectable locally advanced pancreatic cancer [85].

## Surgical Approaches

Surgical treatment, either curative or palliative, should be aimed at alleviating pain and maintaining function. It may also preserve or even restore neurological function, and reveal histology if uncertain. During surgery for curative resection, a tumor may be found unresectable and instead palliative debulking is performed. Nerve-sparing techniques and careful dissection around nerves with avoidance of ischemia, use of non-muscle splitting techniques, intraoperative radiofrequency lesioning or cryoneurolysis should be used to prevent emergence of postoperative neuropathic pain. Radiation therapy needs to be carefully timed in relationship to surgery to prevent poor wound healing and development of fistulas. After surgery, a multidisciplinary team should assure adequate rehabilitation, decrease disability and increase in quality of life after procedures that lead to change in anatomy (radical neck dissection, colostomy). Radiation therapy after surgery may enhance pain control in patients in whom there is recurrence of the primary tumor and may also help control tumor regrowth in patients with microscopically positive margins. Prospective palliative surgery should also be considered to pre-empt development of a fracture in a pathologic bone and of spinal cord compression in a patients with progressive weakness [1].

*1) Metastatic bone disease* may require surgery for treatment of an impending or existing pathologic fracture or for alleviating disabling pain. Approximately 10-30% of patients with metastasis in the long bones will develop a pathologic fracture that will require surgery [2]. Restoration of function in a fractured humerus for instance is a main goal of surgery. After resection, tumors may be reconstructed with prostheses or with cemented nailing [86]. Postoperative radiation may be given to reduce the risk of disease progression that would decrease the stability of the surgical fixation [2].

*2) Spinal epidural and leptomeningeal metastases* occur at a late stage of systemic disease, and the prognosis is generally poor. They are a medical emergency as lack of timely treatment leads to cord compression and irreversible cord dysfunction. Breast, prostate, lung cancer, multiple myeloma, renal cell cancer and melanoma are the most common to metastasize to the epidural space. The mechanism of epidural metastasis may be by direct extension from adjacent vertebral metastases (e.g. to the brachial or lumbosacral plexus), from the thorax (through the intervertebral foramina) and by blood dissemination. Surgery should be performed in selected cases of spinal leptomeningeal metastases, in patients with rapid neurologic deterioration, in patients with tumor progression in a previously irradiated area, for stabilization of spine in patients with vertebral metastases, and in patients who are still ambulatory with controlled systemic disease. It should be followed by adjuvant therapy [87]. Steroids and radiation therapy are an adjunct of surgery. Pain relief in patients with spinal cord compression may be achieved in 73% of patients after radiotherapy alone; this can also restore ambulation in 64% and sphincter tone in 33% of patients with partial spinal block. In patients with complete spinal block, the outcome is poorer, with only 27% improvement in motor function and 58% in pain [2].

*3) Neuroablation* may be considered for incidental (movement-related) pain refractory to medication, radiation, or surgery.

- a. Peripheral neurectomy may be used for multi-level intercostal neuralgia, for a paraspinal tumor involving nerves distal to the neural foramen and to certain cranial nerves (trigeminal or glossopharyngeal) in case of cancer-induced neuralgias; these nerves may be ablated by radiofrequency or chemical neurolysis
- b. Dorsal rhizotomy can lead to paralysis of an extremity therefore it may be considered only in patients with thoracic or abdominal pain or in patients with a paretic limb.
- c. Anterolateral cordotomy (spinal tractotomy) lesions the fibers of the spinothalamic tract in the anterolateral funiculi of the spinal cord. It leads to selective loss of pain and temperature sensation 2- 3 levels below the lesion, in the contralateral limb. It is recommended in unilateral, somatic pain below the midcervical dermatomes. For patients with visceral pain or bilateral pain, bilateral cordotomy is needed for pain control, but this may lead to respiratory failure, and therefore commissural myelotomy may be preferred. The classic approach is a C1-2 cordotomy (by CT guidance and under local anesthesia) but is contraindicated in patients with impaired pulmonary function or a previous cordotomy on an opposite side. In these cases, a computed tomography (CT)-guided transdiscal low cervical cordotomy (C4-5 or C5-6) with radiofrequency [88] or an open cordotomy (performed via a laminectomy at lower cervical or thoracic levels) are indicated. The open cordotomy is also indicated in cases where the percutaneous cordotomy has failed or in patients who are poorly cooperative. Complications include bowel, bladder or sexual dysfunction, ataxia, paresis and sleep apnea. Cordotomy may offer relief still present at 6 months of follow-up.
- d. Commissural myelotomy interrupts the polysynaptic afferent nociceptive pain system in the middle of the spinal cord. It is indicated in patients with bilateral pain,

midline pain or pelvic/ perineal pain. The CT based approach is performed at the cervicomedullary junction. The open approach is via a multilevel laminectomy, exposure of the appropriate levels of the lumbar or sacral segments of the spinal cord and a midline incision. Complications include temporary dysesthesias and limba apraxia [1].

e. Hypophysectomy leads to pain relief through an unknown mechanism, in both hormonally dependent and independent tumors. It can be performed either via a chemical or surgical transsphenoidal approach. Most commonly it is indicated for bilateral diffuse, refractory pain from metastatic disease. Pain relief may be immediate. Complications include lesions of the optic nerves and chiasm, pituitary failure requiring hormonal substitution, headaches, other cranial nerve dysfunctions, and CSF leak [1].

Surgical treatment of metastatic lesions in the lumbar spine improves neurological and ambulatory function, significantly reducing axial spinal pain in 94% of cases after one month [89]. Single-dose radiosurgery for solitary spinal metastases can achieve rapid and durable pain control [90].

*4) Neuromodulation (neuroaugmentation)* in cancer pain is effective if directed towards the deep brain structures that contain endogenous opioids (endorphins) such as the periaqueductal and periventricular greay areas, the limbic system and the pituitary gland. Spinal cord stimulation is only anecdotally effective in cancer-related pain [1].

*5) Neuraxial opioid infusion (epidural and intrathecal)* may be considered for cancer pain refractory to conventional oral medications and cordotomy. The treatment can be successful by the addition of opioids to the intrathecal regimen [91]. Tolerance to neuraxial opioids may occur faster than that to oral or rectal opioids. Risks of catheter insertion and subsequent medication delivery include meningitis, epidural abscess, pruritus or urinary retention. Neuraxial (epidural or intrathecal) catheter placement is contraindicated in the presence of cord compression [1]. Epidural metastasis decreases the efficacy of epidural analgesia due to fibrotic changes and mechanical obstruction by the tumor and may be associated with complications due to decreased compliance of the epidural space [92]. The epidural space may undergo fibrosis after 9-12 months of continuous epidural infusion, which can lead to increasing back pain with decrease in treatment efficacy or backup of solutions with fluid accumulation under the subcutaneous tissue. For a treatment lasting more than 3 months, the cost-effectiveness is in favor of intrathecal drug delivery systems. De Leon-Casasola [92] recommends a polyanalgesic intrathecal drug trial for the patients who have already been on opioid and co-adjuvant therapy (morphine, bupivacaine and clonidine). Long-term complications include granuloma formation that may cause a neurologic deficit by local compression. This has been reported in patients who had high doses of intrathecal morphine >20-25 mg/day for longer than 4 months. Treatment is surgical decompression.

## Conclusion

While a number of clinical modalities have been used for the treatment of cancer-related pain and these treatments are often effective, the emergence of side effects may limit their use for the effective treatment of severe cancer pain. For many cases of intractable cancer pain, the current treatment modalities remain insufficient. Moreover, there are still significant issues regarding the classification of cancer pain as nociceptive, neuropathic, or both, which directly influences the clinical choice of treatment regimen. While there has been extensive basic science research on cancer-related pain conditions, new cancer pain treatment modalities are to be developed to improve the clinical management of cancer pain.

## References

[1] Jacox A, Carr D.B., Payne R. et al. Management of cancer pain. *Clinical Practice Guideline* No 9. AHCPR Publication No 94-0952. Rockville, MD.

[2] Miaskowski C, Cleary J, Burney R et al (2005). Guideline for the management of cancer pain in adults and children. *APS Clinical Practice Guideline Series*, No3. Glenview, IL: American Pain Society.

[3] Caraceni A, Zecca E, Bonezzi C et al. Gabapentin for neuropathic cancer pain: a randomized controlled trial from the gabapentin cancer pain study group. *J. Clin. Oncol.* 2004; 22:2909-17.

[4] Bosnjak S, Jelic S, Susnjar S, Luki V. Gabapentin for relief of neuropathic pain related to anticancer treatment: A preliminary study. *Journal of Chemotherapy.* 2002, 14(2): 214-9.

[5] Bruera E, Roca E, Cedaro L, et al. Action of oral methylprednisolone in terminal cancer patients: a prospective randomized double-blind study. *Cancer. Treat. Rep.* 1985;69:751-754.

[6] Ettinger A.B., Portenoy R.K. The use of corticosteroids in the treatment of symptoms associated with cancer. *Journal of Pain and Symptom Management* 1988; 3(2): 99-103.

[7] Nelson KA, Park KM, Robinovitz E, et al. High-dose oral dextromethorphan versus placebo in painful diabetic neuropathy and postherpetic neuralgia. *Neurology.* 1997;48:1212-1218.

[8] Pud D, Eisenberg E, Spitzer A, et al. The NMDA receptor antagonist amantadine reduces surgical neuropathic pain in cancer patients: a double blind, randomized, placebo controlled trial. *Pain.* 1998;75:349-354.

[9] Nikolajsen L, Hansen PO, Jensen TS. Oral ketamine therapy in the treatment of postamputation stump pain. *Acta Anaesthesiol. Scand.* 1997;41:427-429.

[10] Sang CN, Booher S, Gilron I, Parada S, Max M.B. Dextromethorphan and memantine in painful diabetic neuropathy and postherpetic neuralgia. Efficacy and dose response trials. *Anesthesiology.* 2002; 96(5): 1053-61.

[11] Fogelholm R, Murros K. Tizanidine in chronic tension-type headache: a placebo controlled double-blind cross-over study. *Headache.* 1992;32:509-513.

[12] Eisenach JC, DuPen S, Dubois M, et al. Epidural clonidine analgesia for intractable cancer pain. The Epidural Clonidine Study Group. *Pain.* 1995;61:391-400.

[13] Rowbotham MC. Topical analgesic agents. In: Fields HL, Liebeskind JC, eds. *Pharmacological Approaches to the Treatment of Chronic Pain: New Concepts and Critical Issues.* Seattle, IASP Press, 1994, pp 211-229.

[14] Galer BS, Rowbotham MC, Perander J, Friedman E. Topical lidocaine patch relieves postherpetic neuralgia more effectively than a vehicle topical patch: results of an enriched enrollment study. *Pain.* 1999;80:533-538.

[15] Menegaldo L. The subcutaneous administration of a NSAID in palliative care. *Clin. Ter.* 1992 Oct;141(10):273-8.

[16] Kuttan R, Sudheeran PC, Josph CD. Turmeric and curcumin as topical agents in cancer therapy. *Tumori.* 1987 Feb 28;73(1):29-31.

[17] Schubert MM, Newton RE. The use of benzydamine HCl for the management of cancer therapy-induced mucositis: preliminary report of a multicentre study. *Int. J. Tissue. React.* 1987;9(2):99-103.

[18] Momo K, Shiratsuchi T, Taguchi H, Hashizaki K, Saito Y, Makimura M, Ogawa N. *Preparation and clinical application of indomethacin gel for medical treatment of stomatitis.* Yakugaku Zasshi. 2005 May;125(5):433-40.

[19] Befort K, Filiol D, Decalliot FM, Gaveriaux-Ruff C, Hoehe MR. A single nucleotide polymorphic mutation in the human mu-opioid receptor severely impairs receptor signaling. *J. Biol. Chem.* 2001; 276:3130-7.

[20] Zhou HH, Sheller JR, Nu HE, Wood M, Wood AJ. Ethnic differences in response to morphine. *Clin. Pharm. Ther.* 1993: 54:507-13.

[21] Pleym H, Spigset O, Kharasch ED, Dale O. Gender differences in drug effects: implications for anesthesiologists. *Acta Anesthesiol. Scand.* 2003: 47:241-59.

[22] Kloke M. Gaps and junctions beween clinical experience and theoretical framework in the use of opioids. *Support Care Cancer.* 2004; 12:749-51.

[23] Bolan EA, Tallarida RJ, Pasternak GW. Synergy between mu and opioid ligands: evidence for functional interactions among mu opioid receptor subtypes. *J. Pharmacol. Exp. Ther.* 2002; 303: 557-62.

[24] Walsh D, Rivera NI, Davis MP et al. Strategies for pain management: Cleveland Clinic Foundation Guidelines for opioid dosing for cancer pain. *Support Cancer Ther.* 2004; 1:157-64.

[25] Quigley C. Hydromorphone for acute and chronic pain. *Cochrane Database Syst. Rev.* 2002; 1: CD0003447.

[26] Dean M. Opioids in renal failure and dialysis patients. *J. Pain Sympt. Manage.* 2004; 28: 497-504.

[27] Donner B, Zenz M, Tryba M, Strumpf M. Direct conversion from oral morphine to transdermal fentanyl: A multicenter study in patients with cancer pain. *Pain.* 1996; 64(3): 527-34.

[28] Sloan PA, Moulin DE, Hays H. A clinical evaluation of transdermal therapeutic system fentanyl for the treatment of cancer pain. *J. Pain Sympt. Manage.* 1998; 16(2): 102-11.

[29] Clark AJ, Ahmedzai SH, Allan LG et al. Efficacy and safety of transdermal fentanyl and sustained release oral morphine in patients with cancer and chronic non-cancer pain. *Curr. Med. Res. Opin.* 2004; 20:1419-28.

[30] Ahmedzai S, Brooks D. Transdermal fentanyl versus sustained release oral morphine in cancer pain: prefernce, efficacy, and quality of life. *J. Pain Sympt. Manage.* 1997; 13:254-61.

[31] Van Seventer R, Smit JM, Schipper RM et al. Comparison of TTS-fentanyl and with sustained release oral morphine in the treatment of patients not using opioids for mild-to-moderate pain. *Curr. Med. Res. Opin.* 2003; 19:457-69.

[32] Mercadante S, Casuccio A, Angello A et al. Morphine versus methadone in the pain treatment of advanced cancer patients. Followed up at home. *J. Clin. Oncol.* 1998; 16: 3656-61.

[33] Davis MP, Walsh D, Lagman R, LeGrand S B. Controversies in pharmacotherapy of pain management. *Lancet Oncol.* 2005; 6:695-704.

[34] Ripamonti C, Bianchi M. The use of methadone for cancer pain. *Hematol. Oncol. Clin. North. Am.* 2002; 16:543-55.

[35] McCaffery M, Martin L, Ferrell BR. Analgesic administration via rectum or stoma. *Journal of Enterostomal Therapy Nursing.* 1992; 19(4): 114-21.

[36] Hanks GW, de Conno F, Cherny N et al. Morphine and alternative opioids in cancer pain: the EAPC recommendations. *Br. J. Cancer.* 2001; 95: 587-93.

[37] Krames ES. Practical issues when using neuraxial infusion. *Oncology.* 1999; 13 (suppl1): 37-44.

[38] Lazorthes YR, Sallerin BA, Verdie JC. Intracebroventricular administration of morphine for control of irreducible cancer pain. *Neurosurgery.* 1995; 37(3): 422-8.

[39] Horvath G, Kekesi G, Dobos I, Klimscha W, Benedek G. Long-term changes in the antinociceptive potency of morphine or dexmedetomidine after a single treatment. *Anesth. Analg.* 2005 Sep;101(3):812-8.

[40] Chu LF, Clark DJ, Angst MS. Opioid tolerance and hyperalgesia in chronic pain patients after one month of oral morphine therapy: a preliminary prospective study. *J. Pain.* 2006 Jan;7(1):43-8.

[41] Gardell LR, King T, Ossipov MH, Rice KC, Lai J, Vanderah TW, Porreca F. Opioid receptor-mediated hyperalgesia and antinociceptive tolerance induced by sustained opiate delivery. *Neurosci. Lett.* 2005 Dec 9.

[42] Koppert 2005. Opioid-induced analgesia and hyperalgesia. *Schmerz.* 2005 Oct;19(5):386-90, 392-4.

[43] Van Elstraete AC, Sitbon P, Trabold F, Mazoit JX, Benhamou D. A single dose of intrathecal morphine in rats induces long-lasting hyperalgesia: the protective effect of prior administration of ketamine. *Anesth. Analg.* 2005 Dec;101(6):1750-6.

[44] Simonnet G. Complexity and physiology of the analgesic effects of opioids. *Rev. Med. Suisse.* 2005 Jun 22;1(25):1682-5.

[45] Sakurada T, Komatsu T, Sakurada S. Mechanisms of nociception evoked by intrathecal high-dose morphine. *Neurotoxicology.* 2005 Oct;26(5):801-9. Epub 2005 Jun 4.

[46] Roque M, Martinez MJ, Alonso P, Catala E, Garcia JL, Ferrandiz M. Radioisotopes for metastatic bone pain. *Cochrane Database Syst. Rev.* 2003;(4):CD003347.

[47] Finlay IG, Mason MD, Shelley M. Radioisotopes for the palliation of metastatic bone cancer: a systematic review. *Lancet Oncol.* 2005 Jun;6(6):353-4.

[48] Hellman RS, Krasnow AZ. *J Palliat Med.* Radionuclide therapy for palliation of pain due to osteoblastic metastases.1998 Fall;1(3):277-83.

[49] Robinson RG, Blake GM, Preston DF, et al. Strontium-89: treatment results and kinetics in patients with painful metastatic prostate and breast cancer in bone. *Radiographics.* 1989; 9: 271–81.

[50] Lee CK, Aeppli DM, Unger J, et al. Strontium-89 chloride (Metastron) for palliative treatment of bony metastases: the University of Minnesota experience. *Am. J. Clin. Oncol.* 1996; 19: 102–07.

[51] Baziotis N, Yakoumakis E, Zissimopoulos A, et al. Strontium-89 chloride in the treatment of bone metastases from breast cancer. *Oncology.* 1998; 55: 377–81.

[52] Anderson PM, Wiseman GA, Dispenzieri A, et al. High-dose samarium-153 ethylene diamine tetramethylene phosphonate: low toxicity of skeletal irradiation in patients with osteosarcoma and bone metastases. *J. Clin. Oncol.* 2002; 20: 189–96.

[53] Serafini AN, Houston SJ, Resche I, et al. Palliation of pain associated with metastatic bone cancer using samarium-153 lexidronam: a double-blind placebo-controlled clinical trial. *J. Clin. Oncol.* 1998; 16: 1574–81.

[54] Sartor O, Reid RH, Hoskin PJ, et al. Samarium-153-Lexidronam complex for treatment of painful bone metastases in hormonerefractory prostate cancer. *Urology.* 2004; 63: 940–45.

[55] Tian J, Cao L, Zhang J, et al. Comparative analysis of patients not responding to a single dose of 153Sm-EDTMP palliative treatment for painful skeletal metastases. *Chin. Med. J.* 2002; 115:824–28.

[56] Turner JH, Claringbold PG. A phase II study of treatment of painful multifocal skeletal metastases with single and repeated dose samarium-153 ethylenediaminetetramethylene phosphonate. *Eur. J. Cancer.* 1991; 27: 1084–86.

[57] Maxon HR 3rd, Schroder LE, Thomas SR, et al. Re-186(Sn) HEDP for treatment of painful osseous metastases: initial clinical experience in 20 patients with hormone-resistant prostate cancer. *Radiol.* 1990; 176: 155–59.

[58] Liepe K, Hliscs R, Kropp J, et al. Dosimetry of 188Rehydroxyethylidene diphosphonate in human prostate cancer skeletal metastases. *J. Nucl. Med.* 2003; 44: 953–60.

[59] Palmedo H, Guhlke S, Bender H, et al. Dose escalation study with rhenium-188 hydroxyethylidene diphosphonate in prostate cancer patients with osseous metastases. *Eur. J. Nucl. Med.* 2000; 27: 123–30.

[60] Li S, Liu J, Zhang H, et al. Rhenium-188 HEDP to treat painful bone metastases. *Clin. Nucl. Med.* 2001; 26: 919–22.

[61] Liepe K, Hliscs R, Kropp J, et al. Rhenium-188-HEDP in the palliative treatment of bone metastases. *Cancer Biother. Radiopharm.* 2000; 15: 261–65.

[62] Chen S, Xu K, Yao D, et al. Treatment of metastatic bone pain with Rhenium-188 hydroxyethylidene disphosphate. *Med. Princ. Pract.* 2001; 10: 98–101.

[63] Nilsson S, Larsen RH, Fossa SD, Balteskard L, Borch KW, Westlin JE, Salberg G, Bruland OS. First clinical experience with alpha-emitting radium-223 in the treatment of skeletal metastases. *Clin. Cancer Res.* 2005 Jun 15;11(12):4451-9.

[64] Claude L, Rousmans S, Carrie C, Breteau N, Dijoud F, Gentet JC, Giammarile F, Jouve JL, Kind M, Marec-Berard P, Mascard E, Bataillard A, Philip T. Standards and options for the use of radiation therapy in the management of patients with osteosarcoma. Update 2004. *Bull. Cancer.* 2005 Oct 1;92(10):891-906.

[65] Gerszten PC, Germanwala A, Burton SA, Welch WC, Ozhasoglu C, Vogel WJ. Combination kyphoplasty and spinal radiosurgery: a new treatment paradigm for pathological fractures. *J. Neurosurg. Spine.* 2005 Oct;3(4):296-301.

[66] Stang A, Celebcioglu S, Keles H, von Seydewitz C, Malzfeldt E. Dtsch *Med. Wochenschr.* Minimally-invasive regional treatment of a symptomatic ischial metastasis using radiofrequency ablation and osteoplasty. 2005 May 13;130(19):1195-8.

[67] Gerszten PC, Burton SA, Welch WC, Brufsky AM, Lembersky BC, Ozhasoglu C, Vogel WJ. Single-fraction radiosurgery for the treatment of spinal breast metastases. *Cancer.* 2005 Nov 15;104(10):2244-54.

[68] Mut M, Schiff D, Shaffrey ME. Metastasis to nervous system: spinal epidural and intramedullary metastases. *J. Neurooncol.* 2005 Oct;75(1):43-56.

[69] Mehta M, Bradley K. Radiation therapy for leptomeningeal cancer. *Cancer Treat. Res.* 2005;125:147-58.

[70] Callstrom MR, Charboneau JW, Goetz MP, Rubin J, Atwell TD, Farrell MA, Welch TJ, Maus TP. Image-guided ablation of painful metastatic bone tumors: a new and effective approach to a difficult problem. *Skeletal Radiol.* 2005 Oct 5;1-15.

[71] Lee J, Hodgson D, Chow E, Bezjak A, Catton P, Tsuji D, O'Brien M, Danjoux C, Hayter C, Warde P, Gospodarowicz MK. A phase II trial of palliative radiotherapy for metastatic renal cell carcinoma. *Cancer.* 2005 Nov 1;104(9):1894-900.

[72] Degen JW, Gagnon GJ, Voyadzis JM, McRae DA, Lunsden M, Dieterich S, Molzahn I, Henderson FC. CyberKnife stereotactic radiosurgical treatment of spinal tumors for pain control and quality of life. *J. Neurosurg. Spine.* 2005 May;2(5):540-9.

[73] Roos DE, Turner SL, O'Brien PC, Smith JG, Spry NA, Burmeister BH, Hoskin PJ, Ball DL; Trans-Tasman Radiation Oncology Group, TROG 96.05. Randomized trial of 8 Gy in 1 versus 20 Gy in 5 fractions of radiotherapy for neuropathic pain due to bone metastases (Trans-Tasman Radiation Oncology Group, TROG 96.05). *Radiother. Oncol.* 2005 Apr;75(1):54-63. Epub 2004 Oct 28.

[74] Bagi CM. Targeting of therapeutic agents to bone to treat metastatic cancer. *Adv. Drug. Deliv. Rev.* 2005 May 25;57(7):995-1010. Epub 2005 Apr 13.

[75] Park HC, Seong J, An JH, Kim J, Kim UJ, Lee BW. Alteration of cancer pain-related signals by radiation: proteomic analysis in an animal model with cancer bone invasion. *Int. J. Radiat. Oncol. Biol. Phys.* 2005 Apr 1;61(5):1523-34.

[76] Sevcik MA, Luger NM, Mach DB et al. Bone cancer pain: the effects of the bisphosphonate alendronate on pain, skeletal remodeling, tumor growth and tumor necrosis. *Pain.*2004; 111:169-80.

[77] Urch C. The pathophysiology of cancer-induced bone pain: current understanding. *Palliat. Med.* 2004; 18:267-74.

[78] Roodman G. D. Mechanisms of Disease: mechanisms of bone metastasis. *N. Engl. J. Med.* 2004; 350:1655-1664, Apr 15, 2004.

[79] Body JJ, Diel IJ, Bell R et al. Oral ibandronate improves bone pain and preserves quality of life in patients with skeletal metastases due to breast cancer. *Pain.* 2004; 111:306-12.

[80] Heidenreich A, Ohlmann C, Body JJ. Ibandronate in metastatic bome pain. *Semin. Oncol.* 2004; 31 (suppl 10): 67-72.

[81] Marx RE, Sawatari Y, Fortin M, Broumand V. Bisphosphonate-induced exposed bone (osteonecrosis/osteopetrosis) of the jaws: risk factors, recognition, prevention, and treatment. *J. Oral Maxillofac. Surg.* 2005 Nov;63(11):1567-75.

[82] Martinez MJ, Roque M, Alonso-Coello P, Catala E, Garcia JL, Ferrandiz M. Calcitonin for metastatic bone pain. *Cochrane Database Syst. Rev.* 2003;(3):CD003223.

[83] Allaf ME, Varkarakis IM, Bhayani SB, Inagaki T, Kavoussi LR, Solomon SB. Pain control requirements for percutaneous ablation of renal tumors: cryoablation versus radiofrequency ablation--initial observations. *Radiology.* 2005 Oct;237(1):366-70. Epub 2005 Aug 26.

[84] Ono K, Danura T, Koyama Y, Hidaka H. Combined use of paravertebral block and general anesthesia for breast cancer surgery. *Masui.* 2005 Nov;54(11):1273-6.

[85] Yamaguchi K, Kobayashi K, Ogura Y, Nakamura K, Nakano K, Mizumoto K, Tanaka M. Radiation therapy, bypass operation and celiac plexus block in patients with unresectable locally advanced pancreatic cancer. *Hepatogastroenterology.* 2005 Sep-Oct;52(65):1605-12.

[86] Bickels J, Kollender Y, Wittig JC, Meller I, Malawer MM. Function after resection of humeral metastases: analysis of 59 consecutive patients. *Clin. Orthop. Relat. Res.* 2005 Aug (437):201-8.

[87] Deinsberger R, Regatschnig R, Kaiser B, Bankl HC. Spinal leptomeningeal metastases from prostate cancer. *Acta Neurochir.* (Wien). 2005 Nov 30.

[88] Raslan AM. Percutaneous Computed Tomography-Guided Transdiscal Low Cervical Cordotomy for Cancer Pain as a Method to Avoid Sleep Apnea. *Stereotact. Funct. Neurosurg.* 2005 Oct 17; 83(4):159-164.

[89] Holman PJ, Suki D, McCutcheon I, Wolinsky JP, Rhines LD, Gokaslan ZL. Surgical management of metastatic disease of the lumbar spine: experience with 139 patients. *J. Neurosurg. Spine.* 2005 May; 2(5):550-63.

[90] Ryu S, Rock J, Rosenblum M, Kim JH. Patterns of failure after single-dose radiosurgery for spinal metastasis. *J. Neurosurg.* 2004 Nov;101 Suppl 3:402-5.

[91] Souter KJ, Davies JM, Loeser JD, Fitzgibbon DR. Continuous intrathecal meperidine for severe refractory cancer pain: a case report. *Clin. J. Pain.* 2005 Mar-Apr;21(2):193-6.

[92] De Leon-Casasola O.A. Interventional procedures for cancer pain management: when are they indicated? *Cancer Investigation.* 2004; 22 (4): 630-4.

*Chapter XVII*

# Complementary and Alternative Medicine in Pain Management

### *Lucy Chen*
MGH Pain Center, Massachusetts General Hospital, Harvard Medical School

## Abstract

Complementary and alternative medicine is considered as a group of healthcare practices and products that are not part of conventional medicine (western medicine). The practice of complementary and alterative medicine can be dated back to ancient histories and has grown at a remarkable pace in western countries since 1970's, partially because of the advancement of basic science research in this field. Complementary and alternative medicine has been used either in combination with conventional medicine or as an independent treatment modality. As an example of how basic science research has helped the translation of alternative medicine into a better and more effective clinical practice, acupuncture will be specifically discussed in this chapter and up-to date evidence on the effect of acupuncture in treating many pain conditions will be reviewed in relation to the role of translational pain research. Although there are many positive developments in complementary and alternative medicine, both preclinical and clinical research on this topic faces a number of challenges. It can be anticipated that complementary and alternative medicine is likely to play a growing and positive role in clinical pain management.

## Introduction

Complementary and alternative medicine is considered a group of healthcare practices and products that are not part of the conventional medicine (western medicine). The practice of complementary and alterative medicine can be dated back to ancient histories and has grown at a remarkable pace in western countries since 1970's, partially because of the advancement of basic science research in this field. Complementary and alternative medicine has been used either in combination with the conventional medicine or as an independent treatment modality. A variety of practices are included in complementary and alternative medicine, which can be divided into five major categories based on the information provided by the National Center of Complementary and Alternative Medicine (see Table 1).

Most recently, "integrative medicine" has been used as a term to describe a discipline that combines conventional mainstream therapies with complementary therapies. This treatment discipline appears to be supported by some evidence indicating its safety and effectiveness. Integrative medicine not only is becoming part of the medical practice but also is taught as a course in many medical schools. Integrative medicine may have a unique role in clinical pain management because of the multi-dimensional nature of pain experiences. Among many different modalities of complementary and alternative medicine, acupuncture is perhaps the most studied both preclinically and clinically and is one of the most commonly practiced modality of alternative medicine. Due to the broad range of complementary and alternative medicine, it is impossible to cover each modality in this chapter. As an example of how basic science research has helped the translation of alternative medicine into a better and more effective clinical practice, acupuncture will be specifically discussed in this chapter and up-to date evidence on the effect of acupuncture in treating many pain conditions will be reviewed in the context the role of translational pain research.

**Table 1. Categories of Complementary and Alternative Medicine**

| | |
|---|---|
| Alternative medicine: | Homeopathic medicine, Naturopathic medicine, Ayurueda, Traditional Chinese medicine (Herbs, acupuncture, massage, etc) |
| Mind-body interventions: | Patient supporting groups, Cognitive-behavioral therapy, Meditation, Mental healing, Art/Music/Dance therapies |
| Biologically based therapies: | Herb products, Food/vitamins, Dietary supplement, Natural products (e.g., shark cartilage) |
| Manipulative and body based methods: | Chiropractic manipulation, Osteopathic Manipulation, Massage |
| Energy therapies: (Biofield therapies): (Bioelectromagnetically based therapies): | Qi gong, Reiki, Therapeutic touch Pulse field, Magnetic field, Alternating-current, Direct-current |

## History

Acupuncture is one of the most ancient healing arts and a significant component of the health care system in China for at least 3000 years. The United States Food and Drug Administration (FDA) estimated in 1993 that Americans make 9 to 12 million visits per year to acupuncture practitioners and spend more than 500 million dollars annually on acupuncture treatments. In 1997, there were 385 million recorded patient visits to primary care physicians. However, 630 million recorded visits were made to alternative medicine practitioners. In a nationwide survey published in 1998 (Journal of American Medical Association), it was reported that office visits for alternative therapy were twice as many as those for primary care and that money spent on alternative medicine was nearly equal to the out-of-pocket expenditures for conventional medical care [1]. Indeed, many medical conditions may be effectively treated using acupuncture as summarized in a document published by the World Health Organization (WHO) in 2002 [2].

In 1996, FDA classified acupuncture needles as medical equipment subject to the same strict standards for medical needles, syringes and surgical scalpels. Given the dramatic increase in the use of acupuncture as a modality of alternative medicine, the National Institutes of Health (NIH) organized a Consensus Development Conference on Acupuncture in 1997. This conference noted that acupuncture has been practiced by medical physicians, dentists, non-MD acupuncturists, and other practitioners. This conference also recognized that the extensive practice of acupuncture may be in part due to a low incidence of adverse effects as compared with many drugs and other commonly accepted medical procedures for the same conditions.

# **Definition of Acupuncture**

Acupuncture involves the subcutaneous insertion of fine sterilized needles at specific points (so-called Acupoints). In the ancient medical system in China, maintaining human health is considered to be achieved through a delicate balance between two opposing but inseparable principle elements: *Yin* and *Yang*. Yin represents 'cold, slow, and passive elements', whereas Yang represents 'hot, fast, and active elements'. Accordingly, internal organs of human beings are also divided along the Yin and Yang system. This ancient theory of Chinese medicine suggests that health can be achieved by maintaining the human body in a 'balanced state of *Yin* and *Yang*' and that an internal imbalance of *Yin* and *Yang* is responsible for a disease state.

Traditional Chinese medicine also stipulates that *qi* (i.e., vital energy, pronounced as 'chee') is the life force or energy that sustains and influences health. Maintaining a balance between the opposing forces of *Yin* and *Yang* is considered to be the basis for a healthy flow of *qi*. As such, any disturbance of the *Yin* and *Yang* system would cause the disrupted flow of *qi*, thereby becoming the basis for a disease state or pain. Acupuncture treats a state of disease or pain through adding *qi* or releasing the excessive flow of *qi* in order to restore the normal balance of the *Yin* and *Yang* system. Because *qi* is thought to flow through specific pathways (so called meridians consisting of 12 main meridians and 8 secondary meridians) in a human body, an effective acupuncture treatment requires that acupuncture needles be placed into those Acupoints located along the meridians as shown in lines in fig 1.

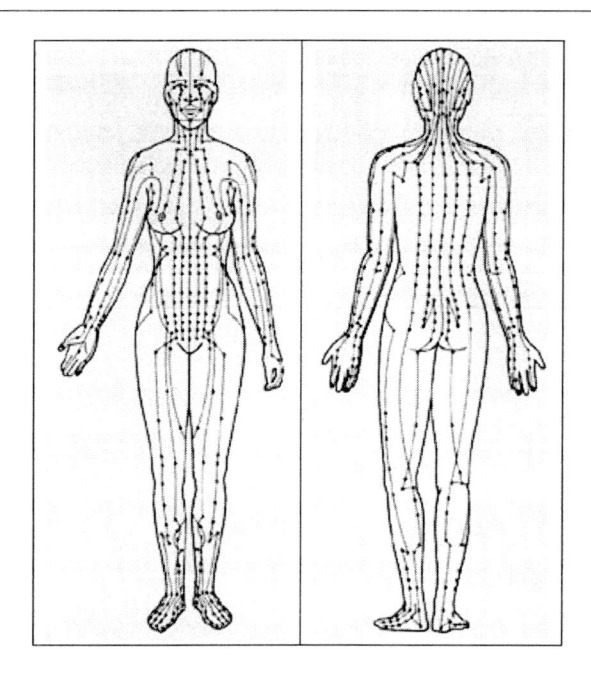

Figure 1.

## Basic Science and Clinical Studies of Acupuncture

Although acupuncture has been used for many thousands of years, the mechanisms of acupuncture remain largely elusive. A large number of studies in humans and animals have demonstrated that acupuncture produces diverse biological effects on the peripheral and central nerve system leading to the production and release of humoral factors, neurotransmitters, and other chemical mediators.

*Peripheral nervous system* -- An intact peripheral nerve system appears to be necessary for the analgesic effects of acupuncture, because the analgesic effects can be abolished if the acupuncture site is affected by posthepetic neuralgia or intervened with local anesthetics [3, 4].

*Humoral factors* – It was reported as early as in the mid 1970s that acupuncture resulted in a significant increase in the endogenous endorphin production and the effect of acupuncture was blocked by the opioid receptor antagonist naloxone [5]. It is believed that humoral factors may mediate acupuncture analgesia by releasing substances into the cerebrospinal fluid after acupuncture. This notion was supported by a cross-perfusion experiment in which acupuncture-induced analgesic effects were replicated in the recipient rabbit that received the cerebrospinal fluid from the donor rabbit with acupuncture [6]. Electric acupuncture (EA) also has been shown to alter the condition of polycystic ovaries induced by steroids through regulating ovarian nerve growth factors [7].

*Central nervous system* -- Earlier studies have showed that EA at different frequencies could have different effects on the synthesis and release of neuropeptides in the central nervous system. For example, EA at the frequencies of 2 Hz and 100 Hz had differential effects on the preproenkephalin mRNA expression in the brain [8]. EA at 100 Hz markedly increased the preprodynorphin mRNA levels, while EA at 2 Hz had no such effects [8]. Moreover, an μ-opioid receptor antagonist or antiserum against endorphin blocked acupuncture analgesia induced by EA at 2 Hz but not at 100 Hz [9]. In addition, EA induced an increase in cholecystokinin-like immunoreactivity within the medial thalamic area after EA [10] and EA enhanced and restored the activity of natural killer cells suppressed by the hypothalamic lesion [11].

Neuroimaging techniques including functional magnetic resonance imaging (fMRI) and positron emission tomographic (PET) scan have been used to understand the effects of acupuncture on the human brain activity. NIciception can activate neuronal activity in periaqueductal gray, thalamus, hypothalamus, somatosensory cortex, and prefrontal cortex regions in human brain [12], which was attenuated by the sensation of 'de-qi' after acupuncture [13]. As compared to manual acupuncture, EA, particularly at a low frequency, produced more widespread fMRI signal changes in the anterior insula area as well as in the limbic and paralimbic structures [14]. These findings are further supported by the data indicating that stimulation of different Acupoints evoked both signal increases or decreases in different areas within the central nerve system [15], suggesting that there might be some correlations between the effects of acupuncture and neuronal changes within the brain.

*Neurotransmitters* – A large body of evidence indicates that acupuncture significantly affects the production and release of neurotransmitters including epinephrine, norepinephrine, dopamine, and 5-hydroxytryptamine [16]. Specifically, stress-induced increases in norepinephrine, dopamine, and corticosterones were inhibited by EA, a process blocked by the opioid receptor antagonist naloxone, suggesting that the EA effects on the release of neurotranmitters are likely to be mediated through endogenous opioids [17]. Similar results were observed in a number of animal studies examine acupuncture analgesia [18-22]. Of interest to note is that using so-called 'Bi-digital O-ring Test Imaging Technique', researchers found that each meridian was connected to a representative area in the cerebral cortex [23], suggesting that the meridian system defined in the theories of Chinese medicine might have connections to distinct brain regions.

A number of studies have indicated the functional significance of acupuncture-induced changes in neurotransmitters. For instance, EA at different frequencies (2, 10, or 100 Hz) elicited reliable analgesic effects and such effects could be at least partially blocked by a serotonin receptor antagonist [24]. The effects of acupuncture on the neurotransmitter release may depend on the EA frequency, because many brainstem regions could be selectively activated by EA at both 4 Hz and 100 Hz, whereas other regions could only be activated by EA at 4 Hz [25]. Interestingly, the analgesic effect of EA at 4 Hz was mediated through endogenous opioids [25], while the analgesic effect of EA at 2 Hz may involve substance P as its mediator [26].

Besides its effect on acupuncture analgesia, the EA-induced modulation of neurotransmitter release may also mediate other therapeutic effects of acupuncture. There is evidence that EA at 100 Hz could protect axotomized dopaminergic neurons from degeneration by suppressing the axotomy-induced inflammatory responses [27], raising the possibility that acupuncture might be tried to treat certain neurological disorders such as Parkinson's disease [28]. Another example is that the excitatory effects on gastrointestinal mobility following EA or moxibustion in rats was abolished by serotonin inhibitors [29], indicating that serotonin may be a critical mediator of many acupuncture effects such as gastric emptying and analgesia. Similarly, the reduced production of nitric oxide within the gracile nucleus after acupuncture has been shown to mediate the effect of acupuncture on reversing bradycardia [30].

## Acupuncture as a Clinical Tool

Pre-acupuncture evaluation – Evaluating patients for acupuncture includes the following aspects: 1) observing a patient's appearance by looking at the patient's tongue such as its shape, color, and texture; 2) asking questions regarding the patient's chief complaints, symptoms, and general medical conditions; and 3) feeling radial pulses for information concerning the internal organ system. Conventional medical examinations such as inspection, palpation, auscultation, percussion, range of motion of the extremities, reflexes, and neurological examinations are also used to obtain patient's information.

Selection of Acupoints -- Acupoints are usually chosen based on the practitioner's assessment of the particular imbalance between Yin and Yang that needs to be restored. Since the formulation of an acupuncture treatment is often highly individualized, which is largely based on the practitioner's philosophical constructs, subjective and intuitive impression about the patient's condition, a practitioner may select different Acupoints at each treatment session based on the patient's particular complaints, symptoms and presentations at the time of treatment. This explains why a repeat evaluation of the patient's condition is needed at each session to formulate an acupuncture treatment plan.

Acupuncture techniques -- After the needle insertion into an Acupoint, the sensation of 'de-qi', which is a feeling of achy, swollen, tingling, numbness and/or heaviness at the insertion site, is thought to be necessary for obtaining a therapeutic effect. An acupuncture needle may remain in place for 15-30 minutes through the manual or electrical stimulation. In some cases, radiant heat from a lamp or Moxa (burning herbs) can be applied to the top of an acupuncture needle to obtain additional effect. Of interest to point out is that there were many different styles of acupuncture techniques including traditional Chinese acupuncture, Korean hand acupuncture, Japanese acupuncture, scalp and ear acupuncture, each of which remains in practice in many parts of the world.

The above discussion on the clinical issues of acupuncture suggests that preclinical studies on acupuncture and its mechanisms need to mimic the clinical practice of acupuncture in order to maximize the gain of preclinical studies.

## Current Clinical Data on the Effectiveness of Acupuncture

Clinical trials on the efficacy of acupuncture have their unique issues such as individualization, placebo controls, and the crossover design. Nevertheless, an increasing number of clinical trials on acupuncture treatments have provided positive information, particularly on the role of acupuncture in clinical pain management. It is encouraging to see that more randomized; controlled clinical studies have replaced anecdotal case reports. Some of these trials are discussed below on several clinical pain conditions such as low back pain, neck and shoulder pain, and headache.

*Low back pain* -- Chronic low back pain is a common health problem associated with high medical expenses and disability. Although there are many medical treatment options, long-term effects from these medical treatments remain limited. Recently, acupuncture has become one of the most frequently used alternative therapies for treating low back pain. In a randomized, placebo-controlled clinical trial with a 9 month follow up period, Leibing and associates recruited 131 patients with non-radiating low back pain for at least 6 months. These patients were divided into three groups (control, acupuncture, or sham acupuncture). Patients in the control group only received physical therapy for 12 weeks, and patients in other two groups received 20 sessions of either acupuncture or sham acupuncture in addition to physical therapy over 12 weeks. The results indicated that acupuncture was superior to physical therapy regarding pain intensity, pain-related disability, and psychological distress. When compared with sham acupuncture, acupuncture was also superior in reducing psychological stress [31].

In another study, a long-term benefit including returning to work, quality of sleep, and reduced use of analgesics from 8 weeks of acupuncture on low back pain was observed in 50 patients, which lasted up to 6 months [32]. Of interest to note is that both acupuncture and transcutaneous electrical stimulation (TENS) showed significant effects on pain management, but acupuncture was more effective than TENS in the improvement of lumbar spine range of motion [33]. In addition, the duration of acupuncture in a single session appears to be an independent parameter critical to the treatment outcome. For example, a 30-min acupuncture session was more effective than a 15-min session, whereas a 45-min session did not further improve the outcome [34].

*Chronic neck and shoulder pain* -- The results from the treatment of chronic neck and shoulder pain using acupuncture are rather promising. In recent studies, acupuncture produced a prolonged effect (for at least three years) on reducing chronic pain in the neck and shoulder with a concomitant improvement in pain-related activity impairment, depression, anxiety, sleep quality, and quality of life [35,36]. These results are further supported by clinic trials of acupuncture on chronic neck pain with sample sizes from 115 to 177 patients, which demonstrated that acupuncture was superior to controls in reducing neck pain and improving range of motion [37-42]. Moreover, acupuncture has been shown to be effective in treating balance disorders caused by the cervical torsion after whiplash injury [43]. Since whiplash injury is often associated with chronic neck and shoulder pain, these data suggest that acupuncture may be a promising alternative approach for the treatment of whiplash injury-related conditions.

*Headaches* -- Despite the recent advancement in the diagnosis and treatment of different headache disorders, headaches are a common cause for patients to seek medical assistance. Although selective serotonin receptor agonists such as sumatriptan have effectively treated millions of migraine sufferers, there are still at least 30% of migraine patients who do not respond to serotonin receptor agonists. Alternatively, acupuncture has become a new modality of treatment for patients suffering from tension headache, migraine, and other types of headaches [44]. For many patients, acupuncture not only has a similar, if not better, efficacy as compared with sumatriptan in preventing full migraine attack but also unique benefits over serotonin receptor agonists because of its minimal side effects [45]. As a prophylactic treatment for migraine without aura, repeated acupuncture treatment for 2-4 months resulted in a significantly lower number of attacks than the oral therapy with flunarizine [46]. These clinical outcomes appear to be well supported in a comprehensive review that included 27 clinical trials evaluating the efficacy of acupuncture in the treatment of primary headaches (migraine headache, tension headache, and mixed forms), which concluded that the majority of these clinical trials (23 out of 27 trials) showed favorable outcomes in the treatment of headaches [47].

*Other pain conditions* -- Several studies have shown that patients who received acupuncture prior to operation had a lower pain level, reduced opioid requirement, a lower incidence of postoperative nausea and vomiting, and lower sympathoadrenal responses [48-51]. Acupuncture also has been used for the labor pain management. For instance, parturients (90 patients in one study) who received acupuncture during labor significantly reduced the need for epidural analgesia with better relaxation but no negative effects on delivery as compare with the control group [52, 53].

Acupuncture also has been shown to provide some improvement in the function and pain relief as compared to sham acupuncture or controls [54]. In addition, acupuncture was beneficial in treating fibromyalgia and rheumatoid arthritis in several small-scale clinical trials [55], and large-scale clinical trials on these pain conditions may be warranted to further evaluate the effectiveness of acupuncture. Similarly, chronic lateral epicondylitis (tennis elbow) may benefit from the acupuncture treatment in part due to the effect of acupuncture on the improvement in the range of motion and reduction in pain on exertion [56, 57]. In some cases, the effects of acupuncture on tennis elbow lasted up to one year after ten sessions of acupuncture [56, 57].

Besides its analgesic effects, acupuncture has been used for the treatment of many other conditions. For example, a number of clinical trials strongly support a therapeutic role of acupuncture (either needle acupuncture or applying acupressure to the relevant Acupoints) in postoperative nausea and vomiting, as compared to antiemetics such as droperidol and zolfran (58). An increasing number of patients are turning to acupuncture either to supplement or replace conventional treatment for depression, anxiety, obesity, spinal cord injury, insomnia, premenstrual syndrome, menopause symptoms, infertility, allergy, quitting smoking, and detoxication from opioids or other drug addiction, as summarized in a document published by the World Health Organization (WHO) in 2002 (2). Table 2 lists the recommended clinical pain conditions that may be treatable by acupuncture (2).

**Table 2.**

| Pain conditions for which acupuncture has been shown to be effective in controlled trials: |
|---|
| - Headaches |
| - Knee pain |
| - Low back pain |
| - Neck pain |
| - Dental pain and temporomandibular dysfunction |
| - Facial pain and craniomandibular dysfunction |
| - Postoperative pain |
| - Rheumatoid arthritis |
| - Arthritis of the shoulder |
| - Renal colic |
| - Tennis elbow |
| - Sciatica |
| - Sprain |
| *Pain conditions for which the therapeutic effect of acupuncture remains to be confirmed through more controlled clinical trials:* |
| - Abdominal pain (acute gastroenteritis or acute gastrointestinal spasm) |
| - Cancer pain |
| - Earache and pruritus |
| - Eye pain due to sub-conjunctival injection |
| - Fibromyalgia and fasciitis |
| - Labor pain |
| - Pain due to endoscopic examination |
| - Pain due to thromboangitis obliterans |
| - Chronic prostatitis |
| - Radicular and pseudoradicular syndrome |
| - Reflex sympathetic dystrophy |
| - Acute spine pain and stiff neck |

# Conclusion

In recent years, an increasing number of physicians have integrated complementary and alternative medicine such as acupuncture into their practices. Many medical schools in the United States have already added courses on integrated (alternative) medicine. Third-party reimbursements for alternative medicine have increased because of the increasing demand from patients. More encouraging is that the National Center for Complementary and Alternative Medicine (NCCAM) has funded a considerable number of research projects related to complementary and alternative medicine including acupuncture, opening an important branch of translational pain research.

Despite many positive developments complementary and alternative medicine, both preclinical and clinical research on this topic faces a number of challenges. Taking acupuncture as an example, although many studies on acupuncture treatment have been published, the scientific merits in some of these studies may be limited by the study design and non-standardized acupuncture practices. Perhaps it is difficult to keep meaningful blindness to patients in a clinical trial on alternative medicine despite the innovative study designs using non-specific needling (i.e. placing an acupuncture needle at an Acupoint not intended for the treatment) or sham needling. In many cases, it is difficult to entirely rule out a placebo effect in many clinical trials of alternative medicine. As discussed in volume one of this book series, a placebo effect by itself may be an active element of many pain treatments. Another issue related to the preclinical and clinical studies of alternative medicine such as acupuncture is that the effect of alternative medicine is highly individualized even for the same pain condition, making it difficult to establish a standard of positive treatment outcome.

Nonetheless, efforts are being made to standardize clinical trials on complementary and alternative medicine. This is certainly an interesting area of translational pain research that may open new opportunities both for pain research and clinical pain management. It can be anticipated that complementary and alternative medicine is likely to play a growing and positive role in clinical pain management.

# References

[1] Eisenberg DM, Davis RB, Ettner SL, et al. Trends in alternative medicine use in the United States 1990-1997, result of a follow up national survey. *JAMA*. 1998 Nov. 11; 280(18) 1569-75.

[2] *WHO* Acupuncture review and analysis of report on controlled clinical trials. 2002. www.who.int.

[3] Bowsher D. Mechanism of acupuncture. In: Filshie J, White A, eds. *Medical acupuncture*. Edinburgh, Scotland: Churchill Livingstone; 1998:69-80.

[4] Chiang CY, Chang CT. Peripheral afferent pathway for acupuncture analgesia. *Sci. Sin.* 1973; 16:210-217.

[5] Mayer DJ, Price DD, Rafii A. Antagonism of acupuncture analgesia in man by the narcotic antagonist naloxone. *Brain Res.* 1977; 121:368-372.

[6] Han JS, Terenius L. Neurochemical basis of acupuncture analgesia. *Annu. Rev. Pharmacol. Toxicol.* 1982; 22:193-220.

[7] Stener-Victorin E, Lundeberg T, Cajander S, et al. Steroid induced polycystic ovaries in rats: effect of electro-acupuncture on concentrations of endothelin-1 and nerve growth factor (NGF), and expression of NGF mRNA in the ovaries, the adrenal glands and the central nervous system. *Reprod. Biol. Endocrinol.* 2003 Apr 8; 1(1): 33.

[8] Guo HF, Wang XM, Tian JH, et al. 2Hz and 100 Hz electro-acupuncture accelerate the expression of genes encoding three opioid peptide in the rat brain. *Sheng Li Xuo Bao* 1997 Apr; 49(2): 121-7.

[9] Huang C, Wang Y, Chang JK, et al. Endomorphine and mu-opioid receptors in mouse brain mediate the analgesic effect induced by 2 Hz but not 100 Hz electroacupuncture stimulation. *Neurosci. Letter.* 2000;Nov.24; 295(3): 159-62.

[10] Xu M, Aiuchi T, NakayaK, et al, Effect of low frequency electric stimulation on in vivo release of cholecystokinin like immunoreactivity in medial thalamus of conscious rat. *Neurosci. Letter.* 1990 Oct; 118(2): 205-7.

[11] Hahm ET, Lee JJ, Lee WK, et al. Electroacupuncture enhancements of natural killer cell activity suppressed by anterior hypothalamic lesions in rats. *Neuroimmunomodulation.* 2004; 11(4): 268-72.

[12] Hsieh JC, Stahle-backdahl M, Hagermark O, et al. Traumatic nociceptive pain activates the hypothalamus and periaqueductal gray: a positron emission tomography study. *Pain.* 1995; 64:303-314.

[13] Hui KK, Liu J, Marina O, et al. The integrated response of the human cerebro-cerebellar and limbic system to acupuncture stimulation at ST 36 as evidenced by fMRI. *Neuro Image.* 2005;Sep; 27(3): 479-96.

[14] Napadow V, Markris N, Lin J, et al. Effects of electroacupuncture versus manual acupuncture on the human brain as measured by fMRI. *Hum. Brain. Mapp.* 2005; Mar; 24(3): 193-205.

[15] Yan B, Li K, Xu J, et al. Acupoint-specific fMRI patterns in human brain. *Neurosci. Letter.* 2005;Aug 5; 383(3): 236-40.

[16] Hou JG, Liu HL, He TX et al. Study of the acupuncture effect on monoamine transmitters in rabbit plasma and brain tissue by high performance of liquid chromatography with electrochemical detection. *Se. Pu. 2002*; Mar; 20(2): 140-3.

[17] Han JS, Yoon SH, Cho YW, et al. Inhibitory effects of electroacupuncture on stress response evoked by tooth-pulp stimulation in rats. *Physio. Behav.* 1999; Apr; 66(2): 217-22.

[18] Zhou Y, Wang Y, Fang Z, et al. Influence of acupuncture on blood pressure, contents of NE, DA, 5-HT of SHR and interrelation between blood pressure and whole blood viscosity. *Zhen. Ci. Yan. Jiu.* 1995; 20(3): 55-61.

[19] Wang H, Jiang J, Can X. Change of norepinephrine release in rats nucleus reticularis paragigantocellularis lateralis in acupuncture analgesia. *Zhen. Ci. Yan. Jiu.* 1994; 19(1): 20-5.

[20] Wang Y, Wang S, Zhang W. Effects of naloxone on changes of pain threshold and contents of monoamine neurotransmitters in rat brain induced by EA. *J. Tradi. Chin. Med.* 1991; Dec; 11(4): 286-90.

[21] Zhu JM, He XP, Cao XD. Changes of release of beta-endorphin like immunoreactive substance and nor-adrenaline in rabbits preoptic area during acupuncture analgesia. *Sheng. Li. Xue. Bao.* 1990; Apr; 42(2): 188-93.

[22] Zhu J, Xia Y, Cao X. Effects of noradrenaline and dopamine in preoptic area on acupuncture analgesia. *Zhen. Ci. Yan. Jiu.* 1990; 15(2): 117-22.

[23] Omura Y. Connections found between each meridian and organ representation area of corresponding internal organ in each side of the cerebral cortex; release of common neurotransmitters and hormones unique to each meridian and corresponding acupuncture point and internal organ after acupuncture electric stimulation, mechanical stimulation (include shiatsu), soft laser stimulation or Qi Gong. Acupuncture Electro *Thera. Res.* 1989; 14(2) 155-86.

[24] Chang FC, Tsai HY, Yu MC, et al. The central serotonergic system mediates the analgesic effects of electroacupuncture on Zusanli (ST36) acupoint. *Biomed. Sci.* 2004; Mar-Apr; 11(2): 179-85.

[25] Lee JH, Beitz AJ. The distribution of brain stem and spinal cord nuclei associated with different frequencies of electroacupuncture analgesia. *Pain.* 1993; Jan; 52(1): 11-28.

[26] Shen S, Bian JT, Tian JB, et al. Frequency dependence of substance P release by electroacupuncture in rat spinal cord. *Sheng. Li. Xiu. Bao.* 1996; Feb; 48(1): 89-93.

[27] Liu XY, Zhou HF, Pan YL, et al. Electroacupuncture stimulation protects dopaminergic neurons from inflammation-mediated damage in medial forebrain bundle transected rats. *Exp. Neurol.* 2004 Sep; 189(1) 189-196.

[28] Park HJ, Lim S, Joo WS, et al. Acupuncture prevents 6-hydroxy dopamine induced neuronal death in the nigrostriatal dopaminergic system in rat Parkinson's disease modal. *Exp. Neurol.* 2003 Mar; 180(1) 93-8.

[29] Sugai GC, Freire Ade O, Tabosa A, et al. Serotonin involvement in the electroacupuncture and Moxibustion induced gastric emptying in rats. *Physiol. Behav.* 2004 Oct; 82(5): 855-61.

[30] Chen S, Ma SX. Nitric oxide in gracile nucleus mediates depressor response to acupuncture (ST 36). *J. Neurophysiol.* 2003 Aug; 90 (2): 780-5.

[31] Leibing E, Leonhardt U, Koster G, et al. Acupuncture treatment of chronic low back pain – a randomized blinded, placebo-controlled trial with 9-month follow up. *Pain.* 2002 Mar; 96(1-2): 189-196.

[32] Molsberger AF, Mau J, Pawelec DB, et al. Does acupuncture improve the orthopedic management of chronic low back pain – a randomized, blind, controlled trial with 3-month follow up. *Pain.* 2002 Oct; 99 (3): 579-87.

[33] Carlsson CP, Sjolund BH. Acupuncture for chronic low back pain: a randomized placebo-controlled study with long term follow up. *Clin. J. of Pain.* 2001 Dec; 17(4): 296-305.

[34] Grant DJ, Bishop-Miller J, Winchester J, et al. A randomized comparative trial of acupuncture versus transcutaneous electrical nerve stimulation for chronic back pain in the elderly. *Pain.* 1999 July; 82(1): 9-13.

[35] Hamza M, Ghoname E, White P, et al. Effect of the duration of electrical stimulation on the analgesic response in patients with low back pain. *Anesthesiology.* 1999 Dec; 91(6): 1622-7.

[36] He D, Veiersted KB, Hostmark AT, et al. Effect of acupuncture treatment on chronic neck and shoulder pain in sedentary female workers: a 6-month and 3 year follow up study. *Pain.* 2004 Jun; 109(3): 299-307.

[37] He D, Hostmark AT, Veiersted KB, et al. Effect of intensive acupuncture on pain related social and psychological variables for women with chronic neck and shoulder pain- an RCT with six month and three year follow up. *Acupuncture. Med* 2005 June; 23(2): 52-61.

[38] White P, Lewith G, Prescott P, et al. Acupuncture versus placebo for the treatment of chronic mechanical neck pain: a randomized controlled trial. *Ann. Intern. Med.* 2004 Dec 21; 141(12): I26.

[39] Bloss Feldt P. Acupuncture for chronic neck pain – a cohort study in an NHS pain clinic. *Acupuncture. Med.* 2004 Sep; 22(3): 146-51.

[40] Konig A, Radke S, Molzen H, et al. Randomized trial of acupuncture compared with conventional massage and sham laser acupuncture for treatment of chronic neck pain – range of motion analysis. *Z. Orthop. Ihre. Grenzgeb.* 2003 Jul-Aug; 141(4): 395-400.

[41] Giles LG, Muller R. Chronic spinal pain: a randomized clinical trial comparing medication, acupuncture and spinal manipulation. *Spine.* 2003 July15; 28 (14): 1490-502.

[42] Irnich D, Behrens N, Molzen H, et al. Randomized trial of acupuncture compared with conventional massage and sham laser acupuncture for treatment of chronic neck pain. *BMJ.* 2001 June 30; 322(7302): 1574-8.

[43] Fattori B, Ursino F, Cingolani C, et al. Acupuncture treatment of whiplash injury. *Int. Tinnitus. J.* 2004; 10 (2): 156-60.

[44] Alexander Mauskop. Alternative therapies in headache. *Med. Clinics of North America* 2001 July; 85(4).

[45] Melchart D, Thormaehlen J, Hager S, et al. Acupuncture versus placebo versus sumatriptan for early treatment of migraine attacks: a randomized control trial. *J. Intern. Med.* 2003 Feb; 253(2): 181-8.

[46] Allais G, De Lorenzo C, Quirico PE, et al. Acupuncture in the prophylactic treatment of migraine headache without aura: a comparison with flunarizine. *Headache.* 2002 Oct; 42(9): 855-61.

[47] Manias P, Tagaris G, Karageorgiou K. Acupuncture in headache: a critical review. *Clin. J. Pain.* 2000 Dec; 16(4); 334-9.

[48] Kotani N, Hoshimoto H, Sato Y, et al. Preoperaive intradermal acupuncture reduces postoperative pain, nausea and vomiting, analgesic requirement and sympathoadrenal response. *Anesthesiology.* 2001 Aug; 95(2) 349-56.

[49] Lin JG, Lo MW, Wen YR et al. The effect of high and low frequency electroacupuncture in pain after lower abdominal surgery. *Pain.* 2002 Oct; 99(3): 509-14.

[50] Sim EK, Xu PC, Pua HL et al. Effects of electroacupuncture on intraoperative and postoperative analgesic requirement. *Acupuncture Med.* 2002 Aug; 20(2-3): 56-65.

[51] Wan SM, Kain ZN. P6 acupoint injections are as effective as droperidol in controlling early postoperative nausea and vomiting in children. *Anesthesiology.* 2002 Aug; 97(2); 359-66.

[52] Ramnero A, Hanson U, Kihlgren M. Acupuncture treatment during labor – a randomized controlled trial. *BJOG.* 2002 June; 109(6): 637-44.

[53] Skiland E, Fossen D, Heiberg E. Acupuncture in the management of pain in the labor. *Acta Obstet. Gynecol. Scand.* 2002 Oct; 81(10): 943-8.

[54] Berman b, Lao L, Langenberg p, et al. Effectiveness of acupuncture as adjunctive therapy in osteoarthritis of the knee. *Ann. Intern. Med.* 2004 Dec; 141(12): I20.

[55] Berman B, Swyers J, Ezzo J. The evidence for acupuncture as a treatment for rhematology conditions. *Rheumatic Disease clinics of North America* 2000 Feb; 26(1): 103-15.

[56] Fink M, Wolkenstein E, Luennemann M, et al. Acupuncture in chronic epicondylitis: effects of real or sham acupuncture treatment: a randomized controlled patient-and

examiner- blinded long term trial. *Forsch. Komplementarmed. Klass Natur.heilkd.* 2002 Aug; 9(4): 210-5.

[57] Tsui P, Leung MC. Comparison of the effectiveness between manual acupuncture and electroacupuncture on patients with tennis elbow. *Acupuncture Electro. Ther. Res.* 2002; 27(2): 107-17.

[58] Alkaissi A, Evertsson K, Johnson VA, et al. P6 acupressure may relieve nausea and vomiting after gynecological surgery: an effectiveness study in 410 women. *Can. J. Anesth.* 2002 Dec; 49(10): 1034-9.

# Index

## A

acceptance, 97, 179, 182
access, 12, 13, 242, 281, 286
accounting, 128
accumulation, 5, 126, 127, 309
acetaminophen, 117, 160, 161, 166, 286, 296
acetic acid, 156
acetylcholine, 58, 103, 178, 186
achievement, 155
acid, 9, 10, 22, 25, 46, 48, 59, 60, 61, 64, 65, 66, 67, 73, 74, 75, 76, 80, 84, 85, 128, 129, 150, 153, 156, 157, 160, 166, 191, 215, 241, 243, 260, 273, 297, 303
acidosis, 10
ACTH, 135, 241
action potential, 3, 32, 40, 50, 97, 105, 189, 200, 203, 223, 224, 236
activation, 10, 13, 15, 19, 20, 21, 26, 45, 46, 47, 48, 49, 51, 52, 55, 56, 57, 58, 59, 60, 62, 63, 67, 70, 71, 73, 74, 75, 80, 84, 85, 86, 89, 90, 92, 95, 97, 99, 100, 101, 102, 104, 106, 143, 148, 149, 162, 165, 173, 174, 176, 178, 184, 186, 206, 208, 223, 224, 225, 226, 229, 230, 237, 241, 244, 254, 255, 257, 258, 280, 299, 301, 306
adaptation, 91, 107
addiction, 109, 111, 113, 129
additives, 296
adenoma, 164
adenosine, 192, 204, 270
ADH, 135
adhesion, 59
adjunctive therapy, 329
administrators, 282
adolescence, 222, 286
adolescents, 244, 287

adrenal glands, 326
adrenaline, 174, 185, 327
adrenoceptors, 173, 175, 176, 178, 184, 186
adult population, 159
adulthood, 8, 222, 226, 247, 251
adults, 161, 165, 210, 217, 218, 223, 224, 225, 227, 239, 241, 242, 243, 244, 261, 264, 265, 266, 267, 293, 310
adverse event, 29, 37, 112, 113, 122, 158, 161, 164, 215, 262, 264, 265, 267, 268, 269
aetiology, 16, 152, 216, 291
affect, 48, 52, 54, 59, 62, 128, 129, 140, 166, 195, 203, 208, 213, 224, 225, 226, 231, 236
affective dimension, 208
affective experience, 212
afferent nerve, 26, 177
age, 28, 109, 118, 124, 158, 159, 222, 223, 224, 225, 227, 228, 229, 230, 231, 236, 237, 238, 242, 243, 244, 245, 246, 248, 269, 292, 293
agent, 28, 29, 31, 32, 33, 34, 36, 38, 48, 50, 61, 125, 129, 131, 136, 171, 178, 193, 198, 215, 270, 271, 286, 296, 307
age-related, 231, 246, 292, 293
aggression, 74
agonist, 33, 48, 57, 59, 60, 61, 62, 65, 73, 80, 89, 90, 95, 99, 100, 102, 125, 127, 173, 178, 225, 251, 260, 263, 268, 275, 279, 296
AIDS, 30, 35, 40
airways, 170
alcohol, 28, 124, 158, 284, 296, 306
alcohol abuse, 284
alcohol consumption, 158
algorithm, 131, 211, 299
alkaloids, 166
allergy, 271, 324

# Index

alternative, viii, 32, 34, 47, 63, 64, 65, 90, 100, 102, 242, 246, 255, 297, 299, 302, 304, 312, 317, 318, 319, 323, 325, 326
alternative medicine, viii, 317, 318, 319, 325, 326
alternatives, 26
alters, 92, 100, 102, 104, 149
amendments, 181
amenorrhea, 135
American Psychiatric Association, 210, 217, 218
amino acids, 46, 56, 66, 73, 139
ammonium, 193
amplitude, 50, 223
amputation, 83, 243
amygdala, 12, 225, 228, 241, 280
analgesic, viii, 4, 8, 9, 13, 18, 25, 26, 27, 29, 31, 32, 33, 35, 39, 40, 41, 43, 62, 63, 71, 76, 77, 82, 84, 85, 87, 90, 94, 97, 101, 105, 110, 111, 112, 113, 116, 121, 122, 123, 124, 125, 126, 127, 128, 129, 130, 132, 133, 134, 139, 143, 151, 155, 157, 161, 179, 190, 191, 192, 222, 229, 230, 232, 235, 241, 245, 261, 279, 286, 287, 289, 292, 293, 296, 297, 298, 299, 300, 302, 303, 306, 311, 312, 320, 321, 324, 326, 327, 328, 329
analgesic agent, 231, 296
anastomosis, 174
anatomy, 247, 307
anesthetics, 16, 149, 179, 187, 189, 192, 195, 200, 202, 204, 205, 206, 242, 243, 298, 300, 320
angina, 181, 268, 283
angiotensin II, 171
animals, 2, 3, 5, 11, 12, 13, 50, 54, 57, 58, 89, 90, 174, 198, 227, 241, 244, 246, 278, 279, 281, 285, 287, 293, 320
anisotropy, 250
ANOVA, 199
ANS, 170, 177, 182
antagonism, 46, 50, 63, 75, 78, 85
antibody, 15, 54, 92
anticholinergic, 28, 214, 286, 298
anticonvulsant, 14, 28, 29, 30, 31, 34, 38, 297
antidepressant, 191, 196, 205, 209, 210, 211, 212, 213, 214, 215, 218, 273, 298
antidepressant medication, 211, 213, 215
antidiuretic hormone, 135, 144
antiemetics, 324
antigen, 66
anti-inflammatory agents, 117
anti-inflammatory drugs, viii, 155, 157, 164, 165, 166, 230, 261, 276, 296

anxiety, 2, 12, 29, 39, 62, 121, 129, 134, 190, 192, 204, 207, 208, 211, 212, 213, 216, 218, 284, 323, 324
anxiety disorder, 204, 207, 212, 213, 216
aplastic anemia, 34
apoptosis, 160, 245, 306
appetite, 255, 297
apraxia, 309
aptitude, 144
arousal, 2
arteries, 261
artery, 268, 269, 275, 283, 290
arthritis, 49, 66, 211
articular cartilage, 160, 165
assessment, 4, 5, 34, 36, 41, 84, 110, 115, 118, 122, 123, 132, 136, 137, 140, 165, 179, 212, 231, 232, 239, 241, 243, 250, 272, 285, 322
assessment tools, 84, 115
association, 87, 90, 94, 96, 98, 104, 106, 107, 133, 140, 169, 177, 252, 256, 271, 291
assumptions, 239
asthma, 209
asymptomatic, 34, 161
ataxia, 308
attacks, 34, 162, 163, 254, 255, 256, 258, 259, 260, 261, 263, 264, 265, 266, 267, 269, 271, 272, 273, 275, 324, 329
attention, 9, 57, 109, 135, 213, 246, 256
attitudes, 109, 137, 281, 285
attribution, 212
autoantibodies, 172
autonomic nervous system, 169, 170, 172, 177, 182, 246, 289
autopsy, 247
availability, 93, 98, 269, 287, 299
avoidance, 256, 307
awareness, 299
axonal degeneration, 193

# B

back pain, 33, 41, 42, 113, 117, 121, 134, 138, 140, 141, 155, 161, 166, 284, 285, 288, 292, 294, 309, 323, 325, 328
balanced state, 319
barriers, 196, 203, 285
basic research, 25, 36, 41, 46, 63, 291
basilar migraine, 275
Beck Depression Inventory, 214

behavior, 17, 21, 22, 52, 54, 60, 61, 70, 72, 76, 118, 122, 124, 126, 136, 140, 151, 152, 153, 173, 185, 186, 207, 213, 216, 218, 227, 244, 245, 305
behavioral change, 176, 255
behavioral medicine, 116
beneficial effect, 178
benzodiazepine, 29, 230
bias, 279, 285, 287
binding, 26, 31, 48, 49, 56, 57, 59, 60, 65, 66, 75, 76, 80, 89, 95, 106, 128, 141, 189, 193, 195, 196, 197, 203, 204, 205, 206, 230, 243, 296, 305
bioavailability, 126, 127, 128, 203
biosynthesis, 160
birth, 67, 225, 227, 230, 235, 236, 241, 244, 246, 249
birth weight, 236, 246
bladder, 170, 292, 307, 308
bleeding, 10, 158
blind spot, 258
blocks, 22, 34, 53, 57, 76, 105, 171, 180, 182, 183, 189, 200, 280, 306, 307
blood, 34, 61, 118, 126, 152, 158, 162, 163, 170, 171, 176, 177, 178, 181, 182, 188, 228, 245, 254, 256, 257, 258, 259, 261, 268, 272, 275, 282, 284, 302, 303, 308, 327
blood dyscrasias, 34
blood flow, 162, 170, 171, 178, 182, 188
blood pressure, 158, 181, 282, 327
blood vessels, 61, 162, 176, 177, 254, 256, 257, 258, 259, 268, 275
blood-brain barrier, 126, 245
bloodstream, 300
body, 13, 27, 35, 124, 126, 163, 170, 174, 179, 210, 212, 223, 227, 240, 243, 284, 289, 302, 303, 304, 305, 318, 319, 321
body fat, 124
body weight, 35, 210
bone cancer, 11, 12, 20, 21, 22, 23, 313
bone marrow, 10, 303
boredom, 209
bowel, 279, 283, 284, 289, 290, 291, 292, 307
boys, 249
brachial plexus, 243, 249
bradycardia, 322
bradykinin, 14, 58, 148, 152, 175
brain, 1, 3, 8, 12, 14, 21, 38, 56, 64, 66, 67, 70, 90, 96, 101, 102, 103, 104, 105, 125, 145, 152, 162, 192, 207, 212, 221, 228, 230, 231, 234, 236, 240, 244, 245, 247, 250, 251, 257, 260, 272, 277, 280, 281, 284, 288, 289, 296, 309, 320, 321, 326, 327, 328
brain activity, 212, 272
brain stem, 328
brainstem, 80, 225, 228, 230, 240, 246, 248, 258, 261, 321
breakdown, 9
breast cancer, 9, 302, 307, 313, 315
breast carcinoma, 304
buccal mucosa, 127
bundle branch block, 214, 298
burning, 7, 27, 28, 35, 322

# C

caffeine, 192, 261, 262, 273
calcitonin, 29, 56, 66, 236, 258, 306
calcium, 8, 15, 18, 25, 26, 29, 30, 31, 35, 36, 40, 46, 59, 60, 65, 69, 73, 74, 80, 148, 151, 186, 192, 226, 229, 233, 297, 303
calcium channel blocker, 15, 31, 36, 186
caliber, 236
cancer, viii, 1, 2, 9, 10, 11, 13, 19, 20, 21, 22, 27, 28, 30, 38, 40, 82, 86, 109, 110, 111, 114, 115, 116, 117, 124, 128, 131, 132, 133, 134, 135, 137, 138, 140, 141, 142, 143, 144, 145, 182, 209, 244, 295, 296, 297, 298, 299, 302, 303, 304, 305, 306, 307, 308, 309, 310, 311, 312, 313, 314, 315
cancer cells, 10, 19
candidates, 30, 304
capillary, 141
capsule, 159, 297
carbon, 190
carcinoma, 11, 304, 314
cardiac surgery, 248
cardiovascular disease, 269
cartilage, 159, 160, 161, 165, 318
cast, 173
catabolism, 305
catalyst, 305
catalytic properties, 99
catecholamines, 171, 174, 175, 241, 291
catheter, 181, 301, 307, 309
cation, 10
Caucasians, 129
cDNA, 71
cell, 4, 7, 10, 11, 19, 26, 51, 52, 59, 80, 87, 97, 100, 104, 106, 148, 150, 151, 157, 165, 175, 176, 193, 222, 226, 233, 235, 236, 245, 258, 304, 308, 314
cell body, 148

cell death, 165, 245
cell line, 11
cell membranes, 106
cell signaling, 104
central nervous system, 1, 2, 30, 34, 45, 46, 55, 71, 80, 151, 158, 247, 259, 280, 281
cerebral blood flow, 162
cerebral cortex, 257, 321
cerebral function, 282
cerebrospinal fluid, 55, 141, 304, 320
cervix, 291
channels, 1, 3, 4, 5, 6, 7, 8, 15, 16, 25, 26, 29, 30, 31, 32, 34, 35, 40, 41, 49, 52, 56, 57, 59, 65, 66, 68, 74, 148, 151, 152, 189, 191, 192, 196, 197, 200, 201, 202, 203, 204, 205, 206, 231, 237, 297
chemical properties, 147
chemical structures, 190
chemokines, 10
chemoprevention, 164
chemotherapy, 9, 298, 301, 303, 304
childhood, 43, 213, 222, 246
children, 37, 43, 221, 222, 229, 231, 232, 239, 243, 244, 246, 247, 248, 249, 250, 251, 310, 329
China, 318, 319
Chinese medicine, 318, 319, 321
CHO cells, 96, 105
cholera, 96, 106
chondrocyte, 160
chromatography, 121
chronic illness, 114
circulation, 55, 152, 179, 256, 272, 275, 300
circumcision, 243, 249
citalopram, 191, 211, 217
classes, 7, 9, 14, 27, 48, 62, 64, 75, 91, 149, 157, 203, 210, 274, 296
classification, 115, 216, 273, 278, 310
clinical depression, 207, 208
clinical judgment, 116, 120
clinical presentation, 171, 209, 244, 253, 282
clinical syndrome, 173
clinical trials, 15, 27, 29, 30, 31, 32, 33, 34, 37, 79, 80, 81, 112, 125, 158, 161, 164, 182, 187, 191, 219, 239, 261, 265, 268, 274, 278, 279, 286, 287, 302, 322, 324, 325, 326
cloning, 98, 104
closure, 241
cluster headache, 43, 264
CNS, 4, 7, 8, 45, 46, 57, 71, 75, 85, 88, 116, 139, 149, 151, 153, 158, 163, 189, 191, 192, 199, 200, 204, 223, 224, 228, 230, 232, 259, 272, 275

cocaine, 119, 120, 251
coding, 1, 12
cognition, 134, 284
cognitive dysfunction, 285
cognitive impairment, 134, 214, 255
cognitive process, 2
cognitive processing, 2
cohort, 216, 288, 328
colic, 282
collateral, 170
colon, 19, 283, 291
colon cancer, 19
colostomy, 300
combination therapy, 14, 28, 33, 35, 295
commitment, viii
common bile duct, 291
communication, 115, 285
community, 286
comorbidity, 207, 216, 291
compartment syndrome, 114
complement, 240, 278
complexity, 87, 100, 244, 246
compliance, 110, 121, 178, 309
complications, 110, 158, 179, 209, 282, 299, 306, 309
components, 46, 60, 63, 73, 90, 160, 170, 208, 228, 243, 257
composition, 49, 69, 224
compounds, 48, 128, 133, 151, 190, 192, 203, 302
computed tomography, 308
concentration, 26, 99, 132, 171, 189, 193, 195, 196, 197, 200, 201, 202, 209, 224, 241, 259, 265, 267
conception, 169
concrete, 119
conditioning, 196
conduct, 120
conduction, 32, 205, 206, 250, 298
confidence, 112
confidence interval, 112
confusion, 191, 299
connectivity, 226
conscious awareness, 248
consensus, 15, 109, 131, 137, 151, 209, 268, 271, 278
consent, 239
constipation, 10, 28, 35, 111, 113, 132, 133, 134, 135, 143, 191, 214, 215, 279, 290, 299, 300, 301
consulting, 272
consumption, 29, 31, 39, 83, 84, 110, 137, 287, 303
context, 109, 207, 213, 318

continuity, 87
control, 2, 3, 5, 6, 7, 14, 21, 26, 27, 28, 34, 36, 37, 41, 42, 46, 48, 50, 53, 58, 61, 63, 66, 74, 77, 102, 107, 110, 114, 135, 137, 143, 147, 151, 161, 162, 170, 172, 173, 180, 182, 184, 186, 188, 199, 216, 225, 226, 234, 236, 242, 243, 254, 280, 284, 288, 294, 297, 300, 304, 305, 307, 308, 309, 312, 314, 315, 323, 324, 329
control group, 323, 324
controlled studies, 81, 215, 240, 265, 288, 306
controlled trials, 110, 113, 158, 159, 160, 163, 180, 183, 298, 306
convergence, 281, 282, 283
conversion, 153, 192, 300, 311
conviction, 88, 213
cooling, 174, 185
coping, 2, 281, 284, 288
coping strategies, 2
coronary artery disease, 269
coronary heart disease, 164, 282
correlation, 12, 38, 41, 70, 159, 172, 248
cortex, 80, 208, 212, 222, 225, 229, 230, 240, 245, 258, 272, 280, 282, 321, 327
cortical neurons, 57, 73, 240
corticosteroid therapy, 297
corticosteroids, 158, 310
cortisol, 135, 241
coupling, 56, 57, 58, 70, 89, 91, 92, 95, 96, 97, 100, 103, 106, 174, 175, 176, 177, 186, 230
cox-2 inhibitor, 22
cranial nerve, 309
critical period, 244
criticism, 132, 173
crossing over, 132
crying, 222, 243
crystals, 303
CSF, 10, 304, 309
cues, 212
culture, 161, 193, 208, 278
culture media, 161
cycles, 192, 247, 255
cyclooxygenase, 19, 22, 55, 71, 139, 149, 150, 153, 155, 156, 157, 163, 164, 165, 166, 237, 270
cytochrome, 127, 129, 215, 242, 246
cytokines, viii, 55, 56, 150, 152, 160, 161, 163, 166, 305

## D

daily living, 122, 123

damage, 2, 3, 4, 8, 10, 143, 148, 159, 174, 176, 221, 227, 228, 231, 242, 285, 328
death, 7, 210, 328
decay, 224
decision making, 118
decisions, 117, 122
defects, 203
deficit, 5, 304, 309
definition, 242, 248
degenerative joint disease, 117
degradation, 89, 100, 160, 165
delirium, 191
delivery, 132, 181, 265, 300, 302, 305, 309, 312, 324
delusions, 210
demand, 289, 325
dementia, 297
demographic data, 130
denial, 213
density, 46, 53, 54, 56, 57, 63, 69, 72, 89, 102, 175, 225, 227, 230, 241, 262, 306
Department of Health and Human Services, 217
dephosphorylation, 95, 105
depolarization, 18, 51, 62, 80, 225, 228, 236, 257, 258
depression, 2, 10, 12, 88, 114, 121, 126, 140, 162, 176, 191, 203, 204, 207, 208, 209, 210, 211, 212, 213, 216, 217, 218, 228, 242, 258, 299, 301, 323, 324
depressive symptomatology, 216
depressive symptoms, 207, 208, 211
deprivation, 246
derivatives, 156, 183, 193, 195, 204, 205, 262
dermis, 175
desensitization, 87, 88, 89, 90, 95, 100, 101, 105, 301
desire, 269
destruction, 9, 10, 11, 14, 15, 20, 21, 22, 160, 181, 182, 226, 304
detection, 9, 172, 327
developing brain, 237
developmental change, 222
diabetes, 27, 37
diabetic neuropathy, 27, 28, 30, 32, 35, 37, 63, 77, 219, 244, 310
diacylglycerol, 56, 59
Diagnostic and Statistical Manual of Mental Disorders, 210, 217
diagnostic criteria, 162, 210, 213, 218, 255, 289
dialysis, 311
diarrhea, 129, 211, 215

dieting, 210
differential diagnosis, 283
differentiation, 19, 254
diffusion, 250
directionality, 92
disability, 36, 112, 113, 161, 166, 207, 208, 210, 213, 218, 255, 261, 264, 271, 285, 288, 307, 323
disappointment, 7
discharges, 32, 186, 199, 200, 203
discipline, 318
discomfort, 179, 209, 212
discrimination, 3, 65
discs, 161, 166
disease progression, 15, 160, 306, 307
disequilibrium, 255
disorder, 1, 162, 166, 170, 207, 208, 209, 210, 211, 212, 213, 214, 215, 216, 217, 218, 219, 254, 255, 256, 257, 282, 291
disposition, 293
dissociation, 102, 201
distress, 114, 122, 191, 208, 210, 285, 288, 296, 323
distribution, 5, 8, 49, 64, 66, 124, 233, 243, 279, 302, 307, 328
diuretic, 158
divergence, 88, 282
diversity, 91
division, 162
doctors, 213, 275
dogs, 160, 205
domain, 47, 48, 65, 69, 74, 119, 123, 150
dominance, 222
dopamine, 69, 92, 103, 104, 107, 175, 192, 257, 321, 327, 328
dorsal horn, 4, 5, 6, 7, 8, 11, 12, 13, 14, 20, 21, 22, 45, 46, 49, 50, 51, 52, 53, 55, 56, 57, 58, 59, 60, 61, 62, 63, 66, 67, 68, 69, 70, 73, 75, 76, 80, 84, 94, 147, 148, 149, 152, 178, 223, 224, 225, 226, 227, 228, 230, 232, 233, 234, 235, 236, 237, 242
dorsolateral prefrontal cortex, 280
dosage, 27, 112, 128, 141, 264, 265, 266, 267
dosing, 13, 14, 30, 37, 83, 84, 125, 127, 131, 178, 231, 240, 242, 266, 267, 274, 297, 303, 311
down-regulation, 102, 106, 259
drug abuse, 130, 142
drug action, 85, 86
drug addict, 107, 324
drug addiction, 107, 324
drug carriers, 203
drug delivery, 30, 132, 143, 203, 265, 309
drug dependence, 137

drug design, 203
drug history, 124
drug metabolism, 128, 222
drug targets, 15
drug therapy, 30
drug treatment, 11, 14, 208, 216, 261
drug use, 38, 130, 142, 286, 292
drugs, 2, 3, 6, 8, 9, 21, 25, 26, 27, 29, 34, 37, 42, 48, 68, 100, 110, 116, 129, 130, 142, 149, 156, 165, 166, 177, 178, 179, 189, 190, 193, 195, 198, 203, 204, 205, 206, 215, 262, 275, 279, 286, 287, 290, 297, 298, 299, 305, 319
dry eyes, 31
DSM, 210, 217, 218
DSM-IV, 210, 217, 218
ductus arteriosus, 241
dura mater, 162
durability, 297
duration, 2, 11, 31, 32, 36, 97, 111, 118, 124, 125, 126, 127, 128, 132, 135, 149, 159, 161, 172, 178, 180, 187, 193, 194, 195, 205, 223, 255, 258, 271, 297, 302, 303, 323, 328

# E

edema, 28, 29, 50, 139, 297, 301, 306
EKG, 298
elderly, 28, 127, 144, 216, 217, 246, 328
electrodes, 182
electrolyte, 9
electron microscopy, 240
electrons, 302
emergence, 8, 21, 92, 93, 100, 104, 307, 310
emission, 273, 275, 321
emotion, 242, 284
emotional experience, 242
emotional state, 12
employment, 207, 213, 216, 288
enantiomers, 127
encoding, 92, 94, 103, 153, 326
endocrine, 135
endometriosis, 282, 291
endoscopic retrograde cholangiopancreatography, 291
endothelial cells, 149, 152
energy supply, 284
England, 16, 155, 248
enlargement, 50, 51
enrollment, 311
enthusiasm, 270

environment, 10, 17, 124, 148, 212, 222, 246, 278, 284
environmental factors, 5
enzymes, 87, 100, 124, 126, 150, 157, 246
epicondylitis, 329
epidemic, 281
epidemiology, 28, 130, 216, 277, 292
epidural hematoma, 181
epilepsy, 3, 31, 78, 182, 203, 297
epinephrine, 171, 184, 321
epithelial cells, 22
equipment, 319
ester, 104
estrogen, 255
ethical issues, 180, 232
ethylene, 190, 303, 313
etiology, 114, 159, 184, 191, 244
Europe, 261, 263, 302
evidence, 10, 11, 12, 13, 14, 27, 28, 37, 45, 46, 57, 58, 62, 64, 71, 72, 79, 80, 81, 87, 90, 93, 95, 96, 97, 106, 111, 113, 116, 123, 125, 130, 132, 134, 141, 149, 158, 159, 160, 162, 166, 171, 172, 173, 174, 178, 179, 180, 181, 182, 188, 192, 193, 196, 207, 210, 226, 228, 231, 232, 236, 244, 246, 254, 261, 268, 269, 271, 272, 273, 285, 287, 297, 298, 299, 302, 306, 311, 317, 318, 321, 329
evolution, 155, 183, 185
examinations, 322
exchange transfusion, 241
excitability, 3, 12, 21, 26, 40, 51, 148, 149, 151, 152, 162, 186, 223, 224, 225, 258
excitation, 51, 56, 61, 126, 162, 176, 185, 224, 225, 226, 235, 241
excitotoxicity, 51
excretion, 135, 273
exercise, 7, 61, 138, 288, 291
exertion, 255, 324
expenditures, 319
exposure, 88, 89, 91, 94, 97, 98, 99, 100, 102, 106, 140, 221, 225, 226, 227, 231, 241, 245, 251, 255, 279, 290, 309
expression, 3, 4, 7, 8, 11, 12, 17, 18, 20, 32, 52, 55, 56, 57, 69, 78, 94, 102, 103, 128, 148, 149, 150, 151, 152, 158, 160, 165, 176, 177, 224, 225, 226, 229, 230, 233, 237, 279, 320, 326
extrapolation, 8
extravasation, 162, 227, 258
extrusion, 234

# F

facial expression, 222
factor analysis, 289
failure, 36, 126, 127, 143, 217, 246, 301, 308, 309, 315
faith, 209
false negative, 212
false positive, 179
family, 45, 46, 54, 57, 58, 59, 60, 71, 72, 73, 95, 104, 109, 119, 120, 123, 124, 209, 210, 213, 255, 269
family environment, 213
family history, 120, 210, 255, 269
family members, 123
fatal arrhythmia, 192
fatiguability, 211
fatigue, 29, 191, 210, 212, 215, 255, 257, 282
FDA, 28, 30, 31, 34, 262, 269, 318, 319
fear, 213, 284
feces, 127
feedback, vii
feelings, 212, 257
females, 135, 255, 277, 278, 279, 280, 281, 283, 285, 286, 287
femur, 11
fetal growth, 245
fetus, 241, 248
fever, 9, 149
fibers, 16, 34, 40, 49, 72, 80, 151, 152, 162, 170, 174, 175, 176, 177, 182, 185, 233, 240, 258, 301, 305, 308
fibroblasts, 159, 165
fibromyalgia, 29, 33, 39, 113, 169, 282, 324
fibrosarcoma, 11
fibrosis, 309
filtration, 242
first generation, 306
fish, 193
fitness, 135
fixation, 303, 307
flavor, 91
flexor, 50, 62
flight, 284
fluctuations, 279
fluid, 30, 126, 309, 320
fluoxetine, 191, 219
focusing, 130
food, 162, 257, 300
foramen, 308

forebrain, 52, 75, 78, 291, 328
fractures, 306
freedom, 9, 266, 269
freezing, 242
friends, 123, 124
functional MRI, 250, 272

## G

ganglion, 32, 54, 97, 148, 170, 172, 175, 176, 178, 179, 180, 181, 185, 186, 187, 236, 273, 307
gastric mucosa, 150
gastroenteritis, 325
gastrointestinal tract, 9, 158, 170, 265, 266, 279, 283, 300
GDP, 89
gel, 311
gender, viii, 8, 124, 210, 213, 277, 278, 279, 281, 282, 284, 285, 286, 287, 288, 289, 291, 292, 294
gender differences, viii, 8, 277, 278, 281, 282, 285, 286, 287, 288
gender effects, 286
gene, 5, 7, 8, 12, 19, 29, 47, 48, 54, 56, 57, 66, 94, 148, 150, 151, 152, 153, 155, 223, 227, 235, 236, 241, 252, 258, 279, 280, 290
gene expression, 12, 148, 150, 227, 235, 279
general anesthesia, 307, 315
generalized anxiety disorder, 212, 213, 218
generation, 4, 13, 21, 93, 169, 170, 177, 183, 184, 185, 200
genes, 8, 56, 66, 98, 148, 149, 158, 160, 326
genetic defect, 203
genetic disease, 203
genetic factors, 285, 299
genetics, 124, 278, 280
genome, 8
genotype, 257, 280, 290
Georgia, 38
gestation, 240, 241
gland, 11
glaucoma, 215
glial cells, 26, 158, 280
glioma, 101, 192
glutamate, viii, 26, 29, 35, 45, 46, 48, 49, 58, 59, 60, 64, 65, 66, 69, 70, 72, 73, 75, 79, 80, 149, 224, 230, 233, 237, 241, 272, 301
glutamate receptor antagonists, viii, 72
glycine, 48, 49, 60, 65, 73, 76, 80, 224, 241
glycosylation, 106
goals, 8, 117, 119, 120

gold, 121, 180
gracilis, 69
graduate students, vii
grants, 64
graph, 6
groups, 33, 36, 46, 113, 121, 125, 133, 135, 148, 162, 163, 178, 197, 198, 246, 282, 287, 288, 306, 318, 323
growth, 10, 19, 22, 135, 144, 147, 148, 151, 159, 165, 223, 224, 227, 240, 241, 247, 251
growth factor, 10, 147, 148, 151, 159, 165, 227, 240, 251
growth hormone, 135, 144, 241
growth rate, 19
guanine, 105, 106
guidance, 179, 308
guidelines, 116, 117, 131, 137, 166, 181, 242, 273
guilt, 210
gut, 279, 283

## H

hair follicle, 234, 247
half-life, 125, 126, 127, 128, 215, 242, 267, 297, 303, 306
hallucinations, 210, 255, 257, 297, 299
hands, 159, 179
harm, 27, 113
HE, 105, 250, 311
head and neck cancer, 301
headache, 33, 36, 38, 41, 43, 162, 163, 211, 215, 253, 254, 255, 256, 257, 261, 262, 264, 265, 266, 267, 271, 272, 273, 275, 310, 323, 329
headache,, 211, 215, 258, 323
healing, 158, 318
health, 46, 108, 109, 110, 112, 115, 130, 137, 182, 207, 208, 213, 216, 248, 278, 281, 282, 285, 286, 288, 289, 318, 319, 323
health care, 108, 109, 110, 115, 278, 281, 282, 285, 286, 288, 289, 318
health care professionals, 278
heart disease, 210, 268
heart rate, 198, 228
heat, 6, 10, 20, 52, 148, 171, 174, 184, 237, 241, 287, 322
heating, 236
hemorrhage, 243
hepatic failure, 296
hepatitis, 143
heritability, 239

herniated, 161, 166
heroin, 107
herpes, 28, 244
herpes zoster, 28, 244
heterogeneity, 271
high blood pressure, 282
hip, 31, 140, 166
hip replacement, 31, 140
hippocampus, 59, 69, 75, 80, 226
histamine, 191, 192, 275
histology, 307
HIV, 27, 28, 35, 38, 43
homeostasis, 170, 259
hopelessness, 207, 209, 212, 213
hormone, 135, 280, 287, 289, 306
hot spots, 302
housing, 278
hub, 12, 74
human animal, 244
human brain, 228, 229, 321, 327
human experience, 244, 281
human subjects, 231, 259
humility, 155
hybrid, 101, 106
hybrid cell, 101, 106
hybridization, 71
hydrogen, 165
hydrogen peroxide, 165
hydrolysis, 97, 107, 127, 303
hydronephrosis, 233, 236
hydrophobicity, 190
hydroxide, 303
hydroxyapatite, 303
hydroxyl, 128
hypercalcemia, 306
hyperesthesia, 76
hyperglycemia, 144
hypersensitivity, 9, 28, 54, 63, 67, 70, 71, 74, 76, 77, 83, 84, 116, 133, 139, 143, 148, 149, 152, 153, 163, 231, 235, 238, 244, 257, 285
hypersomnia, 210
hypertension, 129, 158, 269
hypertrophy, 11, 105
hypochondriasis, 213, 218
hypotension, 214
hypotensive, 298
hypothalamus, 228, 241, 321, 327
hypothesis, 54, 55, 58, 59, 60, 90, 151, 170, 171, 173, 186, 190, 191, 192, 199, 200, 204, 254, 257, 275, 281, 284, 287

hypoxia, 185
hysterectomy, 29

# I

IASP, 51, 62, 70, 183, 219, 271, 278, 290, 291, 293, 311
iatrogenic, 143
ibuprofen, 77, 159, 161, 163, 166, 167, 296
identification, 8, 20, 87, 88, 143, 147, 254, 278
identity, 92
IL-6, 55, 152
ileum, 101
immobilization, 173
immune system, 132
immunodeficiency, 244
immunoprecipitation, 53, 57, 96, 98
immunoreactivity, 4, 16, 20, 105, 234, 235, 276, 321, 326
impotence, 135
imprinting, 232
in situ hybridization, 70, 245
in vitro, 54, 57, 94, 127, 139, 157, 161, 162, 189, 192, 193, 196, 236, 249
incentives, 213
incidence, 27, 28, 29, 30, 34, 35, 129, 130, 131, 133, 134, 158, 175, 176, 181, 243, 244, 296, 304, 319, 324
inclusion, 112, 180
indecisiveness, 210
India, 38
indication, 29, 35, 215, 300, 304
indicators, 96
indirect effect, 126, 170
individualization, 322
induction, 13, 54, 55, 58, 66, 67, 71, 73, 75, 80, 84, 85, 118, 126, 129, 139, 149, 150, 151, 152, 153, 160, 164, 166, 235
inefficiency, 255, 257
inequality, 195, 288
infancy, 222, 247
infants, 221, 222, 226, 227, 228, 229, 231, 233, 235, 236, 242, 243, 245, 246, 247, 250, 251
infection, 28, 150, 181, 244, 301
inferences, 4, 90
inferiority, 299
infertility, 299, 324
inflammation, 4, 7, 11, 12, 15, 19, 21, 45, 47, 50, 52, 53, 54, 55, 56, 57, 58, 59, 60, 62, 63, 64, 67, 68, 70, 72, 76, 77, 80, 81, 82, 83, 85, 116, 133, 139,

148, 149, 150, 151, 152, 153, 157, 158, 161, 162, 171, 175, 221, 226, 227, 228, 231, 233, 235, 236, 254, 257, 258, 259, 281, 306, 328
inflammatory cells, 151
inflammatory mediators, 147, 148, 152, 165, 227
inflammatory responses, 158, 321
inflation, 280
influence, 36, 90, 109, 134, 135, 149, 171, 174, 221, 223, 225, 227, 231, 242, 243, 246, 274, 278, 279, 282, 285, 299
information processing, 135
infrared spectroscopy, 229
ingestion, 296
inhibition, 14, 19, 22, 48, 65, 69, 76, 90, 92, 93, 100, 103, 105, 106, 129, 139, 151, 152, 154, 155, 157, 158, 163, 164, 165, 177, 191, 192, 224, 225, 226, 230, 234, 235, 237, 240, 251, 259, 261, 275, 280, 281
inhibitor, 22, 58, 59, 60, 156, 158, 161, 165, 178, 214, 215, 263
initiation, 45, 54, 58, 102, 118, 161, 200, 210, 259, 298, 302
injections, 13, 33, 172, 174, 184, 204, 237, 242, 306, 329
injury, 4, 7, 8, 13, 15, 16, 17, 18, 20, 21, 27, 28, 31, 32, 33, 35, 38, 41, 45, 46, 47, 50, 51, 52, 54, 55, 56, 57, 61, 62, 64, 67, 68, 71, 72, 75, 76, 78, 80, 81, 82, 83, 84, 85, 145, 148, 149, 150, 151, 153, 158, 171, 172, 173, 175, 176, 177, 181, 184, 185, 186, 200, 222, 226, 227, 228, 235, 236, 242, 243, 249, 284, 285, 286, 288, 297, 323, 324, 329
inositol, 59, 106
input, 4, 11, 12, 36, 49, 50, 55, 56, 61, 63, 67, 71, 83, 149, 170, 224, 226, 233, 234, 239
insertion, 89, 182, 225, 309, 319, 322
insight, 229
insomnia, 190, 214
instability, 243, 246
instruments, 115, 214
integration, 207, 228
integrity, 57, 60
intensity, 2, 9, 16, 33, 34, 35, 36, 41, 49, 82, 83, 96, 110, 112, 115, 118, 119, 122, 138, 148, 172, 179, 226, 255, 256, 261, 262, 264, 265, 266, 267, 270, 271, 274, 283, 286, 287, 323
intensive care unit, 232, 243
interaction, 10, 30, 48, 56, 57, 58, 63, 89, 93, 96, 106, 107, 171, 175, 177, 242, 245, 266, 267, 303

interactions, 17, 20, 29, 34, 48, 58, 65, 72, 84, 100, 128, 141, 151, 165, 175, 183, 282, 283, 284, 286, 300, 301, 311
interest, 4, 7, 29, 31, 33, 35, 210, 231, 241, 244, 259, 278, 321, 322, 323
interface, 98
interference, 29, 114, 135, 300
interleukin-8, 159
interleukins, 10, 152, 161
internalization, 48, 74, 89, 95, 100, 101, 105, 106
interneurons, 224, 230
interpretation, 120, 184, 191, 216, 222, 278, 287
interstitial cystitis, 283, 291
interval, 298
intervention, 152, 211, 244, 274, 285
interview, 123, 211, 213
intestine, 127
intracranial pressure, 304
intravenously, 259
ion channels, vii, 3, 8, 10, 26, 36, 64, 149, 191, 295
ions, 26, 162, 224
ipsilateral, 11, 51, 53, 244
irradiation, 303, 304, 313
irritable bowel syndrome, 279, 291
ischemia, 50, 60, 173, 185, 257, 268
isolation, 143, 149
isomers, 141, 157
isozyme, 104

## J

jobs, 288
joint damage, 159
joint destruction, 159
joint pain, 159, 283
Jordan, 66
judgment, 118, 207, 269

## K

kidney, 58, 143, 151, 158, 296
kidneys, 133, 170
kinase activity, 107
kinetics, 45, 47, 202, 231, 313
knees, 159, 160
knowledge, 4, 8, 15, 25, 31, 36, 47, 87, 90, 100, 151, 203, 228, 232, 247, 253, 254, 270, 285, 295

## L

labeling, 2, 57, 95, 105, 247, 262, 269

labor, 324, 329
labour, 281
laminectomy, 308
language, 180
laparoscopic cholecystectomy, 292
latency, 5, 62, 63
later life, 221, 231
lateral epicondylitis, 324
lead, 1, 4, 8, 10, 26, 51, 57, 83, 84, 121, 125, 126, 129, 130, 135, 147, 149, 152, 160, 176, 177, 182, 183, 214, 224, 227, 282, 284, 286, 296, 299, 305, 306, 307, 308, 309
learning, 47, 134, 232, 245
leisure, 124
lending, 245
lesions, 11, 175, 248, 285, 302, 303, 307, 308, 309, 327
leukotrienes, 153, 160
liability, 130, 298
libido, 132, 135
life expectancy, 295, 302
life quality, 295
life span, 242, 306
lifespan, 277
lifestyle, 118
lifetime, 130, 209, 211, 212, 214
ligands, 3, 80, 105, 141, 176, 311
likelihood, 262, 266, 267
limbic system, 212, 309, 327
limitation, 82
linkage, 246, 280
links, 2
lipid peroxidation, 133
liquid chromatography, 121, 327
liver, 125, 126, 142, 143, 296, 297
local anesthesia, 55, 205, 232
local anesthetic, 31, 32, 55, 172, 178, 179, 180, 181, 187, 189, 192, 193, 195, 198, 202, 203, 205, 206, 298, 306
localization, 52, 65, 245
location, 5, 32, 147, 149, 256
locus, 89, 102, 103, 107, 229, 280
loss of appetite, 210
lumbar radiculopathy, 285
lumbar spine, 16, 166, 309, 315, 323
lung cancer, 303, 304, 308
lying, 174
lymphoma, 104

# M

macrophages, 10
magnesium, 61, 65, 76, 80, 156
magnetic resonance, 208, 240, 247, 248, 250, 280, 321
magnetic resonance imaging, 208, 240, 248, 280, 321
major depression, 217
major depressive disorder, 207, 208, 209, 210, 211, 212, 213, 214, 215, 218
males, 8, 243, 277, 279, 280, 285, 286, 287
malignancy, 10, 13, 244, 250, 306
management, vii, viii, 16, 25, 26, 29, 31, 32, 34, 35, 36, 37, 38, 41, 42, 43, 46, 63, 80, 84, 87, 88, 109, 110, 111, 113, 115, 117, 124, 125, 132, 140, 142, 143, 144, 152, 160, 165, 182, 186, 187, 204, 205, 207, 248, 253, 254, 259, 260, 261, 269, 270, 275, 281, 286, 296, 310, 311, 314, 315, 326, 328, 329
mandates, 239
mania, 30
manipulation, 8, 46, 76, 94, 318, 329
mapping, 302
marijuana, 119, 120
market, 159, 296
marketing, 268
Marx, 315
masking, 89, 90, 91
mass, 96, 106, 121, 124, 141, 305
mass spectrometry, 121, 141
masseter, 50
matrix, 127, 165, 166
matrix metalloproteinase, 165, 166
maturation, 221, 222, 223, 224, 225, 226, 227, 228, 229, 231, 232, 234, 236, 241, 247
measurement, 134, 174, 217
measures, 29, 135, 138, 212, 241, 262, 269, 274, 287, 288
median, 34, 112, 114, 128
mediation, 73, 74, 97, 105
Medicaid, 28, 38
medication, 35, 41, 119, 124, 160, 179, 207, 211, 214, 215, 242, 254, 261, 264, 266, 267, 268, 269, 270, 274, 286, 295, 296, 300, 308, 309, 329
medulla, 12, 54, 145, 170, 225, 230
MEK, 60
melanoma, 11, 308
membranes, 93, 96, 195, 203
memory, 2, 134, 277

men, 135, 162, 210, 249, 269, 279, 280, 281, 282, 283, 285, 286, 287, 288, 289, 293, 294, 299
meninges, 162, 257
menopause, 324
menstruation, 282
mental health, 118, 121
mental health professionals, 121
meridian, 321, 327
messenger RNA, 151
meta analysis, 246
metabolism, 127, 128, 129, 141, 142, 215, 230, 239, 246, 272, 286
metabolites, 126, 127, 128, 133, 141, 242, 259, 272, 287, 293, 300
metastasis, 9, 19, 33, 302, 304, 307, 308, 309, 314
metastatic disease, 309, 315
methodology, 211
methyl methacrylate, 304
mice, 4, 5, 6, 7, 8, 11, 17, 19, 20, 21, 22, 49, 52, 54, 70, 72, 74, 75, 80, 94, 102, 105, 153, 192, 204, 241, 247, 249, 290, 299
micrograms, 181
microsomes, 128, 142
microspheres, 205
midbrain, 89, 102, 170, 241, 280
migraine headache, viii, 31, 36, 162, 163, 167, 256, 258, 261, 271, 272, 273, 324, 329
migraines, 155, 162, 182
minority, 109, 111, 131, 134
mitogen, 60, 153
MMP, 165
mobility, 181, 304, 321
mode, 16, 48, 273, 284
models, vii, 1, 2, 4, 5, 7, 8, 11, 12, 13, 14, 15, 16, 20, 40, 46, 60, 72, 81, 88, 91, 96, 97, 116, 152, 171, 173, 177, 183, 197, 221, 226, 231, 244, 247, 249, 254, 258, 262, 275, 281, 289, 301, 305
modules, 232
molecular biology, 88, 150, 153
molecular dynamics, 74
molecular mass, 96, 98, 106
molecular structure, 48
molecules, 92, 93, 94, 98, 151, 152
money, 319
monitoring, 29, 31, 116, 129, 142, 178, 179, 291
monoamine oxidase inhibitors, 190
mood, 27, 29, 36, 117, 119, 123, 124, 149, 151, 190, 191, 208, 210, 212, 217, 255, 257, 288
mood change, 257
mood disorder, 190, 191

morbidity, 182, 209, 210, 222, 241, 303, 305
morphine, 13, 14, 20, 21, 22, 28, 29, 30, 31, 35, 39, 63, 74, 76, 77, 85, 87, 88, 89, 90, 91, 92, 93, 94, 95, 96, 97, 98, 99, 100, 101, 102, 103, 104, 105, 106, 107, 110, 111, 112, 113, 114, 115, 117, 123, 125, 126, 127, 128, 129, 130, 131, 132, 133, 134, 135, 137, 138, 139, 140, 141, 143, 144, 145, 215, 229, 230, 234, 237, 243, 245, 246, 248, 252, 286, 287, 290, 293, 296, 299, 300, 301, 309, 311, 312
morphology, 20
mortality, 209, 210, 217, 241
mosaic, 92, 98
mothers, 243, 246, 251
motion, 181, 322, 323, 324, 329
motivation, 5
motor fiber, 179
motor neurons, 158
motor system, 5, 240, 281
movement, 9, 14, 20, 29, 39, 50, 112, 151, 293, 308
MRI, 240, 244, 250, 321
mRNA, 18, 55, 64, 70, 92, 103, 153, 161, 177, 241, 245, 320, 326
mucosa, 127, 265, 266
multidimensional, 87, 115
multiple sclerosis, 27, 35, 38
muscle relaxation, 192
muscles, 284
musculoskeletal system, 284
mutagenesis, 48, 65, 189, 202, 204
mutant, 72, 105, 201, 202, 203
mutation, 7, 18, 94, 203, 311
myelin, 240
myocardial infarction, 158, 296
myoclonus, 144, 145

# N

NADH, 74
narcotic, 33, 87, 100, 102, 326
narcotics, 88
National Health Service, 111
National Institutes of Health, 240, 319
natural killer cell, 321, 327
nausea, 10, 34, 35, 111, 113, 125, 129, 132, 134, 163, 214, 215, 255, 258, 261, 264, 265, 266, 269, 270, 282, 299, 300, 306, 324, 329, 330
NCS, 218
necrosis, 19, 71
needs, 2, 58, 83, 115, 307, 322
negative outcomes, 81

negativity, 209
neonates, 229, 231, 232, 233, 235, 241, 242, 247, 248, 249, 250
nerve, 3, 4, 7, 8, 10, 15, 16, 17, 18, 19, 20, 21, 31, 32, 35, 40, 42, 46, 50, 51, 55, 57, 60, 61, 62, 63, 68, 70, 71, 72, 74, 75, 76, 78, 80, 81, 82, 83, 85, 148, 149, 151, 152, 171, 173, 174, 175, 176, 177, 182, 184, 185, 186, 193, 194, 195, 196, 197, 200, 204, 205, 206, 240, 243, 249, 250, 258, 259, 260, 285, 297, 298, 306, 320, 321, 326, 328
nerve fibers, 149
nerve growth factor, 19, 55, 71, 148, 175, 320, 326
nervous system, 2, 3, 8, 17, 20, 64, 75, 80, 88, 91, 100, 148, 152, 170, 171, 172, 173, 177, 183, 191, 222, 226, 229, 240, 241, 244, 257, 259, 277, 281, 284, 289, 314, 320, 326
network, 12, 91
neural network, 244
neural systems, 2, 240
neuralgia, 17, 27, 28, 33, 35, 37, 38, 39, 40, 42, 77, 81, 82, 86, 112, 138, 169, 172, 181, 184, 219, 244, 298, 308, 310, 311, 320
neurobiology, 222, 229, 232, 272, 290
neuroblastoma, 16, 97, 101
neuroimaging, 247
neurokinin, 61, 149, 258, 301
neuroleptics, 246
neurological disease, 32
neurologist, 112
neuroma, 4, 172, 173, 174, 175, 185, 202, 206
neuron response, 73
neuronal circuits, 235
neurons, 1, 12, 15, 16, 18, 21, 32, 40, 49, 50, 51, 52, 53, 54, 55, 56, 57, 58, 59, 61, 62, 63, 67, 68, 69, 70, 71, 73, 74, 75, 97, 102, 116, 139, 147, 148, 149, 152, 158, 162, 173, 174, 175, 176, 177, 185, 186, 190, 199, 205, 223, 224, 225, 227, 228, 229, 230, 233, 234, 235, 236, 237, 242, 245, 258, 262, 271, 272, 276, 321, 328
neuropathic pain, 3, 4, 7, 8, 9, 13, 14, 15, 16, 17, 18, 20, 25, 26, 27, 28, 29, 30, 31, 32, 33, 34, 35, 36, 37, 38, 40, 41, 42, 43, 54, 61, 70, 76, 81, 82, 85, 86, 87, 107, 110, 112, 113, 114, 116, 125, 132, 138, 139, 140, 145, 148, 171, 173, 176, 177, 178, 179, 182, 183, 185, 186, 187, 190, 192, 197, 199, 200, 202, 203, 204, 205, 206, 207, 209, 214, 215, 218, 219, 239, 240, 244, 245, 249, 254, 257, 259, 285, 297, 298, 299, 300, 307, 310, 314

neuropathy, 11, 12, 15, 16, 17, 22, 27, 28, 32, 33, 34, 35, 37, 38, 39, 41, 42, 43, 57, 71, 76, 81, 134, 138, 186, 219, 247
neuropeptides, 162, 320
neuroticism, 121
neurotoxicity, 193, 205
neurotransmitter, 26, 31, 178, 191, 224, 225, 251, 254, 257, 259, 321
neurotransmitters, 26, 29, 35, 46, 56, 103, 149, 151, 152, 190, 224, 230, 241, 257, 301, 320, 321, 327
neutropenia, 302
neutrophils, 10
nightmares, 215, 297
nitric oxide, 61, 66, 76, 166, 230, 259, 275, 301, 322
nitric oxide synthase, 61, 76, 230, 275
nitrous oxide, 245, 250
NMDA receptors, 45, 46, 49, 51, 52, 57, 58, 59, 60, 61, 62, 63, 64, 65, 66, 69, 73, 74, 76, 78, 79, 80, 81, 82, 83, 84, 224, 233, 241, 251, 299
noise, 255
non-depressed, 212
non-steroidal anti-inflammatory drugs, 9, 155, 164, 286, 293
norepinephrine, 171, 172, 175, 176, 178, 179, 183, 184, 192, 204, 214, 215, 259, 321, 327
normal development, 226
North America, 329
NSAIDs, 9, 14, 29, 116, 149, 150, 151, 152, 155, 156, 157, 158, 159, 160, 161, 163, 164, 230, 261, 296, 298, 299, 301
nuclei, 80, 228, 328
nucleus, 8, 69, 228, 258, 259, 322, 327, 328

# O

obesity, 269, 324
observations, 8, 29, 38, 49, 55, 63, 81, 89, 95, 97, 108, 173, 183, 191, 202, 204, 222, 253, 254, 257, 259, 260, 288, 315
obstruction, 309
obstructive lung disease, 210
occipital regions, 280
occlusion, 61, 171
offenders, 304
oil, 50, 235
older adults, 211, 218, 293
opiates, 88, 120, 141, 144, 251
opioids, 13, 14, 26, 88, 89, 90, 91, 109, 110, 111, 112, 113, 114, 115, 116, 117, 118, 119, 120, 121, 122, 123, 124, 125, 126, 129, 130, 131, 132, 133,

134, 135, 137, 138, 144, 229, 240, 242, 245, 246, 247, 286, 287, 296, 299, 300, 301, 309, 312, 321, 324
optic nerve, 309
optimism, 209
organ, 124, 133, 170, 251, 282, 283, 322, 327
organism, 133, 222, 239, 240, 242, 243, 245
organization, 104, 208, 226, 245, 280
organizations, 137
orientation, 135
osteoarthritis, 128, 158, 159, 164, 165, 166, 286, 329
outline, 193
ovaries, 320, 326
ovulation, 135
oxidation, 128
oxygen, 248

# P

pain, vii, viii, 1, 2, 3, 4, 5, 6, 7, 8, 9, 10, 11, 12, 13, 14, 15, 16, 17, 19, 20, 21, 22, 23, 25, 26, 27, 28, 29, 30, 31, 32, 33, 34, 35, 36, 37, 38, 39, 40, 41, 42, 43, 45, 46, 48, 49, 51, 54, 55, 57, 58, 60, 61, 62, 63, 64, 67, 68, 70, 71, 72, 74, 75, 76, 77, 78, 79, 81, 82, 83, 84, 85, 86, 88, 103, 108, 109, 110, 111, 112, 113, 114, 115, 116, 117, 118, 119, 120, 121, 122, 123, 124, 125, 126, 128, 129, 131, 132, 133, 134, 135, 136, 137, 138, 139, 140, 141, 142, 143, 144, 145, 147, 148, 149, 150, 151, 152, 153, 154, 155, 157, 158, 159, 160, 161, 162, 163, 165, 166, 169, 170, 171, 172, 173, 174, 176, 177, 178, 179, 180, 181, 182, 183, 184, 185, 186, 187, 188, 189, 190, 191, 192, 197, 198, 199, 200, 203, 204, 206, 207, 208, 209, 211, 212, 213, 214, 215, 216, 217, 218, 219, 221, 222, 225, 226, 227, 228, 229, 231, 232, 234, 235, 236, 237, 238, 239, 240, 241, 242, 243, 244, 245, 246, 247, 248, 249, 250, 251, 253, 254, 255, 256, 257, 258, 259, 260, 261, 262, 264, 265, 266, 267, 268, 269, 270, 271, 272, 274, 277, 278, 279, 280, 281, 282, 283, 284, 285, 286, 287, 288, 289, 290, 291, 292, 293, 294, 295, 296, 297, 298, 299, 300, 301, 302, 303, 304, 305, 306, 307, 308, 309, 310, 311, 312, 313, 314, 315, 317, 318, 319, 323, 324, 325, 326, 327, 328, 329
pain management, vii, viii, 25, 26, 29, 30, 32, 33, 36, 37, 79, 84, 110, 131, 154, 155, 189, 191, 192, 203, 204, 222, 232, 247, 277, 281, 286, 287, 288, 289, 294, 295, 299, 306, 311, 312, 315, 317, 318, 323, 324, 326
palliate, 143
palliative, 114, 295, 304, 306, 307, 311, 313, 314
palpation, 11
PAN, 175
pancreatic cancer, 307
pancreatitis, 63, 77
panic attack, 190, 213, 218
paralysis, 308
parameter, 99, 273, 323
parasympathetic nervous system, 177
parenchyma, 162
paresis, 308
paresthesias, 27
paroxetine, 298
particles, 302, 305
passive, 124, 319
pathogenesis, 162, 260
pathology, 7, 161, 207, 213, 216, 282, 296
pathophysiology, 1, 19, 22, 25, 155, 160, 162, 163, 166, 169, 207, 213, 216, 253, 254, 257, 259, 271, 282, 295, 315
pathways, viii, 2, 5, 12, 16, 21, 31, 36, 46, 52, 55, 56, 58, 63, 100, 124, 125, 126, 127, 148, 149, 152, 162, 182, 222, 225, 226, 228, 229, 234, 240, 241, 248, 254, 257, 258, 259, 270, 281, 295, 296, 319
PCA, 31
PCP, 121
PCR, 93
pedigree, 133
peer review, 30, 180
pelvic inflammatory disease, 281
pelvis, 280, 303
peptic ulcer, 158
peptic ulcer disease, 158
peptides, 88, 272
perfusion, 177, 254, 257, 268, 275, 320
perinatal, 227, 240, 242, 245
periosteum, 10, 159
peripheral blood, 178
peripheral nervous system, 8, 26, 240, 245
peripheral neuropathy, 20, 31, 33, 37, 42, 43, 112, 185, 214, 215
peristalsis, 283
permeability, 48, 65, 195, 224
permit, 3, 87, 111
perspective, 8, 88, 90, 281, 285, 289, 292
pertussis, 92, 96, 106
pessimism, 213
PET, 261, 321
PGN, 175

pH, 10, 48, 127, 190, 305
phantom limb pain, 37, 138, 249
pharmacogenetics, 239, 240, 246, 247
pharmacokinetics, 127, 141, 217, 222, 245, 267, 274, 300
pharmacological treatment, 85, 86, 232, 279
pharmacology, 1, 64, 76, 88, 163, 183, 186, 229, 232, 237, 239, 273, 279
pharmacotherapy, 9, 11, 100, 217, 312
phencyclidine, 66, 121
phenol, 306
phenotype, 7, 148, 236
phenytoin, 6, 17
phosphates, 106
phospholipids, 150
phosphorus, 302
phosphorylation, 46, 48, 49, 52, 53, 54, 55, 56, 57, 58, 59, 60, 63, 65, 68, 69, 70, 71, 74, 75, 87, 89, 92, 93, 94, 95, 97, 98, 99, 100, 101, 104, 106, 151
photons, 302
physical activity, 121, 124
physical fitness, 288
physical therapy, 244, 288, 323
physicochemical properties, 195
physiology, 5, 14, 91, 222, 239, 278, 312
pigs, 93
pilot study, 30, 37, 38, 39, 110, 137, 141, 197, 204
placebo, 17, 27, 30, 31, 34, 35, 36, 37, 38, 39, 40, 42, 43, 86, 110, 111, 112, 113, 134, 135, 137, 138, 141, 159, 160, 163, 165, 166, 167, 180, 181, 197, 199, 210, 212, 214, 215, 219, 262, 264, 265, 266, 267, 274, 288, 294, 306, 310, 313, 322, 323, 326, 328, 329
plasma, 93, 95, 125, 126, 127, 128, 151, 162, 163, 171, 175, 183, 189, 197, 200, 202, 204, 243, 245, 258, 273, 303, 327
plasma levels, 245
plasma membrane, 93, 95, 175
plasma proteins, 127, 162, 303
plasticity, 1, 13, 45, 46, 49, 50, 54, 57, 58, 59, 64, 67, 68, 69, 75, 85, 87, 88, 100, 103, 147, 148, 222, 234, 235, 239, 259
platelets, 150
pleasure, 210
pleiotropy, 91
plexus, 89, 97, 99, 101, 102, 180, 244, 301, 307, 308, 315
PM, 66, 73, 78, 142, 166, 183, 184, 185, 249, 313
polarization, 117
polymorphism, 128, 246

polypeptide, 107, 236
poor, 8, 108, 182, 209, 255, 282, 299, 307, 308
population, 6, 35, 38, 109, 130, 131, 161, 163, 182, 210, 218, 239, 245, 255, 256, 280, 285, 286, 287, 291
positive correlation, 111
positron, 41, 261, 268, 275, 321, 327
positron emission tomography, 41, 261, 268, 327
potassium, 8, 18, 102, 230
precipitation, 97
prediction, 252
predictors, 17, 284, 297
prednisone, 297
preference, 117, 261
prefrontal cortex, 208, 212, 321
pregnancy, 284
premature infant, 222, 232
premenstrual syndrome, 324
preparation, 59, 92, 99, 117, 123, 133
pressure, 5, 7, 33, 208, 223, 228, 255, 287, 327
preterm infants, 226, 228, 237, 243
prevention, 39, 43, 83, 152, 248, 259, 290, 315
primary tumor, 307
primate, 72, 174, 176
principle, 319
probability, 12, 130, 159, 264, 265, 266, 267
problem solving, 211
production, 147, 148, 150, 151, 152, 161, 165, 215, 230, 301, 320, 321, 322
prognosis, 109, 114, 118, 295, 308
program, 114
prolactin, 144
proliferation, 105, 245
promoter, 149
propagation, 200
prophylactic, 43, 211, 324, 329
prophylaxis, 30, 31, 38, 304
propranolol, 172, 259, 266
prostaglandins, 10, 55, 153, 158, 163, 165, 175, 272
prostate, 157, 302, 303, 305, 308, 313, 315
prostate cancer, 303, 313
prostate gland, 157
prostatectomy, 31
prostatitis, 283
prostheses, 307
protein kinase C, 48, 56, 68, 69, 74, 76, 97, 105, 107, 148, 228, 259
protein kinases, 46, 48, 54, 57, 58, 63, 246
proteins, 5, 8, 46, 52, 53, 57, 63, 65, 72, 85, 87, 89, 91, 93, 94, 95, 97, 102, 103, 105, 106, 148, 157

protocol, 59, 182, 262, 299
protons, 10, 48, 65
prototype, 125
pruritus, 300, 309
PSD, 57
psychiatric disorders, 190, 204
psychological assessments, 288
psychological stress, 323
psychological variables, 328
psychology, 278
psychopathology, 121
psychotropic drugs, 205
puberty, 222, 286
pulmonary vascular resistance, 251
pulse, 196, 201, 282
pumps, 301
pyramidal cells, 57
pyrimidine, 60

## Q

quality of life, 9, 27, 29, 35, 112, 113, 123, 182, 242, 288, 297, 299, 304, 307, 315, 323
quaternary ammonium, 193

## R

race, 127, 272, 289
radiation, 295, 298, 302, 303, 304, 305, 306, 307, 308, 314
radiation therapy, 295, 304, 307, 308, 314
radical formation, 160
radiculopathy, 292
radiography, 159
radiotherapy, 9, 301, 302, 303, 304, 305, 308, 314
radium, 303, 314
Ramadan, 272, 275, 276
range, 5, 6, 7, 12, 13, 14, 31, 35, 36, 98, 99, 110, 112, 114, 127, 151, 158, 181, 194, 197, 200, 225, 255, 283, 303, 305, 318, 322, 323, 324, 329
rash, 35
rating scale, 112
ratings, 123, 172, 243
reading, 108
reagents, 48
real time, 229
reality, 75, 116, 120
receptive field, 4, 16, 50, 51, 61, 67, 68, 223, 226, 227, 233, 235, 236, 242, 282
receptors, 10, 12, 21, 26, 29, 35, 45, 46, 49, 55, 56, 57, 58, 59, 60, 61, 64, 65, 66, 67, 69, 72, 73, 74,
75, 80, 81, 83, 84, 87, 88, 89, 90, 91, 92, 95, 101, 102, 103, 104, 105, 106, 116, 124, 139, 148, 149, 150, 152, 153, 157, 163, 171, 173, 175, 176, 177, 178, 185, 191, 192, 204, 224, 228, 230, 233, 236, 237, 241, 245, 251, 254, 259, 260, 262, 263, 264, 265, 266, 267, 268, 273, 275, 277, 279, 283, 295, 299, 301, 305, 326
recognition, 48, 150, 239, 257, 278, 288, 315
reconcile, 288
recovery, 29, 39, 111, 182, 194, 244, 258, 287
rectum, 312
recurrence, 163, 262, 264, 265, 266, 267, 268, 269, 270, 307
redistribution, 4
reduction, 3, 8, 9, 22, 26, 27, 28, 29, 30, 31, 32, 34, 35, 36, 50, 56, 96, 112, 135, 161, 163, 166, 170, 171, 173, 180, 182, 210, 211, 214, 215, 226, 243, 246, 260, 261, 264, 283, 302, 303, 324
reflection, 3, 50
reflex sympathetic dystrophy, 183, 186, 187
reflexes, 62, 71, 77, 182, 221, 223, 224, 234, 243, 322
regression, 201, 304
regrowth, 307
regulation, 12, 18, 48, 65, 69, 71, 74, 90, 92, 98, 99, 100, 102, 103, 106, 107, 150, 164, 175, 176, 186, 222, 228, 229, 230, 231, 237, 272
regulators, 103
rehabilitation, 113, 137, 294, 307
rehabilitation program, 113, 114, 294
relationship, 12, 17, 116, 118, 121, 140, 162, 176, 195, 208, 209, 216, 217, 278, 281, 283, 307
relationships, 4, 119, 283, 291, 297
relative toxicity, 205
relaxation, 324
relevance, vii, 92, 94, 95, 96, 103, 104, 278, 280
remission, 210, 211, 217
renal failure, 126, 300, 311
repair, 160
replacement, 85
reproduction, 280
reproductive organs, 278, 281, 292
resection, 295, 315
residues, 48, 53, 54, 56, 65, 101
resolution, 258, 260
respiration, 246, 251
respiratory, 10, 88, 126, 198, 242, 282, 299, 301, 308
respiratory arrest, 198

responsiveness, 7, 50, 93, 98, 99, 100, 104, 115, 148, 173, 177, 180, 185, 246, 287, 290
resting potential, 18, 224
retardation, 210
retention, 126
reticulum, 52, 56
rhenium, 302, 313
rheumatoid arthritis, 151, 153, 164, 171, 324
rhinorrhea, 255
rhythm, 205
risk, 3, 31, 109, 110, 120, 129, 132, 133, 157, 158, 163, 164, 179, 208, 210, 211, 212, 214, 268, 277, 284, 286, 297, 298, 304, 305, 306, 307, 315
risk assessment, 109
risk factors, 269, 277, 284, 286, 315
RNA, 65
RNA splicing, 65
rodents, 4, 279, 280, 287, 290

# S

safety, 30, 110, 111, 113, 128, 133, 134, 137, 138, 141, 143, 159, 162, 166, 214, 240, 242, 247, 261, 268, 270, 274, 275, 300, 302, 305, 312, 318
sales, 286
salicylates, 165
saliva, 127, 163, 265
samarium, 302, 303, 313
sample, 79, 82, 130, 180, 208, 302, 323
sampling, 241
SAP, 71
satisfaction, 269, 270, 271, 274
schizophrenia, 217
school, 124, 245, 251, 318, 325
scores, 36, 112, 132, 134, 180, 181, 243, 288, 303
search, 31, 46, 60, 121, 260, 270
searching, 46, 63
secrete, 10
secretion, 144, 242, 283
sedatives, 28
seizure, 296
selective serotonin reuptake inhibitor, 296
selectivity, 14, 301, 305
self, 107, 120, 122, 212, 214, 234, 244, 264, 278, 286
self esteem, 212
self representation, 278
self-mutilation, 244
self-organization, 234

sensation, 3, 12, 17, 28, 63, 147, 171, 199, 200, 203, 222, 242, 282, 283, 292, 308, 321, 322
sensations, 174, 249, 283
sensing, 5, 10
sensitivity, 12, 21, 22, 48, 49, 50, 58, 59, 65, 74, 78, 84, 121, 147, 148, 149, 151, 152, 157, 171, 172, 174, 175, 176, 177, 178, 185, 186, 224, 225, 227, 233, 235, 236, 239, 240, 245, 249, 254, 257, 272, 279
sensitization, 10, 12, 15, 45, 50, 51, 52, 54, 56, 58, 60, 66, 67, 70, 71, 72, 75, 83, 84, 86, 148, 151, 152, 162, 163, 166, 167, 175, 176, 177, 221, 227, 228, 230, 231, 233, 236, 243, 244, 254, 257, 258, 261, 262, 270, 282, 291
sensory symptoms, 256, 279
sensory systems, 240, 277
series, 38, 40, 142, 180, 289, 326
serotonin, viii, 190, 191, 192, 214, 215, 225, 234, 241, 246, 253, 254, 259, 260, 273, 274, 279, 290, 296, 298, 321, 323
sertraline, 211, 217
serum, 141, 153, 265, 267, 268, 300
services, 281
severity, 9, 29, 31, 36, 113, 114, 129, 131, 159, 207, 211, 213, 216, 244, 285, 286, 289, 291
sex differences, 278, 287, 289, 293
sex steroid, 279, 280
shape, 322
shaping, 226
shares, 11
sharing, 119
sheep, 72, 193, 197
side effects, 3, 8, 10, 13, 27, 28, 29, 31, 34, 35, 36, 46, 63, 109, 110, 111, 125, 126, 127, 131, 132, 133, 134, 135, 136, 150, 151, 155, 157, 179, 181, 191, 203, 206, 214, 266, 268, 279, 287, 293, 296, 297, 298, 299, 300, 306, 310, 324
sign, 209, 210, 282
signaling pathways, 58, 73, 149
signalling, 1, 69, 106, 224, 226, 228
signals, 12, 26, 104, 150, 180, 314
simulation, 182
Singapore, 153
sinus, 255, 273, 276
siRNA, 68
sites, 9, 26, 48, 51, 52, 54, 66, 70, 71, 75, 80, 148, 164, 172, 189, 190, 193, 195, 204, 205, 230, 282, 288, 296, 301, 302, 303, 304
skeletal muscle, 16
skeleton, 9, 19, 302, 306

skills, 285
skin, 50, 55, 62, 67, 170, 171, 172, 173, 174, 176, 178, 179, 184, 187, 197, 216, 223, 226, 227, 235, 236, 241, 242, 247, 249, 282, 291, 300
sleep disturbance, 28, 29, 212, 299
smoking, 158, 324
SNS, 16, 17, 18, 170, 171, 177, 237
social institutions, 278
social support, 210
sodium, 3, 4, 6, 7, 8, 15, 16, 18, 25, 26, 30, 32, 34, 35, 36, 40, 41, 56, 148, 151, 152, 200, 205, 206, 237, 274, 296
solubility, 243
somatic nervous system, 170
somnolence, 28, 29, 111
SPA, 234
Spain, 1
species, 2, 11, 80, 96, 106, 205, 222, 239, 242, 281, 284, 287
specificity, 3, 6, 92, 93, 105, 177
spectrum, 4, 100, 114, 131, 213, 277
speech, 256
speed, 108
sphincter, 308
spinal anesthesia, 193
spinal cord, 2, 3, 4, 6, 7, 8, 11, 12, 17, 18, 20, 22, 27, 28, 33, 35, 38, 41, 42, 45, 49, 52, 53, 55, 57, 58, 59, 66, 67, 68, 69, 70, 71, 72, 74, 76, 84, 86, 94, 96, 99, 105, 116, 138, 145, 147, 148, 149, 152, 153, 154, 158, 164, 170, 177, 178, 181, 182, 183, 186, 188, 222, 223, 224, 225, 226, 227, 228, 230, 233, 234, 235, 236, 237, 240, 241, 248, 258, 273, 281, 286, 291, 293, 301, 302, 304, 305, 307, 308, 324, 328
spinal cord injury, 17, 33, 35, 38, 41, 42, 69, 86
spine, 159, 161, 240, 304, 308, 325
Sprague-Dawley rats, 11
stability, 288, 307
stabilization, 308
stable angina, 291
stages, 171, 183, 193, 240, 254
standards, 132, 215, 278, 319
stellate, 187, 307
steroids, 290, 306, 320
stigma, 212
stimulus, 2, 3, 4, 5, 12, 17, 49, 50, 51, 54, 61, 148, 149, 184, 223, 227, 233, 241, 242, 245, 280, 281, 282, 283, 284
stoichiometry, 93
stoma, 300, 312

stomach, 127, 215
stomatitis, 311
strain, 285, 287, 292
strategies, 3, 88, 91, 92, 100, 110, 115, 117, 132, 217, 253, 254, 270, 288, 301
strength, 50, 62, 171, 181, 263, 266
stress, 124, 150, 151, 171, 173, 208, 227, 241, 242, 246, 248, 255, 279, 280, 284, 290, 321, 327
stressors, 279
stretching, 10, 258, 297
striatum, 69, 80, 245
stroke, 30, 32, 78
stroma, 305
strontium, 302
subcutaneous injection, 264, 268
subcutaneous tissue, 283
substance abuse, 118, 120, 129, 210
substance use, 118
substitution, 65, 134, 299, 309
substrates, 246
success rate, 36
suicidal ideation, 210
suicide, 209, 210, 213
suicide attempts, 210, 213
Sun, 69
superiority, 269
supply, 10, 170, 176, 286
suppository, 261
suppression, 68, 163, 234, 258
surgical intervention, 9
surveillance, 268
survival, 75, 87, 100, 132, 143, 217, 295, 301, 303, 306, 307
susceptibility, 126, 246
sweat, 179
sweat test, 179
Sweden, 286
swelling, 170
sympathectomy, 176, 178, 180, 181, 182, 185, 187
sympathetic denervation, 176
sympathetic fibers, 170, 176, 177, 186
sympathetic nervous system, viii, 169, 170, 171, 172, 173, 177, 181, 183, 184, 284
symptom, 6, 162, 207, 210, 211, 216, 256, 261, 270, 283, 289, 295, 297, 304
symptomatic treatment, 37, 284
symptoms, 3, 4, 5, 6, 15, 16, 27, 28, 30, 33, 35, 38, 39, 84, 110, 122, 129, 143, 148, 152, 161, 163, 166, 180, 198, 203, 207, 208, 209, 210, 211, 212, 213, 216, 217, 254, 255, 256, 257, 264, 268, 269,

270, 272, 277, 279, 281, 282, 283, 284, 289, 291, 297, 304, 310, 322, 324
synapse, 170
synaptic plasticity, 52
synaptic strength, 47
synaptic transmission, 52, 57, 62, 69, 73, 74, 225
synchronization, 224
syndrome, 27, 28, 34, 35, 39, 41, 81, 112, 113, 129, 133, 138, 143, 144, 149, 151, 162, 169, 170, 173, 181, 183, 184, 185, 186, 187, 188, 189, 209, 210, 215, 216, 243, 244, 246, 250, 252, 282, 289, 290, 291, 292, 325
synovial membrane, 165
synovitis, 159
synthesis, 93, 94, 97, 98, 129, 149, 152, 153, 155, 157, 158, 187, 230, 272, 305, 320
systemic change, 151
systems, 1, 2, 31, 52, 58, 63, 76, 88, 98, 132, 143, 149, 150, 177, 192, 222, 225, 226, 230, 237, 241, 251, 259, 280, 281, 284, 288, 289, 301, 305, 309

# T

tachycardia, 129, 170, 243
tachypnea, 129
tactics, 270
tactile stimuli, 255
targets, 1, 2, 14, 43, 46, 48, 87, 89, 100, 147, 148, 191, 192, 204, 228, 253, 270, 279, 282
taxonomy, 213
technology, 245
temperament, 249
temperature, 7, 10, 170, 174, 178, 179, 187, 256, 282, 308
tennis elbow, 324
tension, 36, 254, 255, 256, 258, 271, 272, 310, 323
terminally ill, 109
terminals, 3, 7, 49, 66, 116, 147, 148, 151, 152, 175, 176, 177, 179, 223, 225, 227, 240, 254, 258, 259, 260
testosterone, 135, 144, 290
thalamus, 2, 8, 228, 240, 258, 282, 326
theft, 119
theory, 171, 191, 208, 257, 319
therapeutic agents, 31, 36, 260, 270, 314
therapeutic interventions, 170
therapeutic targets, 2, 40, 153, 190, 253, 254
therapeutics, 204, 247, 305
therapy, 2, 28, 31, 35, 74, 108, 109, 110, 111, 112, 113, 114, 115, 116, 117, 118, 119, 120, 122, 123, 125, 129, 131, 132, 133, 134, 137, 138, 139, 140, 142, 143, 144, 147, 164, 191, 192, 198, 211, 250, 271, 274, 275, 286, 288, 297, 298, 301, 302, 307, 308, 309, 310, 311, 312, 313, 314, 315, 318, 319, 323, 324
thinking, 213, 218
thoracotomy, 241
thorax, 308
threat, 181, 212, 284
threats, 248
threshold, 2, 5, 10, 12, 14, 29, 33, 50, 56, 63, 82, 112, 135, 148, 151, 152, 208, 210, 224, 231, 233, 241, 242, 243, 247, 271, 283, 301, 327
threshold level, 12
thresholds, 5, 31, 223, 227, 242, 257, 296
thrombosis, 114
thromboxanes, 153
thyroid, 135
thyroid stimulating hormone, 135
tibia, 11
tides, 141
time, 2, 4, 11, 13, 32, 50, 52, 53, 54, 61, 78, 83, 89, 108, 109, 116, 119, 125, 126, 127, 128, 131, 152, 155, 161, 176, 178, 183, 185, 199, 201, 202, 214, 218, 222, 224, 244, 258, 265, 274, 277, 287, 288, 292, 296, 297, 303, 306, 322
time periods, 89
timing, 114, 118, 214, 224, 226, 242
tin, 322
tissue, 4, 13, 32, 45, 46, 47, 50, 51, 56, 61, 62, 64, 68, 85, 89, 90, 92, 93, 148, 149, 150, 151, 152, 160, 162, 166, 175, 176, 186, 204, 221, 222, 227, 230, 231, 242, 245, 253, 309, 327
TNF, 149, 153, 157, 160, 161
TNF-α, 157
tobacco, 269
toddlers, 243, 249
tonic, 66, 73, 174, 225, 235
tourniquet, 178, 179
toxic effect, 302
toxic side effect, 299
toxicity, 9, 10, 31, 143, 157, 158, 164, 197, 242, 243, 296, 313
toxicology, 120, 129, 140, 142
toxin, 33, 41, 92, 96, 105, 106
tracking, 122
trading, 119
training, 108, 124
transcription, 56, 148, 151, 305
transcription factors, 148

transducer, 6, 93
transduction, 25, 26, 36, 46, 52, 60, 63, 88, 89, 102, 148, 149, 176
transection, 173, 174, 175, 225, 234
transforming growth factor, 19, 305
transition, 246, 284
transitions, 200
translation, 1, 2, 3, 84, 247, 280, 317, 318
translocation, 107
transmission, 1, 2, 3, 4, 5, 6, 7, 12, 25, 26, 30, 31, 32, 36, 57, 73, 76, 152, 170, 171, 176, 182, 189, 200, 203, 224, 233, 237, 240, 243, 245, 254, 259, 276, 279
transport, 129
trauma, 3, 4, 157, 176, 177, 227, 279, 284
trial, 17, 27, 28, 30, 31, 32, 35, 37, 38, 39, 40, 41, 42, 43, 80, 84, 86, 111, 112, 125, 132, 133, 138, 141, 143, 160, 161, 164, 165, 166, 167, 179, 180, 181, 182, 188, 197, 211, 215, 218, 219, 243, 248, 249, 273, 274, 286, 288, 298, 305, 309, 310, 313, 314, 323, 326, 328, 329, 330
tricyclic antidepressant, 214
tricyclic antidepressants, viii, 28, 112, 204, 214, 259, 298
trigeminal nerve, 162, 254, 257, 258, 260
trigeminal neuralgia, 6, 17, 27, 28, 34, 37, 38, 42, 68, 244, 249
triggers, 71, 185, 209, 227, 255, 272
tumor, 19, 20, 22, 55, 157, 160, 161, 165, 295, 303, 304, 305, 306, 307, 308, 309, 314
tumor cells, 305
tumor growth, 22, 314
tumor necrosis factor, 55, 157, 160, 161, 165, 305
tumor progression, 304, 308
tumors, 20, 301, 304, 305, 307, 309, 314, 315
tumour growth, 14
turbulence, 121
turnover, 302
tyrosine, 46, 48, 53, 54, 55, 56, 57, 58, 59, 60, 65, 66, 69, 70, 71, 74, 75, 149, 165

## U

UK, 1, 109, 131, 167, 285
ulcer, 158
uncertainty, 269
underlying mechanisms, 11, 55, 83, 189, 190, 280
United Kingdom, 108, 111
United States, 30, 113, 128, 167, 218, 240, 260, 262, 263, 269, 278, 297, 318, 325, 326

universe, 155
unmasking, 66
urinary retention, 191, 299
urinary tract, 292
urine, 117, 118, 120, 121, 127, 128, 129, 140, 141, 142, 303
usual dose, 264
uterus, 283, 291

## V

vagus, 182, 188
vagus nerve, 182, 188
validation, 13
validity, 12
values, 126, 196, 197, 202
variability, 124, 127, 128, 252, 299, 300
variable, 127, 128, 142, 157, 159, 171, 180, 244, 287
variables, 134, 135, 270
variation, 80, 128, 252, 285
vasculature, 152, 260
vasoactive intestinal peptide, 241
vasoconstriction, 169, 171, 174, 257, 261, 268
vasodilation, 170, 260
vasomotor, 171, 180
vasopressin, 171, 290
vasospasm, 162
vein, 114, 272
velocity, 162
venlafaxine, 211, 214, 215, 217, 218, 219, 298
vertigo, 257
vessels, 162
viscera, 170, 282, 283, 284, 292
viscosity, 327
vision, 162, 256
visualization, 182
vitamins, 318
vomiting, 113, 255, 264, 300, 329, 330
vulnerability, 247

## W

walking, 209, 256
war, 209
water, 174, 243
WDR, 12
weakness, 256, 258, 284, 307
wealth, 96
wear, 13
weight gain, 210
weight loss, 35, 210

well-being, 216
white matter, 228
wild type, 94, 196
wind, 49, 53, 58, 62, 63, 66, 75, 77, 84, 228
withdrawal, 2, 5, 6, 7, 27, 58, 61, 62, 90, 102, 110, 113, 114, 117, 129, 137, 145, 159, 215, 223, 226, 229, 251, 252
women, 85, 135, 210, 269, 278, 279, 281, 282, 283, 284, 286, 287, 288, 289, 290, 292, 294, 299, 328, 330
words, 8, 92, 111, 116, 208, 278
work, vii, 1, 64, 94, 110, 115, 116, 151, 160, 208, 245, 257, 259, 278, 288, 323
workers, 88, 328
World Health Organization, 110, 124, 137, 299, 319, 324
worry, 212, 213, 299
wound healing, 307
wound infection, 181
writing, 109, 129

# Y

yield, 116, 119, 123, 128, 298
young men, 286

# Z

zinc, 48, 65, 69

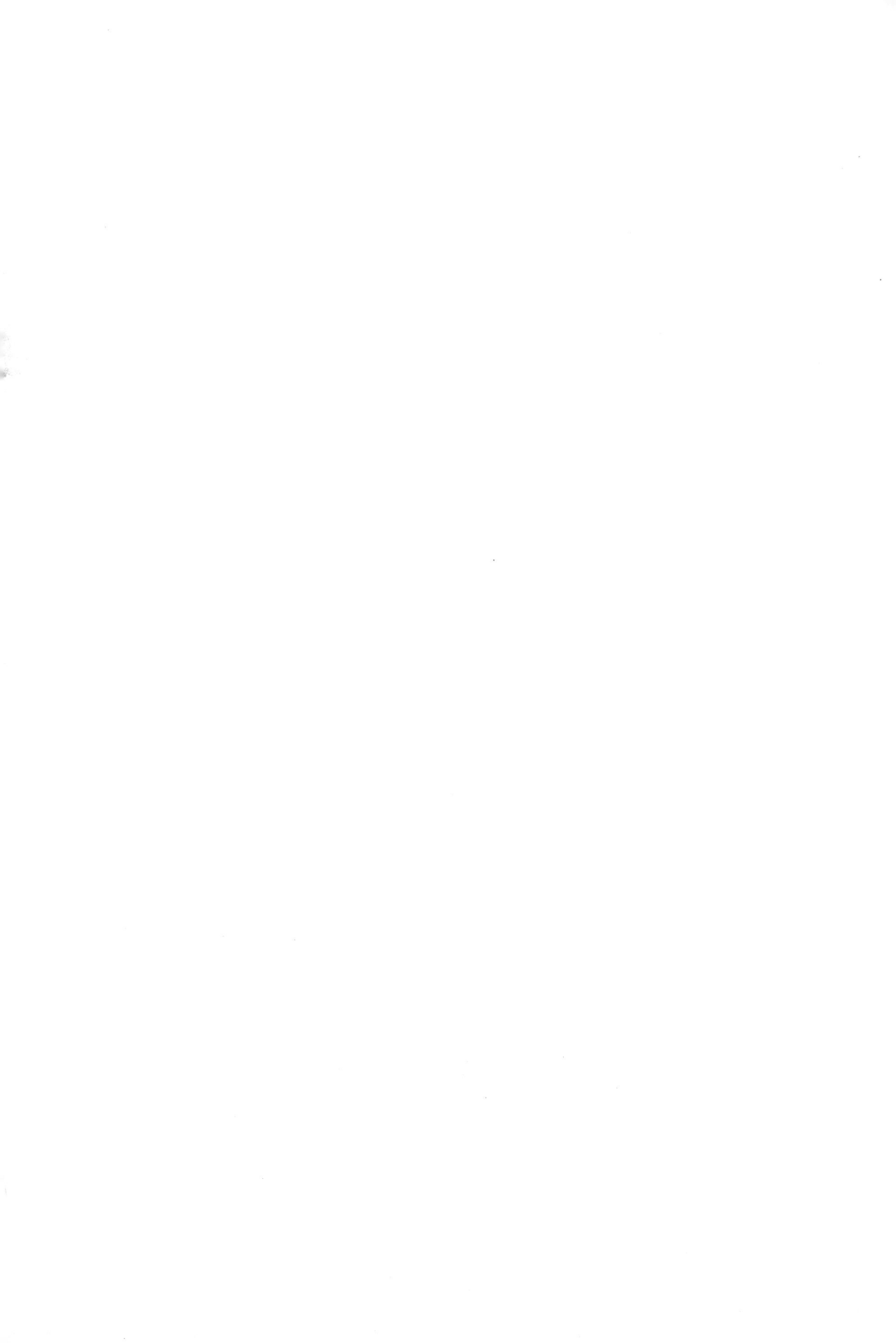